DreamChild Adventures
in Relaxation and Sleep

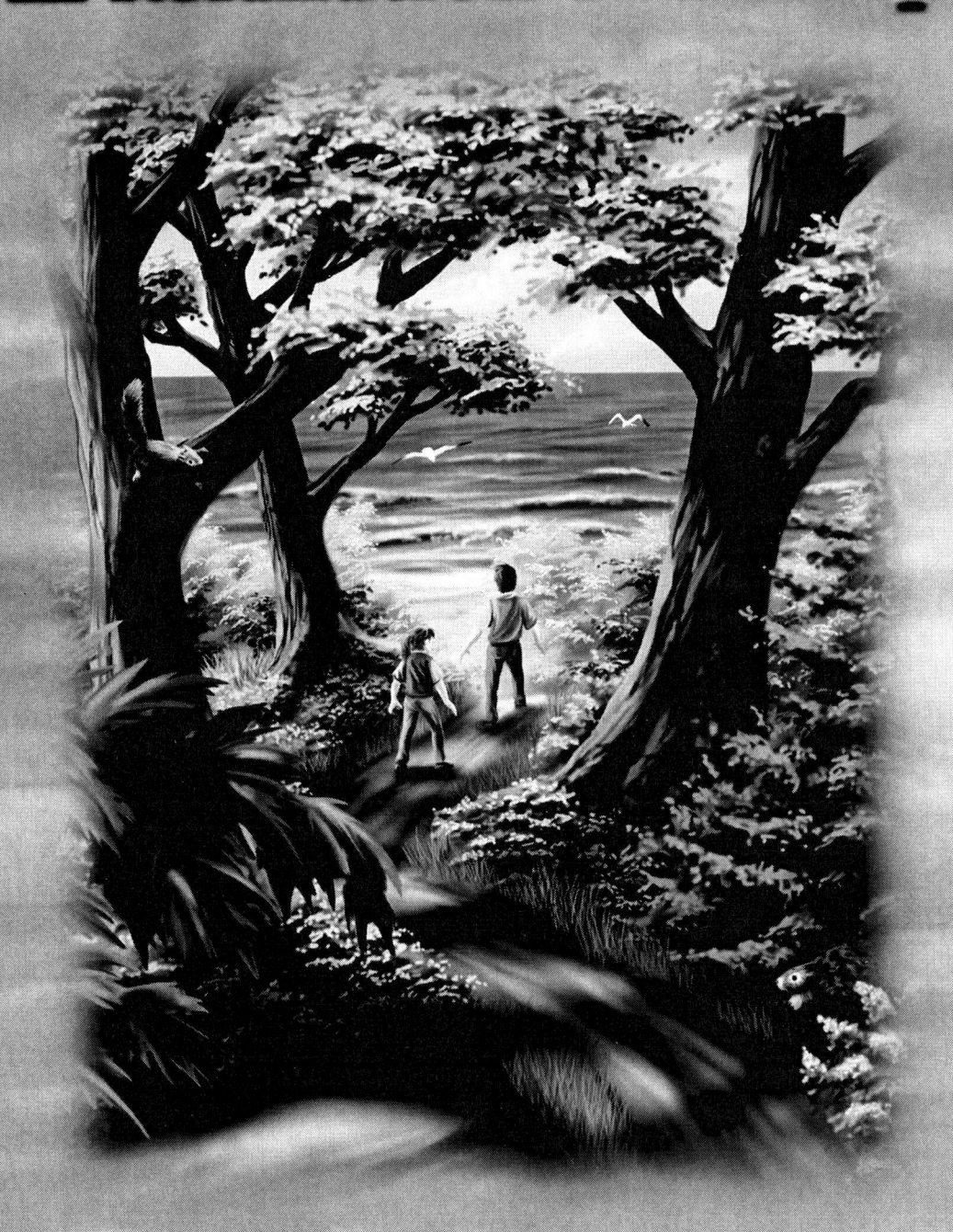

Tom Jackson, M.D.

DreamChild™ Adventures in Relaxation and Sleep
FIRST EDITION

Copyright © 2012 Thomas Jackson, M.D.
Original cover art copyright © 2012 Thomas Jackson, M.D.

All Rights Reserved

Printed and bound in the United States by Circadian Publishing

ISBN 978-0-9825928-1-6
e-book ISBN 978-0-9825928-2-3
Library of Congress LCCN 2010918432

NO PART OF THIS BOOK MAY BE REPRODUCED IN ANY FORM, EXCEPT FOR THE INCLUSION OF BRIEF QUOTATIONS IN REVIEW, OR STORED IN ANY ELECTRONIC RETRIEVAL SYSTEM, WITHOUT PERMISSION IN WRITING FROM THE PUBLISHER.

NOTE: This publication contains the ideas and opinions of its author and is intended to provide helpful and informative material on the subjects addressed. This book and the companion audio programs are not intended to serve as a replacement for professional medical advice or therapy and are sold with the understanding that the author and publisher are not rendering medical, health, or any other kind of personal professional services. The author and publisher specifically disclaim any and all liability arising directly or indirectly from the use or application of any information contained in this book or from use of any of the author's audio programs. The reader should consult his or her medical, health or other competent professional regarding specific problems and before implementing use of the author's audio programs to treat any and all ailments.

For more information, please contact the publisher at:
Circadian Publishing
PO Box 3589
Idyllwild, CA 92549
(877) 659-5322

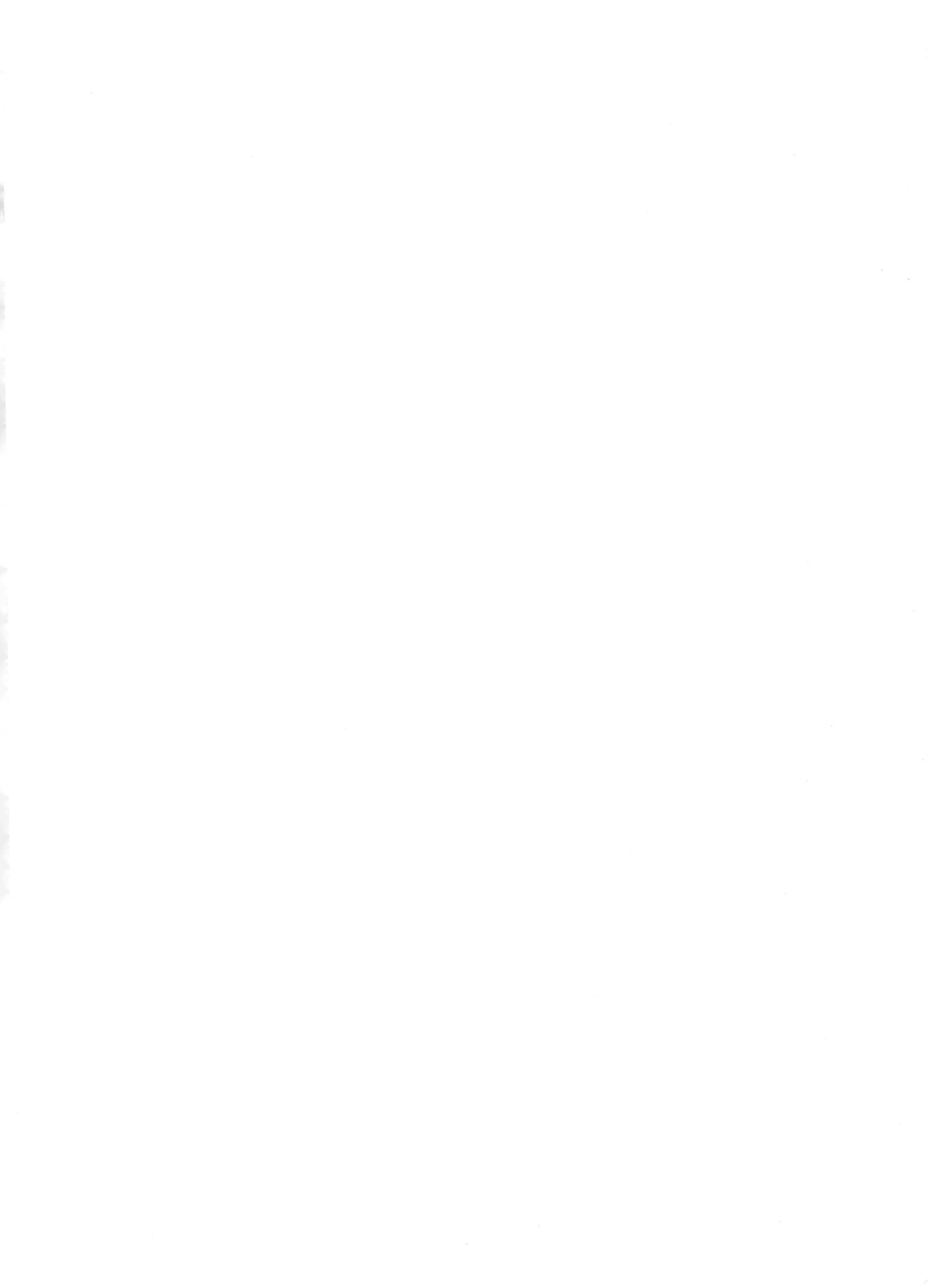

DEDICATION

This book is about people, *first and foremost.*

Specifically, it is about 22 children, and their parents or caregivers, whose very personal and deeply moving stories are revealed as they unfold in the following pages.

It is because of their participation in this process that this book even exists.

For this reason, I dedicate this book to each of these wonderful individuals who so graciously, bravely, and openly spoke of the challenges they and their children faced—and overcame—as they shared intimate details about themselves and their families, in the belief that other children, parents, and caregivers experiencing similar struggles might benefit from their experiences.

I wish each of them a lifetime of nights of deep, restful sleep and invigorating days of blissful relaxation.

ACKNOWLEDGMENTS

I would like to thank Sage Kalmus, my right hand on this project–who, as a blessed result, has now become my good friend–for his brilliant and tireless assistance which was indispensable in the writing of this book.

Nor could this book appear to you in its present form without the meticulous editing of my close friend and colleague, Dick Ridenour. I am a doctor, not a writer, by profession. And it is, in large part, thanks to Dick that the text reads as clearly and coherently as it does.

I also owe a tremendous debt of gratitude to another trusted colleague and dear friend, Chris Alsten, for his invaluable research and continued contribution to the promise of this work.

I sincerely hope each of these great men find that all the hours they devoted to the development of this text have paid off.

Finally, many thanks go to a very talented artist, David Graham, for his beautiful artwork that graces the cover of this book, capturing so vividly the essence of the *DreamChild*™ *Adventures*, and also to Max Herr and his eye for typography, for the layout of the text as well as his masterful graphic design of the titles and text for the front and back covers, skills that knit everything together seamlessly.

Contents

PART I: INTRODUCTION 1

DreamChild Adventures Children's Programs 3
    Who Created It? 3
    How DreamChild Adventures Came About 3
    Why a Companion Book? 3
    The Link Between Sleep and Other Issues 4
    An Inextricable Web 4
    Every Child Is Different 4
    How to Use This Book 5
    Children and Anxiety 6
    The Effects of Stress in Contemporary Society 6
    What is Anxiety? 7
    A Vicious Cycle: Fear of the Imaginary 7
    Age-Appropriate Fears 8
    The Fear of Sleeping Alone 9
    Anxiety in Teens 9
    Signs of an Anxious Child 9
    Consequences of Unresolved Childhood Anxiety 9
    Children, Anxiety, and Sleep 10
    Anxiety and Sleep 10
    A Nightly Struggle 10
    Common Childhood Sleep Problems 10
    The Untold Effects of Sleep 11
    A Turning Point 11
    The Programs 12
        Country Friends 12
        Magic Carpet 13
        Playhouse on the Beach 13
    Benefits Of the DreamChild Adventures Children's Programs 14
    Simple Measures Yield Extraordinary Results 14
    Possible Explanations 14
    A Caveat: Every Child is Different-Revisited 15
    The Fast Track to Success 15
    Research 15
    Adverse Reactions and Side Effects 16
    Participants in the Case Studies 16
    Background on the Case Studies 17
    A Brief Technical Note 17
    Let the Adventures Begin! 17

Part II: Clinical Interviews 19

Chapter 1: Leonard / David 21
Fear of the Dark 24
Symptoms of a Fear of the Dark 24
Causes of a Fear of the Dark 24
The Commonality: Protection 25
Fear of the Unknown 25
The Absence of Light 25
Getting to the Deeper Underlying Issue 25
Common Pitfall: Playing Along With Their Fantasies 26
A Security Tour 26
A Little Compassion Goes a Long Way 26
Fear of the Dark–Case Study 27
A System of Rewards 27
Other Fear-of-the-Dark Solutions to Try 27
Remember, Compassion 28

Chapter 2: Kenneth / Alicia and Pamela 29
Television 35
The Common Picture 35
Television and Other Issues 36
Television and Sleep 36
Common Pitfall: Appeasement 36
Daytime Television Viewing 37
Duration of Television Viewing 37
Nighttime Television Viewing 37
The Problem of Content 37
The Problem of Technology 38
A Television in Their Bedroom 38
What the Medical Experts Say 38
Reading: The Television Cure 39
Good Television Viewing Habits 39

Chapter 3: Alan / Bobby 41
Resistance to Reading 48
Hearing Stories versus Reading Them 48
The Later Repercussions of Resisting Reading 48
What's a Parent to Do (And Not to Do)? 48
Approaches to the Common Reasons Children Resist Reading 49
Teaching by Example: Do You Resist Reading? 50
How to Read to (or with) Your Child to Encourage Reading 50
A Little Encouragement Goes a Long Way 51
The DreamChild Adventures Programs and Reading 51

Chapter 4: Iris / Beatrice and Melissa 53
Academic Performance 55
The Connection Between Sleep and Academic Performance 56
The Effects of Sleep Deprivation on Learning 56
The Harm of Sleep Deprivation to Social Development 56
The Effect of Sleep Deprivation on the Brain 56
Why Children Need More Sleep, Not Less 57
Parental Perceptions on Their Children's Sleep 57
Statistics on Sleep and Academic Performance 57
Academic Subjects Most Adversely Affected by Poor Sleep Patterns .. 57
How Much Sleep Does a School-Age Child Require? 57
Common Pitfall: "When I was Your Age..." 58
Common Misconception: Making Up for Lost Sleep 58
Does Snoring Affect a Child's Grades? 58
Bedtime Resistance and Poor Academic Performance 58
The Total Picture 58

Chapter 5: Angela / Corey, Zoe, and Molly 59
Children of Divorce 66
The Crisis of Divorce 66
How Divorce Affects Children 67
Common Childhood Sleep Disturbances Related to Divorce 67
Approaching the Challenge of Divorce with Your Child 67
How to Have Open, Honest, and Clear Communication with Your Child
  Around Your Divorce 67
Encourage your Child to Express Her Feelings 68
Give Them Time to Adjust on the Inside Before Life Changes on the Outside .. 68
Addressing your Child's Needs 68
Expect Many Conversations 68
Be Gentle but Honest 69
...And Keep Your Marital Troubles Out of Your Child's Life 69
Full Disclosure-For Your Child's Sake 69
Taking Care of Your Child Means Taking Care of Yourself 69
You're Still the Parent, She's Still the Child 70
Nip the Matchmaker Syndrome in the Bud 70
Compensate for Choices Lost with Choices Gained 70
Compensate for Structure Lost with Structure Gained 71
Common Pitfall: Compensating with Gifts and Liberties 71
Just Because They're No Longer Your Family... 71
Signs of More Serious Trauma to Watch For 71
The Golden Promise: I'll Never Divorce You 72

Chapter 6: Janice / Timothy ... 73

- Sibling Rivalry ... 76
- Influences Affecting Sibling Relationships ... 76
- How Age Affects Sibling Relationships ... 76
- A New Baby's Arrival ... 77
- How Individuality Creates Sibling Rivalry ... 77
- How to Handle Sibling Rivalry ... 77
- Common Pitfall: Refereeing Your Children's Relationships ... 77
- The Critical Caveat: Violence ... 78
- Common Pitfall: Who Started It? ... 78
- Equally Accountable but Not Equal Accountability ... 78
- The One Exception: "Separate Corners!" ... 79
- You Can't Force Love, but You Can Enforce Civility ... 79
- Give Them Nothing to Prove ... 79
- Common Pitfall: Showing Favoritism ... 79
- What's Fair? ... 79
- Get to Know Them as Individuals ... 80
- . . . While Facilitating Positive Siblinghood Scenarios ... 80
- Don't Take the Bait! ... 81
- Positive Reinforcement Is Your Friend ... 81
- Help Them to Help You Help Them ... 81
- Teaching by Example: How Do You and Your Siblings Relate? ... 81
- Indications that Professional Help may be Called For ... 82

Chapter 7: Priscilla / Harry and Chloe ... 83

- Nightmares ... 87
- What Causes Nightmares? ... 87
- Statistics on Nightmares in Children ... 87
- When Are Nightmares Age-Appropriate? ... 87
- Effects of Nightmares on Waking Life ... 88
- The Time Nightmares Are Prone to Occur ... 88
- What Distinguishes a Nightmare Disorder? ... 88
- The Stuff of Children's Nightmares ... 88
- Upon Waking From A Nightmare ... 88
- The Best Cure Is Prevention ... 88
- Other Ways to Help Prevent Your Child from Having Nightmares ... 89
- Monitor Television and Video Games ... 89
- Discuss Daily Stressors ... 89
- Encourage Expression ... 89
- How to Deal With a Child's Nightmare in the Moment of Crisis ... 90
- What Distinguishes Night Terrors from Nightmares? ... 90
- How to Handle a Child's Night Terror While It's Happening ... 91

Are Night Terrors Dangerous to a Child? ... 91
Handling Nightmares and Night Terrors –In a Nutshell ... 91

Chapter 8: Kevin / Kelly ... 93
Death and Dying ... 97
How a Child Perceives Death ... 97
Explaining the Death of a Loved One to a Child ... 97
Common Pitfall: Sheltering Them from the Truth ... 98
How to Have Open, Honest, and Clear Communication
  with Your Child on the Subject of Death ... 98
Everyone Grieves in Their Own Way . . . Children Included ... 98
Emotions Happen: Let Them ... 99
Taking Care of Your Child Means Taking Care of Yourself ... 99

Chapter 9: Vivian / Georgia ... 101
Spanking ... 111
Teaching by Example: You're the Model ... 111
What Spanking Teaches ... 111
A Brief History of Spanking ... 111
A Caveat on Spanking and Child Abuse ... 111
Is Spanking Effective? ... 111
Hitting versus Discipline ... 112
Potential Consequences in Adulthood ... 112
Spanking's Sexual Component ... 112
Potential Physical Damage ... 113
Is It Too Late to Change? ... 113
What the U.N. Convention on the Rights of the Child Says ... 113
A Better Way? ... 113

Chapter 10: Lia /Ana ... 115
Childhood Obesity ... 126
Statistics on Childhood Obesity Today ... 126
Is My Child at Risk? Signs and Symptoms of Childhood Obesity ... 126
Causes of Childhood Obesity ... 126
The Effects of Sleep on Childhood Obesity ... 127
How to Deal With an Obese Child ... 128
Weight Loss versus Weight Maintenance ... 128
Common Pitfalls: Over Fixing ... 128
Healthy Eating Basics ... 129
Exercise and Activity Basics ... 129
Slow and Steady Wins the Race: Making Small, Gradual Changes ... 130
Teaching by Example: Watch Your Own Weight ... 130
The Best Support You Can Give ... 130

Chapter 11: Andrew / Darren 133
   Bedwetting 137
   The Problem of Bedwetting 137
   Causes of Bedwetting 137
   Statistics on Bedwetting 138
   Signs and Symptoms Associated with Bedwetting 138
   Effects of Bedwetting 138
   Long-Term Psychological Consequences of Bedwetting 138
   Won't Children Outgrow Bedwetting? 139
   Common Pitfall: Anger and Frustration 139
   What to Do if Your Child Wets the Bed 139
   Prevention is the Best Cure 139
   How Better Hydration Helps Prevent Bedwetting 140
   Exercises to Prevent Bedwetting 140
   Medications to Treat Bedwetting 140
   The Latest Word on Bedwetting: Alarms 141
   Being Realistic About Timelines for Results 141
   Secondary Enuresis 141
   If Bedwetting Persists 141

Chapter 12: Susan / Heather and Tamara 143
   Pain and Medical Illness 153
   The Mind-Body Connection 153
   The Stress Response versus the Relaxation Response 154
   Visualizing Freedom From Pain 154
   What Else Visualization May Help 155
   Pain and Sleep 155
   How to Help Your Child Relax and Visualize The Pain Away 155

Chapter 13: Howard / Maya 157
   Adult Use of Children's Programs 162
   Stirring Up Emotions 162
   Loss of Self 162
   Reconnecting: With the Child Within and with Mother Nature 163
   Emotional Intelligence 163
   Breaking Down Ego Barriers 163

Chapter 14: Frances / Clarissa, Danielle, and Tanya 165
   Low Self-Esteem 178
   Sleep and Self-Esteem 179
   The Role and Benefits of Self-Esteem 179
   Threats to Self-Esteem 179
   Seven Pillars of High Self-Esteem 179

PART III: OTHER CONSIDERATIONS 181

Chapter 15: Strategies and Solutions for Childhood Insomnia: Sleep Hygiene and Beyond ... 183

Sleep Hygiene 183
Childhood Sleep Problems that Can Be Sourced Back to Poor Sleep Hygiene 184
Benefits of Improving a Child's Sleep Hygiene 184
Guidelines to Good Sleep Hygiene 184
Bedtime Schedule 184
The Body Clock and Circadian Rhythms 184
How to Establish a Bedtime Schedule for Your Child that Works 185
Common Pitfall: Your Own Schedule's Irregularity 185
Optimal Sleep Duration for Children 185
Bedtime Routine 186
Why a Bedtime Routine is So Important 186
What Not to Do 30 Minutes Before Bedtime 186
The Foundation of Good Sleep Hygiene 187
Environmental Sleep Hygiene 187
Daytime Sleep Hygiene 188
Beyond Sleep Hygiene 189
Sleep Associations 189
Nighttime Wakings 190
Rocking Young Children to Sleep 190
Leaving the Light On 190
Relaxation Aids and Sleep Associations 190
Teaching Your Child to Fall Asleep Alone 191
If Your Child Leaves the Bed During the Night 192
Co-sleeping 192
Cultural Opinions on Co-sleeping Over Time 193
The Two Holdouts: U.S. and Europe 193
Separation Anxiety: Necessity or Not? 193
Latest Research on Crying 193
What Ferber's Opponents Say 194
Ferber Counters 194
Ferber's Argument Against the Family Bed 194
What About Security Objects ... Blankets, Teddy Bears? 195
Co-sleeping and Sudden Infant Death Syndrome (SIDS) 195
Parent-Child Sleep Synchronization 195
Other Benefits of Co-sleeping 196
Co-sleeping and Breast-Feeding 196
A Shocking Turnaround: Ferber Rethinks 197
Ultimately, a Choice 197
Making the Family Bed Safe 197

When Not to Co-sleep	198
Co-sleeping and Nighttime Wakings	198
Co-sleeping and Sex	198
Where to Place the Baby in the Family Bed	198
Transitioning a Child from the Family Bed	199
A Two-Week Plan for Weaning Your Child off the Family Bed	199
Medication for Sleep Problems	200
Reasons For and Against Using Medications	200
Sleep Medications for Kids when There's No Emergency?	201
Rebound Insomnia	201
Studies on Sleep Medications in Children	201
Deciding Whether or Not to Medicate	201
Managing a Child on Sleep Medication	201
Specific Medication Used in Pediatric Insomnia	203

Chapter 16: Medical Causes of Sleep Problems ... 207

Chronic Middle Ear Diseases and Sleep	207
Heartburn and Sleep	207
ADHD (ADD) and Sleep	208
Which Came First: The ADHD or the Sleep Disturbances?	208
If Your Child Has Symptoms or a Diagnosis of ADHD	208
The Genetic Component of ADHD	208
The Dietary Component of ADHD	209
Obstructive Sleep Apnea	209
What is Obstructive Sleep Apnea?	209
Signs and Symptoms of Childhood Sleep Apnea	209
When is Sleep Apnea Most Likely to Occur?	210
Diagnosing Childhood Sleep Apnea	210
Does Effective Treatment Exist for Sleep Apnea?	210
Brain Damage and Sleep	210

Chapter 17: Strategies and Solutions for the Problem of Anxiety ... 211

The Sleep-Anxiety Link	211
Fear versus Anxiety Revisited	211
The Stress Response: How Anxiety Works	212
How Children Experience Anxiety	212
The True Root of a Child's Fears	213
Why Reassurance Doesn't Work	213
Common Pitfall: Downplaying It	213
How to Help a Child with Anxiety	214
Talking with Your Child About Anxiety	214
The First, Biggest, and Most Powerful Step in Dealing with Anxiety	214

A Support System 215
Separating the Child from His Anxiety 215
Empowering Children 215
Mission Accomplished? 216
Relaxation 216
The Relaxation Response 217
Benefits of Relaxation for Children 217
Common Relaxation Techniques 218
A Caveat: The Child's Volition 218
The Sleep-Relaxation Link 218
Dietary Relaxation Aids 219
Exercise for Relaxation 219
Anxiety Disorders 219
Digging for the Root Cause of a Child's Anxiety 220
Medical Assistance for Anxiety Disorders 220
Hereditary Anxiety: The Role of Genetics in Childhood Anxiety 221
The Silver Lining on Anxiety's Dark Cloud 221
Better People 221
A Self-Feeding Cycle: For Worse or For Better 222

Chapter 18: Summary: Nature-Deficit Disorder 223
A Web of Interrelationships 223
Nature-Deficit Disorder (NDD) 224
Television, NDD, and Sleep 225
Academic Performance, NDD, and Sleep 226
Childhood Obesity, NDD, and Sleep 227
Self-Esteem, NDD, and Sleep 228
Medical Issues 228
Divorce, NDD, and Sleep 229
The Unseen Perils of Modern City Life 229
Urban versus Natural Environments Put to the Test 230
Therapeutic Properties of Nature 230
A Heartening Realization 231
Back to the Core Question: How to Help a Child Sleep? 231
The DreamChild Adventures 3D Audio Series 231
Conclusion 233
A Personal Invitation 234

APPENDICES 235
Appendix A: A Brief Disclaimer 237
Appendix B: Audio Equipment 239

Appendix C: Hearing Risk 241
   Noise-Induced Hearing Loss in Children 241
   What Causes Hearing Loss? 241
   Statistics on Children's Hearing 241
   Safe-Listening Standards for Children 242
   Variables: The Crux of the Formula 242
   Common Pitfall: Desensitization 242
   How Safe Are Portable Music Players? 243
   The Hand that Giveth . . . How Technology Helps and Hinders 243
   Myths and Facts about Personal Music Players 243
   How to Set the Volume on a Listening Device 244
   A Couple of Caveats 244
   More on Setting the Volume on a Listening Device 245
   A Partial List of Recommended "Kid-safe" Audio Listening Products 245
   Where Technology Leaves Off 246
   Audio Settings and the DreamChild Adventures Programs 246
   Competing Standards for Safe Listening 246
   Other Guidelines for Protecting Your Child's Hearing (and Your Own) 247

Appendix D: Audio Program Scripts 249
   Country Friends 249
   Magic Carpet 256
   Playhouse on the Beach 261

Appendix E: Bibliography 267

Appendix F: 3D AudioMagic Programs Catalogue 273
   3D AudioMagic Program Descriptions 274

Appendix G: Additional Resources 281

Appendix H: Research on the AudioMagic Programs and 3D Living Sound 283

INDEX 297

PART I

INTRODUCTION

DreamChild Adventures
Children's Programs

Dream*Child* **Adventures** *is a series of entertaining* and therapeutic audio programs designed to promote relaxation and sleep in children between the ages of four and twelve.

Who Created It?

I'm Tom Jackson, M.D., and I have been a practicing psychiatrist for the past 30 years. My first involvement with audio recording began in 1978 with the production of popular music. Through this process I developed a love for audio recording and engineering. There followed a 25-year exploration of therapeutic uses of sound. Since the mid-1980s I have utilized an innovative recording technology, *3D Living Sound*™, in the production of my programs. This breakthrough in recording technology creates a multi-dimensional listening experience in which the listener hears sounds as emanating from all around

How DreamChild Adventures Came About

I developed my first therapeutic audio programs for the treatment of anxiety and insomnia to treat adults in my clinical practice. A number of these patients who had experienced personal success used the adult programs with their children, and the results they achieved inspired a new series of programs—*DreamChild Adventures*—designed specifically for children. As it turned out, these new programs seem to speak to the "child in all of us" and, though designed for ages 4-12, they have been enjoyed by people of all ages. The *DreamChild Adventures* incorporate a number of elements including guided imagery, breathing techniques, Neuro-Linguistic Programming (NLP), nature sounds, sound effects, music, poetry, and story telling.

Why a Companion Book?

Throughout my years of clinical practice, I have witnessed the central roles that stress and anxiety play in a wide variety of problems both children and adults experience. By providing people with the means to attain deep states of relaxation, I have enjoyed a unique vantage point from which to view the remarkable benefits many achieve. I invite you to join me and share my intimate perspective as I conduct clinical interviews with caretakers (or therapists) of children who struggled with sleep difficulties and other anxiety-related problems. These people, perhaps like you, often felt confused, frustrated, and desperate for solutions to pressing issues. And yet, as you will discover, the most dramatic benefits frequently extended far beyond the initial problems that motivated program use with these children. I traveled far and wide to record the various sound effects that make up the 3D backgrounds for the programs

The Link Between Sleep and Other Issues

Throughout the process of working with these caretakers, a compelling (if none too surprising) phenomenon became apparent: the programs benefitted these children not only in regards to their sleep-related issues but also appeared to impact a whole constellation of anxiety-related emotional and behavioral issues that these children faced.

Some of these issues are obviously directly related to sleep, such as:

- bedwetting
- nightmares/night terrors
- fear of the dark

But others seemed, at least on the surface, incidental to sleep, such as:

- childhood obesity
- resistance to reading/poor academic performance
- television habits
- defiance
- self-esteem

An Inextricable Web

What these caretakers and I found was that their children's troubles sleeping and the other related problems they encountered were woven inextricably together in a web of cause and effect. Each child faced a different set of problems, many of which the caretakers had not even associated with the child's sleep problems until after they experienced a near-simultaneous improvement in both sets of problems, as they used the programs.

Every Child Is Different

As you proceed through this book, you may find that some case studies call out to you more than others. You may recognize your own child in some of the children we examine, while finding little correlation between your child and some of the others studied herein.

Therefore, you may decide not to read this book all the way through, from cover to cover—though I certainly recommend it. You may instead choose to scan the "complaints" which precede each case for those specific issues most pertinent to those your own child currently faces to find how others have successfully dealt with the same concerns.

Afterwards, you may put this book aside as you explore the solutions it offers (not least of which are the audio programs), picking it up again at some point in the future should any of the other issues broached in the book come up for your child.

With this in mind, let me introduce you to the layout of this book so that you may get the most value out of reading it, whatever your goals.

How to Use This Book

DreamChild Adventures in Relaxation and Sleep is most useful as a companion to the *DreamChild Adventures* 3D audio programs I refer to frequently throughout the book.

Part I is the section you're reading now. It is the Introduction to this book and to the intertwining problems of sleep and anxiety in children, as well to the *DreamChild Adventures* programs as a powerful solution to many of these problems.

Part II presents a series of cases, each of which follows one or more children who suffered sleep problems but who subsequently benefitted from using the audio programs. Each interview with the children's parent, guardian, or therapist (hereafter referred to, for simplicity's sake, as "*caretakers*") is broken up into two basic sections:

- a "*Before*" section describing problems the children experienced prior to using the programs
- an "*After*" section relaying one or more follow-up interviews conducted several days, weeks, or months (and in one case, years) later, detailing the improvements the caretakers noticed after use of the programs.

In addition, after each of the interviews, I include a commentary providing further information and insights into a particular problem associated with the case.

Part III broadens the scope of the conversation to explore traditional strategies and solutions to the problems of sleep and anxiety in children that can work hand-in-hand with the *DreamChild Adventures* children's audio programs to produce maximum results. This section, by no means comprehensive, presents a sweeping overview of some of the ways most commonly recommended by experts to help children relax and sleep well

The **Appendices** includes topics specific to the *DreamChild Adventures* 3D audio programs and the related *3D Living Sound* technology. It includes extensive details about the research conducted on the AudioMagic™ programs and *3D Living Sound* technology, as well as

- a discussion on potential hearing risks associated with some audio listening devices and practices
- a bibliography for this book
- the scripts for the three *DreamChild Adventures* 3D audio programs
- a catalogue of all of the *AudioMagic* programs currently available

If you have a specific topic of interest or pressing issue with a child in your life you wish to investigate, rather than reading the book sequentially, you can look for it in the Table of Contents and go directly to that section

- If it regards a specific sleep problem—like bedwetting, nightmares, or fear of the dark—or an aspect of childhood development only tangentially related (or seemingly unrelated) to sleep—such as academic performance, childhood obesity or sibling rivalry—then you may find it in one of the Interviews or subsequent Commentaries in **Part II**

- If it regards some aspect of sleep, anxiety, or relaxation in general, you will most likely find it in **Part III**
- If it regards the *DreamChild Adventures* children's audio programs or any element of *3D Living Sound* technology, or research on the AudioMagic programs, you will most likely find it in the **Appendice**s.

In presenting the material in this way, I hope to provide you with a deep understanding of the kinds of problems these audio programs can be used to treat, as well as related benefits that may be achieved. By showing you the specific and often sweeping changes these children underwent through their experiences with the programs, my aim is to give you confidence in their potential usefulness and to inspire you to use them with any child in your life who you believe may benefit.

There is no right or wrong way to use this book. There is only your way—what works best for you and the children in your life. I propose through this book to help you and the children you love and care for find your own individual pathway to greater health and happiness

CHILDREN AND ANXIETY

THE EFFECTS OF STRESS IN CONTEMPORARY SOCIETY

How can we explain why one in eight children develops a diagnosable anxiety disorder, and approximately 25% of children and upwards of 40% of adolescents struggle with significant sleep problems? The increasing stress of contemporary society, I believe, plays a major role:

- disrupted homes
- blended families
- both parents working outside the home
- school pressures (including state testing)
- peer pressure to "fit in"
- exposure to violence (virtual and real)
- pressure to perform
- excessive stimulation
- information overload (TV, radio, video games, the Internet)

A recent Harvard study concluded that a single edition of *The New York Times* contains more information than the average person living in the eighteenth century would have been exposed to in an entire lifetime. Think about it. Our brains haven't evolved over the last 300 years, but we now absorb thousands of times more information, and into which our children are immersed at earlier and earlier ages.

But sleep problems don't solely result from the increased stress of contemporary society. A number of other important factors affect sleep, like bedtime routines and situational issues. Likewise, not all anxiety can be blamed on life's stresses. Two children exposed to the same stress will not necessarily react in the same manner. And clearly, some children are predisposed to anxiety, as evidenced by the strong genetic link that research has shown.

WHAT IS ANXIETY?

"We have nothing to fear but fear itself." Never a truer statement was spoken than those famous words uttered by Franklin D. Roosevelt (albeit in a completely unrelated context).

Anxiety is literally the fear of fear—being afraid of being afraid. All the thoughts, feelings, and sensations associated with being afraid—they are the essence of anxiety.

As the books *The Anxiety Cure* and *The Anxiety Cure for Kids* explain, anxiety is the perception of danger where, in reality, no danger is present. While fear is a valuable internal alarm signaling real and immediate danger, as authors Robert L. DuPont, M.D., Founding President of the Anxiety Disorders Association of America, and his daughters Elizabeth DuPont Spencer, M.S.W. and Caroline M. DuPont, M.D. succinctly describe it, anxiety is a "false alarm" responding to imagined danger, that which isn't present except in the mind of the person experiencing the anxiety.

When that false alarm sounds repeatedly, incessantly, it causes a predictable surge of disturbing thoughts and feelings, including: irrational fear, discomfort, self-doubt, and panic.

A VICIOUS CYCLE: FEAR OF THE IMAGINARY

All of these negative by-products of anxiety only serve to escalate anxiety by fueling a vicious cycle of self-defeating avoidance of life. In fact, anxiety may even cause deeper and more lasting anguish than the actual experience of the feared situation would likely produce. That is because, as the DuPonts point out: "Anxiety is a disorder of anticipation." Almost all of the resulting discomfort comes *before* the situation or experience that provoked the anxiety. Anxiety arises from the question, "*What if?*" Anxiety exacerbates, intensifies, and perpetuates those *"what ifs"* to the point that they become a hindrance to a person's proper functioning. The remedy for this spiraling cascade of *"what ifs"* is contained in the realization of *"what is."*

Because anxiety is a fear of what might be, and more, a fear of the physical and emotional experience of fear itself, it is irrational and inappropriate to the situation provoking it. Fear is useful, whereas anxiety is not. Fear alerts us to something which really does require our undivided, alert attention. Anxiety simply causes us to worry that the object of our fear *might* materialize. Fear alerts us to the immediate need to jump out of the way of an oncoming car; anxiety keeps us from going for a walk in the first place because we fear we may be struck by a car. Importantly, in terms of our mental health . . . and this is a crucial point . . . fear does not usually lead to the doubt, insecurity, and low self-esteem that anxiety typically does.

AGE-APPROPRIATE FEARS

Anxiety, then, is any fear that is out of proportion to the given circumstances, and that places unreasonable restrictions on a person's daily experience of life. Applying this to children, that means any fear that is not age-appropriate. In a *WebMD*® feature article, Annie Stuart outlines age-appropriate fears as follows:

Infants/Toddlers
- Loud noises
- Sudden movements
- Large and looming objects
- Strangers
- Separation from parents/guardians
- Changes in environment

Preschool-age children
- Darkness
- Noises during the night
- Masks
- Ghosts, monsters, etc.
- Dogs and other such animals

School-age children
- Spiders
- Snakes
- Storms (thunder, lightning)
- Being left alone at home
- The anger of a trusted authority figure (such as a teacher)
- Illness and injury
- Doctors, shots, hospitals
- Rejection
- Failure

Any of these fears only become problematic when they continue beyond a certain age; that's when they cross over from fear into anxiety. Children with anxiety problems worry about things that simply don't worry most other children of their age.

For example, young children normally fear separation from mommy and daddy when they're taken off to school, and that's appropriate for a very young child, but if a child still experiences that same separation anxiety after several years of school, it ceases to be a reasonable fear and becomes an unreasonable anxiety, as it is no longer appropriate. Anxiety may manifest in young children as excessive clinginess to the trusted adults in their lives.

THE FEAR OF SLEEPING ALONE

As you'll see in many of the children's case studies that follow, another common anxiety children experience with varying degrees of intensity and age-appropriateness is sleeping alone at night. According to a chart in *Help For Worried Kids*, similar to the one above, author Cynthia G. Last, Ph.D. says that six years of age is when the fear of sleeping alone commonly begins in children. I explore this anxiety in great detail, as well as the ongoing debate on how parents can best handle it, in a section on Co-sleeping found in Part III of this book.

ANXIETY IN TEENS

Similarly, in adolescence it is appropriate for teenagers to harbor social insecurities, but as those teens grow into young adults, those social anxieties are no longer appropriate. Older children may deal with anxiety more subversively, such as by simply asserting their unwillingness to do something demanded of them. A lot of disruptive and oppositional behavior, as a matter of fact, has its roots in anxiety.

SIGNS OF AN ANXIOUS CHILD

Anxious children typically avoid speaking up in the classroom and, in extreme cases, try to avoid going to school altogether, devising any excuses they can to get their parents to let them stay home. Anxious children are often homebodies, typical "mama's boys" and "daddy's girls," rarely venturing outside of their comfort zone to take social risks. Anxious children have difficulties socializing with other children and "fitting in" with their peers. Anxiety can cause a child to avoid many of the joyous activities and pleasures of being a child. They often miss out on sleepovers, field trips, and extracurricular activities involving separation from their parents and home.

Children experiencing persistent anxiety feel alienated from their peers and their family alike. Seeing that other people, especially their peers, don't feel the same anxiety they do about things causes anxious children to distrust their own thoughts, feelings, and bodily messages. This naturally leads anxious children to believe there is something wrong with them, fostering shame, self-doubt, and low self esteem. It also leads to the anxious child feeling terribly alone and trapped by their problem, helpless in the face of endless triggers of their anxiety all around them.

CONSEQUENCES OF UNRESOLVED CHILDHOOD ANXIETY

Chronic anxiety can stunt a child's developmental growth, preventing him from maturing into an emotionally healthy young adult. Untreated, anxious children grow into insecure, anxious adults with deep-rooted problems that are increasingly harder to correct the longer they persist.

At the end of this book, I will review some core strategies and solutions for the problem of anxiety, including an in-depth discussion on relaxation. But for the time being, let's look at some of the ways anxiety interferes with mental and physical development through sleep disturbance.

CHILDREN, ANXIETY, AND SLEEP

ANXIETY AND SLEEP

Anxiety can make it hard for a child to study, to sleep, to eat, or even to play, for his mind is consumed by the object of his anxiety. Anxiety consumes an abundance of mental energy, exhausting the person suffering from it, eventually leading to fatigue and, potentially, even depression. Anxiety, in fact, is frequently found to be the precursor to depression, and an anxious child can easily grow into a depressed adult. Incidentally, changes in sleep patterns are another symptom of depression Dr. Last points out, noting that anxious children tend to sleep less and depressed children tend to sleep more.

I could not present a thorough exploration of sleep and relaxation without giving due coverage to anxiety. As Tamar E. Chansky, Ph.D. says in her book, *Freeing Your Child From Anxiety*: "Anyone who has spent a sleepless night watching the numbers flip one by one, hour after hour, on their digital clock knows that sleep and anxiety are diametrically opposed and, for that reason, inextricably linked."

A NIGHTLY STRUGGLE

Perhaps getting your child to bed is a nightly struggle, not to mention getting him to remain in bed and asleep throughout the night. Maybe you have lost sleep yourself from attending to your child's sleep problems during the night. Is it an all too familiar experience to awaken in the morning to a child who is tired and cranky? You, too, may start the day irritable from a lack of deep, restful, uninterrupted sleep. If so, you no doubt spend much of your waking hours concerned that the following night will only bring more of the same.

You certainly don't want to let this concern progress to the point that it blocks your own effectiveness in helping your child. Many caretakers find themselves at their wit's end trying to deal with sleepless children, so you're not alone in this struggle. And, rest assured, you are not only about to gain greater understanding of the problems you face; you will also find answers and solutions that may have eluded you.

COMMON CHILDHOOD SLEEP PROBLEMS

You may be dealing with any number of common sleep problems that can be present to different degrees and in various combinations. In the personal stories to follow, we will encounter a range of sleep problems (and we will share in these patients' struggles and subsequent achievements):

- bedtime resistance
- anxiety about sleep
- sleep onset delay

- nighttime wakings
- inadequate sleep duration
- difficulty waking in the morning
- morning moodiness
- daytime sleepiness

Other related childhood sleep problems we'll explore in the interviews include bedwetting, nightmares, night terrors, and obstructive sleep apnea.

Throughout the clinical interviews you'll encounter children facing sleep problems, each in their own unique way. Reading through the stories, you'll likely gain insights as you recognize elements that also apply to your own experiences with the child you're trying to help.

THE UNTOLD EFFECTS OF SLEEP

Indeed, sleep influences all bodily functions—for good and for bad. Inadequate sleep has been found to contribute to many medical problems and presents an array of deleterious effects on all aspects of daily living. The following are just some of the problems associated with poor sleeping patterns:

- obesity
- diabetes
- anxiety and depression
- impeded physical development
- weakened immune system
- allergies
- infections
- accident proneness
- diminished attention span

A TURNING POINT

But whatever sleeping problems affect your household, definitely do not despair. All of the *DreamChild Adventures* have proven extremely valuable tools for relaxation and sleep. If your child's sleep problems have perplexed and frustrated you, I'm sure an enjoyable, effective solution to those issues will come as a welcome gift for both you and your child.

This book will likely mark a turning point in your struggles. You now have in your hands the information and tools you need to chart a new course to restful sleep for both you and the children you love.

The Programs

The *DreamChild Adventures* include one relaxation program, *Country Friends*, and two sleep programs, *Magic Carpet* and *Playhouse on the Beach*. Both *Country Friends* and *Magic Carpet* are brought to life through a variety of entertaining 3D sound effects that engage the imagination of even the most restless children. Although *Playhouse on the Beach* incorporates only waves in the background, children who don't have the need for more engaging 3D sounds to draw their attention inward may find it ideal for falling asleep. And, best of all, most children really enjoy the programs, which minimizes resistance to listening or going to bed.

Once your child has become familiar with these programs, you might enjoy reading the scripts together as bedtime stories.

Country Friends

Country Friends is a unique relaxation program that offers benefits to children struggling with problems exacerbated by stress or anxiety, such as nervousness, worry, sadness, fear, insecurity, anger, pain, bedtime resistance, and sleep problems. The program can be used any time of day to create greater relaxation, and can as well be used as a wind-down before bedtime, or in conjunction with *Magic Carpet* and *Playhouse on the Beach*.

I encourage you to listen to *Country Friends* yourself also, because your understanding of the experience may help you guide your child to receive the greatest possible benefits. I narrate the story, which starts with a car trip to the countryside. After suggesting that your child close his eyes, the narration guides him through daydreams, his imagination stirred by a medley of sounds: bike riding, skating, swings, slides, horses, cars, airplanes, a train, a circus, and so on. With your child's attention thus drawn inward, the program enters the relaxation phase, as we begin walking down an imaginary pathway through an enchanted forest.

Soon, we come upon a meadow with a farmhouse where we stop for directions to the river that will lead us down to the ocean. We are invited to sit on the porch and are treated to some country hospitality. A bluegrass group named *Harmony Grits* (www.harmonygrits.com) plays a traditional country tune and then two of their original songs, sending us on our way to the soothing lilt of "Down by the River." After a short walk we sit beside the river where we slip into a relaxing meditation with the peaceful sounds of water, wind and birds.

Continuing our walk down the pathway, we discover a pond where we watch images appear upon its surface in reflection; we contemplate poetic words of inspiration and comfort. We then walk further along the path and emerge on a magical beach where the child finds time for imaginary play. *Country Friends* concludes with the suggestion that the child take some of the wonderful feelings he is experiencing with him as he returns home.

MAGIC CARPET

Next, I'd like to introduce *Magic Carpet*, a program designed to make bedtime pleasant for both children and those who care for them. It is a whimsical story-poem brought to life by enthralling *3D Living Sound* effects.

Although most children have little problem with sleep, they may still display varying degrees of resistance to going to bed or make extra requests for attention when it's time to go to sleep. For these children, *Magic Carpet* can make the bedtime ritual much easier and more enjoyable. If your child is accustomed to having you read him a bedtime story, perhaps *Magic Carpet* can stand in when you don't have time to read, or it is inconvenient.

As noted earlier, if your child struggles with a significant sleep problem, you're probably losing sleep, too. You may find yourself trying to help your child work through any number of sleep-related problems, such as a high degree of resistance to going to bed, trouble falling asleep, restless sleep, nightmares, or nighttime wakings from which your child cannot fall back to sleep. The results that others have achieved with the audio programs, and which you will shortly read about, should give you hope that you may solve your child's sleep problems more easily than you imagined. Many children, especially those with severe or habitual sleep problems, may also benefit from additional techniques we'll cover later.

You might enjoy listening to *Magic Carpet* yourself, and your understanding of the program may help you in guiding your child's use. The program begins with a musical introduction, after which I narrate a story told in the form of a poem. Your child goes on a magic carpet ride through various scenes, his imagination stirred by a variety of sounds: city sounds, a parade, a playground, a zoo, farm animals, and so on. After drawing your child's attention inward, the program becomes even more relaxing as it invites your child down a pathway through an enchanted forest. Mother Nature comes to life through various elements (trees, a bird, a stream, and the ocean) and shares words of care and comfort. The pathway emerges on an enchanted beach where your child will build sand castles and watch seagulls fly overhead. The suggestions for relaxation and sleepiness continue as your child is led to discover a playhouse containing a special bed where he may drift to sleep as the background of gently rolling waves gradually fades away.

PLAYHOUSE ON THE BEACH

The final program in this series, *Playhouse on the Beach*, is a sequel to *Magic Carpet* (which I generally recommend for initial use). But if your child has a calmer disposition and doesn't require the livelier format of *Magic Carpet* to hold his attention, you'll certainly find *Playhouse on the Beach* appropriate; some children find it even more relaxing than *Magic Carpet*. Like *Magic Carpet*, however, this program offers an enjoyable bedtime activity that helps children fall asleep.

Playhouse on the Beach takes place on an inviting beach amidst the calls of seabirds and the pleasant roll of ocean waves. The narrator (male or female voice) guides your child to play along the water's edge where he is then invited to float over the surf on a raft and observe the fish below, to ride upon the waves, to gather seashells, to play with the sand. Eventually, he discovers a playhouse containing a chest of toys and games, along with a welcoming bed. The program becomes gradually more restful, drawing your child into sleep with subtle suggestions and the slowly fading sound of waves.

BENEFITS OF THE DREAMCHILD ADVENTURES CHILDREN'S PROGRAMS

Children who use the programs usually experience rapid improvement in a variety of sleep problems. And for this, users have been very grateful, since a search for resolution to a child's sleep problems is the primary reason that most people are drawn to the programs. But as you will discover in the following case reports, additional benefits, which are often reported, are frequently the most exciting rewards of the programs.

Extraordinary improvements should not be completely surprising, considering that research on relaxation therapies with children has been so promising. Children also do as well as, or better than, adults when it comes to learning relaxation techniques. My own work with children has certainly been consistent with this conclusion. In addition, studies show that relaxation therapies can improve not only sleep but academic performance and self-esteem, and can as well reduce hyperactivity, headache frequency/intensity, gastrointestinal complaints, impulsivity, and disruptive behavior.

SIMPLE MEASURES YIELD EXTRAORDINARY RESULTS

Many of the following cases show such dramatic results that I would expect some people, especially professionals, to wonder how "simple" audio programs could possibly have such profound effects. But please hold off judgment regarding what is or isn't possible until after you have experienced the *3D Living Sound* technology for yourself and have had a chance to discover the depth of relaxation that the audio programs can induce.

Despite the supportive research on relaxation therapies and children, the extensive degree of improvement you'll see in the following case studies still remains somewhat difficult to explain.

POSSIBLE EXPLANATIONS

In seeking explanations for the results, one could postulate the timing of program use is a major contributor. Perhaps, by creating a deeply relaxed state in a child as he falls asleep, we are able to "reset" the autonomic nervous system. And this deeply relaxed state, being relatively unperturbed through the night, may take hold to a degree that has not been fully appreciated. Subsequently this new level of relaxation (both physiological and psychological) may stick with a child for much longer, and to a much greater degree, than would normally be expected. And, because anxiety is such a powerful driving force behind so many problems, its resolution may result in a cascading effect which in some cases appears transformative.

Such a theory seems plausible in children, especially considering that their emotional and behavioral problems have not been present so long that they have crystallized into the more resistant, deep-seated patterns often encountered in adults.

The extraordinary benefits some children experience can be at least partially explained by their improvement in sleep alone. Just like anxiety, sleep can have a profound effect on mood, behavior, and performance. And when we consider the possible resulting benefits from dramatically improved sleep and reduced anxiety simultaneously, the results reported may become easier to comprehend.

A Caveat: Every Child is Different-Revisited

In addition to the degree of improvement reported, there is the issue of the percentage of children who can expect to experience such benefits. The results that are reported here are not unusual in the least, but I cannot claim that they represent a precise cross section of users. Interestingly though, those cases that had disappointing results almost always involved children who were resistant to listening or who "didn't like the programs." It's impossible to know what kind of outcomes these children might have achieved if there had been a way to enlist their cooperation. (Even reliable medications are ineffective if patients won't take them.) What I can say is that the cases presented here do represent the kinds of real-life success that I have come to expect when children use the programs regularly.

The Fast Track to Success

Up until now, most solutions to children's sleep problems have involved fairly rigorous adherence to bedtime schedules and routines, along with behavioral interventions, all of which can be quite challenging and demand consistent application. Although most children benefit from the traditional approaches, for many the audio programs offer a relatively easy "short cut" to success.

Still, I do not want to minimize the importance, efficacy, or even necessity of these other valuable techniques, which we will review following the case presentations. You'll also find discussions of certain sleep disorders caused by medical problems which require very specific medical interventions.

Research

Although no formal research has yet been done with program use in children, initial testing at Children's Hospital of Orange County was very encouraging, with reported success involving separation anxiety (when parents leave their children in the hospital) and decreased anxiety associated with medical procedures. The children's programs will soon be introduced to children's hospitals across the country, along with an effort to encourage academic research, in order to quantify the degree of improvement in a number of areas.

The adult audio programs, on the other hand, have undergone extensive formal evaluation. The original relaxation program (*Natural Relaxation 1*) was tested in four separate psychiatric and chemical dependency hospital units and produced an average decrease in anxiety of 52% (comparing anxiety levels immediately before and after program use). On the chemical dependency units, where medications were seldom used, it was possible to measure the effect of this relaxation program over time by measuring daily anxiety levels (before program use), which decreased an average of 32% over three weeks compared to patients who did not use the program. The advantage of statistics is that they are objective and allow for comparisons to other treatment modalities. The numbers, of course, helpful as they are, do not begin to communicate what the results meant to the individuals experiencing decreased anxiety.

Other research conducted on the adult sleep programs includes a successful sleep-training and fatigue reduction program that I developed, along with Dr. Christopher Alsten, for jet-lagged U.S. Air Force pilots, air crews, and shiftworkers, and funded by the USAF. Another study, this on a locked inpatient psychiatric unit, showed a reduction of sleeping pill usage of 98%. A study at the University of California Irvine Medical Center sleep lab, utilizing all-night EEG's, demonstrated improvement in both sleep and emotional states. And in a study funded by the National Institute of Health conducted at the University of California San Francisco, first-time mothers were able to sleep an average of 55 additional minutes per night following childbirth.

This and other related research, a total of ten studies, is laid out in greater depth in Appendix H—Research on the *AudioMagic Programs* and *3D Living Sound*.

ADVERSE REACTIONS AND SIDE EFFECTS

Now I need to don my doctor's hat and address an issue that I have not found problematic, but one we must discuss. In the same manner that I caution my psychiatric patients about the possibility of adverse reactions or side effects to medications, it is my professional duty to take the same approach with relaxation techniques. Researchers have determined that some patients, when undergoing relaxation training, may experience relaxation-induced anxiety, including panic attacks, and what is termed "autogenic discharges," which can include pain, anxiety, palpitations, muscle twitches, and crying. Although users of my programs have reported very mild adverse reactions, such reports have been rare and have never involved children.

If, while using any of these programs, anyone experiences an increase in anxiety or any of the above symptoms, it is advisable to stop listening immediately. Under these circumstances one may wish to try again another time. But if unpleasant experiences recur, program use should be discontinued permanently. There are also reports of adverse reactions to relaxation techniques in people who suffer from psychotic disorders, such as schizophrenia, in which "flights of the imagination" may not be therapeutic and could even exacerbate preexisting hallucinations or delusions. I have, however, used my programs with such patients and have not encountered problems. Nevertheless, it is logical that there may be an increased risk under these circumstances, in which case the programs should only be used under professional supervision and with caution.

PARTICIPANTS IN THE CASE STUDIES

I would like to express my deep appreciation to the people who so generously opened their lives in such intimate and honest ways in order to share their personal experiences. Some of the interviews I conducted were with caretakers of children who were treated and others were with therapists who used the programs to treat children. With permission from these people, I made audio recordings of the interviews, although at the time I had no idea I would eventually include the interviews in a book. The recordings have assured accuracy, though I have changed names and certain details to protect confidentiality.

I present 22 clinical cases in the 14 interviews included this book to help you to understand the potential benefits the programs offer your child. You'll likely recognize some of your own struggles in these narratives; this recognition may provide valuable insights regarding your own solutions. And importantly as well, the successes you read about in these cases may also offer you needed encouragement along the way. At the beginning of each interview, I have provided a summary of the problems each child was experiencing to help you identify those problems most appropriate to your particular situation. Following each interview, I develop additional perspectives on a topic of importance that came up during the interview.

BACKGROUND ON THE CASE STUDIES

Before we begin the interviews, I'll take a moment to explain my original motivation for conducting the interviews. The initial feedback I received regarding children who were using the programs was clearly going to be hard to explain to others. My hope from the beginning was that, someday, more formal clinical research would be conducted with children to provide an accurate analysis of program efficacy. But knowing this might not be done for some time, I wanted to at least obtain in-depth case studies to help illustrate the results that were being reported. I am now very grateful that I made this effort because I believe these stories provide insights that mere statistics cannot begin to convey.

The cases in this book represent the first ones for which I was able to obtain feedback, with the exception of two additional recent interviews I selected because they brought up issues that I felt were important to address.

A BRIEF TECHNICAL NOTE

Lastly, a note on manuscript mechanics: since reading "he or she" and "him or her" seems cumbersome, I simply alternate between the masculine and the feminine gender from section to section.

LET THE ADVENTURES BEGIN!

Quite a few years have passed since I conducted these interviews. In fact, until recently the transcripts were literally gathering dust in the attic of my mountain home in "mile high" Idyllwild, California. I feel fortunate to live in a small town, tucked in a protected alpine valley with towering pines, and surrounded by the majesty of 10,000-foot rocky peaks which, at this moment, are covered with four feet of snow. "For all things there is a time," and the time has finally arrived for me to share these stories with you.

PART II
CLINICAL INTERVIEWS

Chapter 1

Leonard/David

Interviewed:	**Leonard**
Child:	**David, age 7**
Complaints:	*Fear of the dark*
	Difficulty unwinding at night
	Difficulty getting him into bed and staying in bed
	Excessive time to fall asleep
	Many requests to sleep with his parents
	"Impossible" in the morning
	Oppositional behavior
	School problems:
	Excessively sleepy, long naps
	Acting out—fights
	Short attention span

Maybe you can share a little about David and the problems he is having around going to sleep.

> David is seven years old and he's having a lot of problems sleeping in the dark at night with the lights out. I'll have to turn the main light in his room on, because he's afraid there are monsters in there. Nightlights are not enough for him; he'll use a flashlight and I'll find him in the morning with a flashlight on. We also have a lot of trouble with him not being able to wind down at night.

What is the average time it takes him to go to sleep at night?

> From fifteen minutes to three hours.

How many nights a week is it a really difficult task to get him into bed and to sleep?

> Every night we have a problem, but I would say three or four nights a week we really have a problem with it where we'll be struggling with him for two to three hours. Then, once he's in bed, he'll still get up, maybe ten times, and have a million excuses why he needed to get out of bed.

How long has that been going on?

Ever since I can remember—I would say maybe three years.

When you have trouble getting him to go to sleep, what are the typical kinds of things you do to try to solve the problem?

He always wants to fall asleep with me there, in addition to having the lights on. And if I lie down with him, it will take about an hour for him to fall asleep. Sometimes I tell him to get in bed with me, because it seems like the easiest thing to do, although not the best, and then at some point I switch beds after he's asleep.

What kinds of things do you do to get him to go to sleep?

We read books, but it seems like he enjoys the books and then he's just ready for another activity. He doesn't really see it as unwinding or relaxing. The things I do to try to get him to relax don't seem to help in terms of him going to sleep.

Once you get him to sleep, does he sleep okay?

Yes, he sleeps throughout the night, he doesn't wake up.

On bad nights, what is he like in the morning?

He is impossible in the morning. Nothing is right for him; everything is wrong. He doesn't want to eat, he doesn't want to get up, and he doesn't want to get dressed—very oppositional. He even wants me to quit my job so he can stay home and sleep in. I have to physically get him up and march him into the bathroom and splash water on his face and try to get him going. On days like that, he has real problems in school.

What kind of school problems?

Many times, he falls asleep at nap time and sleeps for hours, right through the recess, and partly through class; they have to wake him up.

Why do they let him sleep so long?

His behavior is really a problem and probably that's one of the reasons they let him sleep.

What are the behavior problems?

He acts out, he has fighting issues, he doesn't get along very good with the other kids. Sometimes he'll hit them. Also he has a very short attention span, which his teachers have told me a lot.

≈ • ≈

After Leonard and I spoke a bit more, I gave him the *Magic Carpet* CD and instructed him on its use. One month later, I asked if Leonard would come see me again to discuss his observations of the program's effect, if any, on David.

≈ • ≈

Now, David has been using Magic Carpet for how long?

About a month.

So, can you tell me what happened?

Immediately I noticed, probably the second day, that there were no more questions about, *"Can we turn the lights on?"* He's never asked me that again.

You mean he no longer wants a night light or the main lights on?

No, I just turn the program on and he goes to sleep.

Do you have to prompt him to use the program?

I ask him, sometimes, if he would like to use it, but usually he automatically turns it on, on his own. It's his CD player, so he knows how to operate it without a problem.

Does he usually do it himself?

Yes.

What other changes have you seen in him? What about getting him into bed? And how long does it take to get him to sleep?

It takes no time at all now. I would say about 10 or 15 minutes and I can hear him snoring.

Is there less resistance to getting him into bed?

There is no resistance to getting him into bed now. He gets ready for bed and he goes to bed and turns on the program. Before, it was tooth and nail trying to get him into bed.

So it seems like he has something to look forward to now?

He enjoys listening; he enjoys the music, the sounds of the animals and the water, and those are the words he uses.

Is he always asleep quickly?

It works for him always; within 10 to 15 minutes, and he's asleep, and this has been consistent.

Is he different now when he wakes up in the morning?

He's not nearly as difficult as he used to be. He seems to just get up and go into his routine. He knows he needs to wash up and get dressed. Before I would have to tell him do everything. Now he just does it.

Grouchiness?

Not nearly like he used to be. Sometimes if he has a late night, he might have a problem, but nothing like before.

How are the reports from school?

His teacher says his behavior has done a 180-degree turn. They don't have any problems in terms of behavior anymore. No more fighting; he can complete the activities from beginning to end right along with the other kids; no problems with concentration. And no more excessive sleepiness.

Is he still napping?

No. He doesn't even need a nap. He must be getting much more restful sleep at night compared to before.

Was he napping before, even on good days?

Yes, he's always been a napper, but the two or three hour naps were new.

For you, what is the biggest difference in putting him to bed?

In terms of my own hassle and frustration level, now when he goes to bed, he stays in bed and sleeps.

Thank you very much.

FEAR OF THE DARK

In this interview, Leonard spoke of seven-year-old David's fear of the dark, a problem quite common in children.

SYMPTOMS OF A FEAR OF THE DARK

A variety of symptoms commonly associated with this fear include rapid heartbeat, sweating, rapid breathing or shortness of breath, nausea, and a generalized feeling of dread. In cases of extreme or prolonged fear of the dark, more pronounced symptoms can also be encountered, including temper tantrums, insistence that bright lights, television, or the radio be left on, insistence that a caretaker remain in the room with the child until she falls asleep, or the inability to sleep anywhere outside of the home (such as at a grandparent's or other relative's house, at a friend's sleepover, or on a camping trip).

Left to its own devices, a fear of the dark can fester and build into more severe disruptions in a child's bedtime routines, sleeping habits, and even daytime demeanor. A child whose fear of the dark is not adequately addressed can easily carry this fear into adulthood.

CAUSES OF A FEAR OF THE DARK

Fear of the dark can be caused by any number of factors, often a single event linking the darkness with some sort of emotional trauma. This catalyst could be as simple as a movie, book, or television program, or as dire as being locked in a closet or darkened room by a peer, sibling, or babysitter, or even as complex as witnessing another person, such as a loved one, experiencing a similar fear. All sorts of stressful scenarios can trigger fear of the dark, from a hospital stay to a sudden injury to a divorce, a death in the family, or any other form of parental separation.

Some children are simply more fearful in general than others, whether more genetically susceptible or conditioned through experience, tending towards a heightened sensitivity and more emotional temperament. Some children with this problem are merely mimicking behavior they witness in anxious parental figures, siblings, or other role models in their lives. Similarly, this sort of fearful behavior can be unwittingly encouraged in a more dependent sort of child by a parent's over-protectiveness.

The Commonality: Protection

In all of these cases, there is a common element, namely that the child has a sense—whether consciously or not—that something catastrophic may happen to her in the dark of night.

Whatever the catalyst, the unconscious mind, in attempting to protect the child, can create a profoundly negative association between a particular experience and the environment in which it took place, in this case the dark. When viewed this way, it becomes clear how fear of the dark is actually a protective mechanism of the unconscious mind attempting to keep the child safe.

Fear of the Unknown

One obvious factor in being afraid of the dark is the simple fact that you cannot see well around you when there's no light. As human beings we are all genetically predisposed to fear the unknown, and what is that which we cannot see if not a vivid actualization of the unknown?

When you can't see what is going on around you, the imagination can conjure up all sorts of foreboding and sinister things happening all around, within arm's reach, waiting for just the right moment of vulnerability to strike, especially when you have the heightened imagination of a young child, often barely able (if able at all) to distinguish between fantasy and reality.

The Absence of Light

In the dark, all other senses are heightened as well, so that "things that go bump in the night" could reasonably become any number of insidious threats, and sound, in the mind's ear, far more imposing than they otherwise would, were the sense of sight not impaired by darkness.

The child at this point finds herself alone in bed in a dark room, without the reassuring element of sight. Her predicament is now only amplified by the additional absence of the child's primary source of safety and reassurance, namely her trusted caretakers.

Getting to the Deeper Underlying Issue

This fear of the dark, however, may on the surface seem just that. But parents need to remain alert to the possibility this fear actually masks a deeper emotional issue, such as a fear of death (that if they fall asleep, they may not wake back up), a fear of abandonment (that the parent may not be there when the child awakens), separation anxiety, or a craving for the loving, affectionate sort of attention that a parent often shows when coming back into the room to comfort a child in the throes of this kind of anxiety. If you find any of these the case with your child, discuss these larger issues with her openly.

Reasoning with a child can only go so far, though. While it is certainly worthwhile to explain to the child that there is nothing in the room to fear, don't expect this sort of logic and rationality to completely eradicate an experience that, by its very nature, is founded on the ever-irrational and illogical realm of emotions.

That doesn't mean, however, that you have nothing to gain by talking openly with your child about her feelings. Simply asking your child to discuss her fears with you can go a long way towards assuaging those fears. Your child will usually welcome the opportunity to discuss her perception of reality with you—her protector—who provides acceptance and understanding.

Common Pitfall: Playing Along With Their Fantasies

For this to happen, though, it is crucial that in discussing your child's fears, you avoid giving her the impression that you share those fears. Checking under the bed or looking in the closet for monsters, for example, may suggest that you genuinely think there is a possibility that something terrifying may be lurking nearby.

The child already believes you're invincible; otherwise the monsters would also be under your bed or in your closet. The child needs to believe you understand her fears, not to see you buy into the reality of the fears. If she is convinced that there is something under the bed or in the closet, and your assurance that there can't be anything there is to no avail, you might allow her to look, with you present, in order to convince herself of this truth. Invite her, in other words, to share your invincibility.

A Security Tour

You might also show your child the security systems you've employed in the house, such as deadbolt locks on the doors to the outside (though don't actually lock them at night as it could be a fire hazard) or any alarm systems you may have installed.

And it doesn't hurt to ask your child if there are any measures she can think of for handling the fear. A solution could be as simple as permission to bring a comforting toy or other belonging to bed with her (so long as it isn't physically dangerous to do so, of course).

A Little Compassion Goes a Long Way

In broaching the subject of your child's fear, take extreme care to remain sensitive to the child's experience of the dark and to avoid ridiculing her or impassively dismissing her feelings. Belittling a child for being afraid or showing frustration with repeated outbursts of fear will only exacerbate the negative associations the child already has with the experience.

Fear of the Dark—Case Study

In a 1984 University of Mississippi study on children's fear of the dark, the nighttime experiences of six children prone to fearing the dark were followed incrementally over a period of one year as the parents exposed their children to various fear-reducing techniques, including a fear-reducing game they played with the child each night.

The gist of the fear-reducing game was simple—see if the child could remain alone in a dark (or dimly lit) room for increasing periods of time without undue anxiety. But do practice this great experiment with a child at times of the day or night other than bedtimes, so that there is time to discuss any emotions that arise without infringing on sleep.

Besides the fear-reducing game, the experiment included several other successful techniques. One was the use of positive reinforcement by means of having the parent and child repeat together each night certain affirmations such as: *"I am brave and I can take care of myself when I'm alone or when I'm in the dark."*

In another approach the child received a reward each morning when, without any difficulties, she went to bed, fell asleep, and stayed in bed throughout the night in a progressively dimmer room. Rewards included verbal praise, physical affection (hugs), treats, toys, or tokens.

A System of Rewards

Following this example, you can implement a similar program of rewarding your child for taking even small steps towards confronting her fears, for example, rewarding her for simply remaining quietly in bed and not jumping out (or acting out) the moment you're done tucking her in.

As for the participants of the University of Mississippi study, within two weeks after beginning treatment, all six were able to sleep straight through the night with the lighting in the room set at standard illumination for sleeping or lower.

Other Fear-of-the-Dark Solutions to Try

Other steps to try out in helping free your child from fear of the dark include the following:
- establishing a predictable and reliable bedtime routine
- installing a nightlight in the room or in a visible part of the hallway outside the door
- giving your child a sense of control over her environment by placing a lamp on a bedside table that she may turn on or off on her own
- monitoring television viewing behavior and ensuring that reading material your child is exposed to is appropriate for her age group
- studying the room from the child's perspective to identify any objects that may appear threatening in the dark and then making the necessary adjustments accordingly

Remember, Compassion

Just remember, whatever ways you deal with your child's fear of the dark, an attitude of gentle understanding and sympathy is paramount. Frustration and anger coming from you will likely only aggravate the child's anxiety. A solution to your child's fear of the dark begins with your acceptance that her feelings are genuine and quite real. From that vantage point, all sorts of healing is possible.

CHAPTER 2
KENNETH/ALICIA AND PAMELA

Interviewed:	**Kenneth**
Child:	**Alicia, age 5**
Complaints:	*Difficulty unwinding at bedtime*
	Bedtime resistance and refusal to stay in bed
	Difficulty falling asleep
	Nighttime wakings and difficulty returning to sleep
	Insistence on sleeping with parents
	Hard to awaken in the morning
	Drowsy in the morning after getting up
	Oppositional behavior
	Overactive
	Reckless playing
	Short attention span
	Excessive worrying
Child:	**Pamela, age 8**
Complaints:	*Difficulty getting into bed*
	Refusal to stay in bed
	Nightmares
	Difficulty waking in the morning
	Meanness to brothers and sisters
	Excessive television watching
	Oppositional behavior
	Anger
	Avoidance of reading
	Reading skills below average

≈ • ≈

Would you please explain *a little about the kinds of problems* your girls are having?

Alicia has trouble going to bed at night and getting to sleep.

How long does it take to get her into bed?

Usually about an hour. She is very resistant. She will constantly be coming out and requesting water or something.

How long does it take on average to get her to go to sleep?

I would say, when all the activities are over in the house and things are really quiet and she knows everyone else is in bed then she will mellow out and go to sleep. On the average, I would say it takes her about two hours each night to go to sleep.

How long has that pattern been present?

For about two years.

Any other problems with her sleep, like waking up in the middle of the night?

Yes, she does have some nighttime wakings and then she wants to come in and get in bed with us.

Any other problems at night, like nightmares?

Not really. She doesn't have nightmares. She'll wake up and wander around the house and this happens about two to three times a week.

In those instances, how long does it take on average to get her back to sleep?

A lot of times, if she's not able to get in bed with us, she'll be up and wandering around, and if you don't do anything about it, she'll just stay up for hours making noise and no one gets any sleep.

What is she like in the morning?

In the morning she's sluggish and drowsy. She's hard to wake up.

Is that just when she's had little sleep, or most mornings?

It's her usual pattern. She's pretty much always hard to wake up, until about mid-morning.

Any significant behavior problems, in addition to her sleep problem?

At times she can be very oppositional. She'll have to have things her way; more than usual for a child her age. When her mom wants her to do something, it can take forever to convince her to do it.

Is that about it for her behavior problems? Nothing particularly significant?

Well, as the day goes on, she does tend to become overactive. She's a tomboy, very rough; always has scratches. She plays with the little boys, and she's always really rough. I've also noticed that she has a real short attention span. She'll start playing with her coloring books and just won't stay with it for long. If you give her something to do, she'll forget to do it—things like picking up her toys and putting them away.

Does she have more of a problem with concentration or being hyperactive?

The thing is she's easily distractible. I wouldn't say she's hyperactive, just has a lot of energy.

Any other behavior issues?

Well, yes. Now that you mention it, she's a worrywart. She worries about everything and that makes me worry.

Now how about her stepsister? What's her name?

Pamela, and she is eight years old.

Has she been having any problems?

She started having problems when her mother and father divorced. She is a very angry child. She started having problems learning—poor reading, poor grades. And she started having problems getting along with other kids; she became mean toward her other brothers and sisters. She also suffers from nightmares and it's really hard to get her up in the morning. She wants to watch television all night. And we can't get her to read.

Is it hard to get her into bed?

Yes. It takes a lot of pushing and threatening to get her into bed.

Once in bed, how long does it take her to fall asleep, on average?

She likes to pretend she's asleep; that's her game. She'll turn off the light and everything, but later I'll hear her up and about. I would say it takes one, two, or even three hours most of the time. This is a constant thing, almost every night.

That she'll be up for hours longer than you wanted?

Yes, way past her allotted bedtime. We've thought about taking her to a therapist to see if we can get some help, because her school grades are dropping and they are thinking of putting her into special education classes. This had her mother really upset, to say the least. So we explored the idea that it might have something to do with the separation from her real father because she was very close to him—she was about three or four years old when he left.

Now, regarding her nightmares, about how often would you say they've been happening?

About once a week. She watches those crazy shows on Saturday night and then she'll have nightmares.

And what problem behaviors have you noticed during the day?

She never wants to read, even though I keep telling her that to do anything she's going to have to know how to read, but that never really fazes her. She doesn't even care about bedtime stories. And then there's the problem with her younger siblings. It's like she doesn't even want to be bothered with them. She has no patience with them. Sometimes she'll even strike out at them.

After Kenneth and I talked a while longer, I gave him the *Magic Carpet* CD to try with Alicia and Pamela. About a month later he returned to tell me how it went.

So Alicia began using Magic Carpet how long ago?

About a month and a half.

What has happened during that time, first with her sleep problem?

It has helped especially with her sleep problem and going to bed. She is able to retire with little prompting and that is a great improvement. She is less argumentative and she will follow instructions and obey without a lot of fuss or prodding. She's not oppositional anymore. And although she continues to have a high level of energy, she doesn't come in with all the cuts and scrapes. I think she's beginning to think her activities out; she started to be more aware of what she's doing. She still does everything, but she's more in touch with what she's doing and she's more careful. Not as reckless.

How has her sleep problem changed?

She is able, now, to go to sleep without it being a big ordeal. She likes the program because it entertains her and it makes her sleepy. She cuddles up, and when it's on her eyes close and she starts to drift. I'm really shocked at how easy this has been.

How long does it take her on average to get to sleep now?

Her bedtime right now is 9:00, and within 30 minutes she's asleep.

Does she still wake up in the middle of the night?

Yes, but if she does, it's a legitimate reason. It's not like she used to do, continually.

When she gets up to go the bathroom, does she wake you up and want to get into bed with you?

No. That has stopped.

Does she go back to bed by herself?

Yes, she does. The bathroom is right around the corner from her room and it used to be that somebody would have to get up with her because she was afraid to go back to bed. Now she gets up, goes to the bathroom, and then goes back to her room and gets into bed by herself. That is all new. Maybe it's partly related to just getting older, I don't know, but her behavior has been like this since age three. It was a consistent problem and now it's suddenly gone.

So in terms of when these new behaviors started, when did you think they really began? She started using the program about six weeks ago?

Yes, approximately six weeks.

And how long was it before you noticed these changes?

Well, after she started listening to *Magic Carpet* her sleep was better right away. Maybe it wasn't as good as it is now, but it was better from the start. There were some subtle changes in her behavior right away, too, but that has also just kept improving. When we first started using the program it was a big family event. Everybody got together in a room and put it on and I would tell her to listen to it and see how it made her feel. She did, and she eased off to sleep and it didn't take long. The next night we tried it with her and her sister. Pamela put it on and started listing and before it was over, they were both asleep. By the second week her behavioral changes were starting to become obvious. I'm a skeptic. You have to prove things to me, and at that point I knew for sure something was happening.

So that's the point when it became apparent that real changes were happening.

Right. There were some definite changes; you couldn't miss them. And after the second week, the changes accelerated. Everybody was taking notice, and I was definitely on top of it. I was getting reports about her behavior during the day. She goes to the sitter. The sitter said, "I don't know what is going on with this child, but she has definitely changed." I asked how she had changed and she said, "She used to be reckless and was always accidentally hurting herself, but that's not happening now." This is the kind of feedback I've been getting, so something is happening. I'm assuming that her concentration has improved and she's paying more attention to what she's doing And in the morning, she looks so much more alert now, so much more with it.

In terms of behavior during the day, are there any other changes you noticed?

Well, remember when I told you about her constant worrying?

I do.

I've noticed a change in that. She is much more relaxed now, even though she still has a high energy level. She's mellower, more controlled and balanced. I'm totally in awe of this.

Have you used the program with Pamela, too?

I have.

Has it made a difference for her?

Since listening to the program I think she has done almost a 180-degree turnaround. She's started going to bed when it's her bedtime. Before it was one to three hours after, but now, at the most, it is 30 minutes. But let me tell you about her reading, which is what surprises me most. I can't get over the fact that she is reading so much. Now she has started reading before going to sleep, or she asks someone to read to her, which is new behavior. Another thing, she is attempting to read to her little brother and sister. As you can imagine, this is very unusual because she used to ignore them. Now she is more loving, she shares with them. She even tries to help her little brother when he gets into mischief. She's growing up. This program is helping her grow up; she's starting to act like a normal eight-year-old. Before, her behavior was worse than a two-year-old.

Have you noticed any other changes?

This is a child who never wanted to read and she is now picking up books and is reading on her own. She is not reading up to her age level yet, but she is getting better. And now she's looking forward to going back to school. Last year, she didn't want to go; she hated it. Now she is excited about going to school. My real clue to the school thing is that she is playing school with the other kids. She usually would rather go roller skating, or ride her bike, but now she's able to sit down in a circle with the other kids and play like she's the teacher and she's helping them read and write. She never did that before.

And how has her mood been?

She has seemed happier with herself, more content. She is starting to realize she has a lot of ability. She's a pretty girl, too. She used to think she was ugly, a little chubby. She's starting to feel a lot better about herself.

Has there been any lessening of her nightmares?

There sure has.

What percent change has there been in them?

I would say about 75% better.

You mentioned that you felt the television was related to her nightmares. Is there any change in her television watching?

Now she turns it off when you tell her to without putting up a fight. We used to fight with her practically every night.

Are you saying there is no resistance to turning off the TV now?

None whatsoever. Unless she's sneaking and watching a show and I don't know it. I think some of her sneaking habits have changed. This was part of the problem. I censored what she watched. I do maintain that control—I don't want her watching scary movies. Her choice of programs has improved. She's more into the family shows now.

To your knowledge, she's not sneaking TV at night now?

She has a TV in her room. In the past I threatened to take it away, but I haven't done it. Every once in a while, I will get up and look to see if she has turned it on when she's not supposed to, but she hasn't been doing it.

You're saying she's watching less TV. What percentage less, would you estimate?

I would say 70%. There are some nights when she doesn't watch it at all. She might watch cartoons, early in the afternoon, but after that, I would say from seven to nine there is almost no TV.

What is she doing during that time now that she didn't do before?

She is reading and playing with her brothers and her sisters. She's taking more time with them; she's more patient. I think that is great, because she knows they are not her real brothers and sisters, so to speak, but she's starting to treat them as such. They're getting closer. She's keeping her brother out of trouble because she's giving him more attention. She has her reading and she's into coloring. She has some artistic ability but she wasn't using it before. We knew it was there. I think she wanted to express it, but she couldn't concentrate long enough to do it.

So you're saying you feel her artistic talent is now being expressed?

I think the mood she was usually in kept her from expressing it, because she was always so angry at everything and everybody. Now she has begun to draw and I believe, with some training, she could become a very good artist. It's really exciting to see her blossoming.

Thank you very much for sharing your story.

You're welcome.

Television

Kenneth spoke of his stepdaughter Pamela's excessive television viewing. He also made reference to her reading skills (and thus her grades) having fallen behind those of her peers, and pointed to a profusion of misbehavior occurring to the point where Pamela even had difficulty interacting appropriately with her own family. And of course she was experiencing an exhausting pattern of sleeping difficulties, with the sleep she was able to achieve interrupted by nightmares, and mornings marred by resistance to getting out of bed, followed by morning moodiness. Whether any of these circumstances are related is pure speculation, but beyond speculation, this very combination of circumstances often occurs in children of Pamela's age group.

The Common Picture

Alas, this is an all-too-common picture (and problem) for many families. I've therefore grouped this and the subsequent two interviews together, as the commentaries following each of them are, respectively,

Television, Resistance to Reading, and Academic Performance. In the interview that follows, for example, you'll meet young Bobby, whose near-obsessive television viewing habit was associated with (whether or not the actual cause of) the havoc of his familial relationships, not to mention his academic performance and reading behavior.

Incidentally, as the divorce of Pamela's parents also keyed into her developmental struggles, it seems appropriate that my interview with Brenda and subsequent commentary on Children of Divorce follows. Later in the book I will also discuss nightmares, another prevalent problem from which Pamela and many children, teens, and even adults suffer.

Many of the child subjects of these interviews seemed to have their sleep direly influenced by their television habits. This is an important consideration, particularly because more than 75% of all American children watch television as part of their regular pre-bedtime routine.

Television and Other Issues

Studies have documented that too much TV, especially when associated with poor choice of programs, causes a whole host of problems, including poor academic performance and learning difficulties in general, as well as aggression and even childhood obesity.

Understandably enough, these problems also tie in with too little sleep.

Television and Sleep

After years of extensive worldwide studies, researchers have definitively connected television viewing to the full range of sleep disturbances, starting primarily with bedtime resistance, anxiety around sleep, and sleep onset delay (how long after lying down it takes to actually fall asleep), followed closely by sleep duration, and finally by nighttime wakings, parasomnias (*i.e.*, sleepwalking, night terrors, restless leg syndrome, talking in one's sleep), and daytime sleepiness.

How can one habit do all this?

Obviously, excessive TV watching can affect good sleeping habits by delaying bedtimes. Imposing and enforcing some sort of regularity in your child's bedtime schedule seems to play a large role in facilitating healthy sleep patterns. Watching television tends to get in the way of sleep-inducing routines. And as most children already get insufficient amounts of sleep to begin with, getting to bed later and later, all because they want to watch just one more program, only aggravates any sleep-related problems already present.

Common Pitfall: Appeasement

Parents find it very hard to say, "No," in the face of a simple request for just an extra half-hour, especially when so many parents feel guilty for not spending enough quality time with their children, as it is. But appeasing a child with such leniency certainly doesn't do either the child or the parents any favors.

DAYTIME TELEVISION VIEWING

As it turns out, not only nighttime television viewing impairs sleep. According to a study done in 1975, excessive daytime television viewing was found to cause insomnia and other sleep-related difficulties in children, too (including trouble falling asleep and remaining asleep, as well as trouble returning to sleep after waking up during the night).

DURATION OF TELEVISION VIEWING

The difficulties were most pronounced in kids who watched TV at least three hours a day. As it happens, that's about the average amount of TV that today's children watch. In a given week, the average American child watches around 25 hours of television, about the same amount of time that he spends each week in school. What's more, one-third of households containing at least one child under the age of 6 have the television on *all or most of the time.*

NIGHTTIME TELEVISION VIEWING

As for the effects of the content of nighttime TV viewed by kids, especially those with televisions in their bedrooms, I defer to this poem by esteemed sleep researcher Florence Cardinal:

AND SO TO DREAM

Midnight! Bats fly. Howl of werewolf
Echoes through a crumbling castle.
Ghostly laughter
Haunts deserted hallways.
Mist in clammy tendrils
Rises damply from the swamp.
Grave yards, weeds and molding moss,
Silence shattered by an eerie moan.
Nightmare seeds planted in entranced
And fertile minds—
Children's' bedtime TV horror drama.

THE PROBLEM OF CONTENT

Today's television programming—especially during late-night—is rife with over-stimulating action such as violence and gore. No wonder children have a rough time falling asleep; their little brains are buzzing with all sorts of thoughts, images, and emotions—none of which are very much help to a body and brain attempting to relax.

And even when these children finally do fall asleep, the input from all they've just seen on TV often leaks into their dreams and fills their slumbering minds with nightmares.

THE PROBLEM OF TECHNOLOGY

It's not only the content of the television viewed that causes sleep disturbances, however. It is also the very act of watching television itself, or more explicitly, watching the bright and flashing television screen. Regardless of the quality or content of television programming viewed, the light from the TV screen seems to impede the body's drop in core temperature necessary for properly regulating the circadian rhythms (in this case, 24-hour cycles repeated over and over) involved in both the onset of sleep and patterns of sleep, including the initiation of vital REM-sleep. This phenomenon, incidentally, also explains why people tend to sleep better in cooler rooms.

Further, the brightness of the television screen has another biochemical effect that impedes healthy sleep patterns. A study in Florence, Italy, revealed that watching television actually prohibits the body's production of melatonin, a hormone that promotes sleep.

A TELEVISION IN THEIR BEDROOM

To make matters worse, all of these adverse effects of television on sleep escalate when children have a bedroom television. More than 25% of American children have a television in their bedroom, and over 60% of those children fall asleep with it on at least two nights each week.

We unfortunately find parents too often use television in an attempt to help their children fall asleep, although as we now see, TV turns out to stimulate far more than sedate. Many parents also use television—especially when it's in their child's bedroom—as a way to avoid having to deal with struggles over bedtime. The end result, however, is quite the opposite of what was intended. Children who fall asleep in front of the television tend to have more sleep disturbances and greater long-term bedtime resistance than those who do not. Such a child may grow up dependent on the television to help him fall asleep, a frightening fate when you consider that pre-sleep TV does not promote restful sleep at all. In fact, I frequently treat adults with sleep problems who claim they cannot fall asleep without the TV on—a habit that goes back to childhood.

Studies have even shown that children with a bedroom TV are more prone to smoking, drinking, obesity, trouble in school, both mental/emotional and physical health problems, and—of course—greater risk of sleep disturbances than children without a TV in their rooms.

It's also simply harder for a parent to monitor what and how much a child watches when there's a television in the child's bedroom. One study found kids four to seven years old with TVs in their bedrooms watched an average of nine hours more television per week than peers who had no TV in their rooms.

WHAT THE MEDICAL EXPERTS SAY

In August of 1999, the American Academy of Pediatrics (AAP) recommended that children younger than age two watch absolutely no television at all, explaining that it may interfere with the extensive one-on-one interaction with parents and others that is critical to early brain development.

Reading: The Television Cure

Reading instead of watching television goes a long way toward remedying all the sleep problems discussed above. The commentary on Resistance to Reading following the next interview with Alan about eight-year-old Bobby has much to offer on this subject.

Good Television Viewing Habits

Television, of course, is a fact of contemporary life. For most of us it's not practical to isolate our children from TV, but we can help them develop a healthy relationship with it. After all, there are also healthful, inspiring, and artistic programs that enrich our lives and lift up our spirits. Consider the following:

- Monitor the types of shows your child watches. Cable TV, along with select videos and DVDs, afford a wealth of educational material. Do your best to avoid violent and frightening programming.
- Whenever possible, watch shows with your child and be available to discuss openly the things he sees (*i.e.*, smoking, drinking, sexuality, social/interpersonal relations, peer pressure, ethics and morals, advertising, etc.).
- Limit how much TV your child watches, aiming for two hours or less per day.
- Shut off the TV during mealtimes, and forbid any eating in front of the television.
- Prohibit your child from having the TV on while doing homework.
- Don't allow the TV to be used as background noise. Only permit it to be on when someone in the household is actually watching a specific program.
- Don't use the TV as a babysitter, but rather plan with your child the shows he will watch, scheduling his TV viewing time around these shows (or if you have Tivo, On Demand, or other such technology, then around you and your child's schedules). Keep the TV off the rest of the time.
- Take the television out of your child's bedroom (as well as the computer and video game console).
- Encourage alternatives to watching television at any time of day, including reading, socializing, exercise, and play.
- Enforce a bedtime routine for your child designed around a regular schedule and made up of relaxing activities and loving interactions, rather than allow the TV be the last thing your child sees before going to bed.

Teach by example; follow all these guidelines yourself—you'll sleep better for it, too!

CHAPTER 3

ALAN/BOBBY

Interviewed:	**Alan/Bobby**
Child:	**Bobby, age 8**
Complaints:	*Bedtime resistance*
	Excessive time to fall asleep
	Nighttime wakings
	Outbursts of anger
	Excessive television watching
	Resistance to reading
	Restlessness
	Irritability
	Fearful of physical injury

ಹ • ೊ

Hi, Alan. Please start *by telling me a little about Bobby.*

Bobby is eight and the son of a woman I've been living with for the past three years. He has a number of problems. He is generally fidgety, restless and troublesome. Always wants everyone's attention. Not really abnormal, but to the point of getting on your nerves.

Do you have any difficulty getting him to go to bed at night?

That's an understatement. He generally stays up as long as you do, if you don't insist that he go to bed.

What time would you say you usually get him into bed by?

He'll usually stay up until 10:00 to 10:30.

How long has that been his pattern?

At least since I have known him, which is three years. Even on school nights he won't go to bed. He'll go in his room and raise hell. He'll bang things, make twenty trips to the bathroom or refrigerator, come back in to see what we're watching on TV or ask questions. He'll do anything to stay up.

Does he watch a lot of television?

Oh, does he ever.

What percent of the time would you say he watches TV when he's home?

Almost all the time.

Does he ever read?

No, he isn't reading at all. He'll just stare at the TV blankly, even when there's nothing in particular on, just to watch it, you know. He'll just flip through the channels mindlessly. And God forbid I should tell him to turn it off. He won't listen. He just throws a fit until I give up trying. He doesn't cry; just gets real restless and then angry if I tell him to turn off the TV or that he has to go to bed. About three nights of the week I have to fight with him over this.

How often does he wake up during the night?

Maybe two or three times a week, even after everyone else is asleep he'll just wake us up.

So, two to three times a week, you get awakened and have to put him back to bed?

Yes, sit with him a while.

Are there times when you can't get back to sleep?

No. When I want to sleep, nothing can keep me awake.

What is his mood like during the day?

Honestly? He can be really irritable. His mom says he had that problem when he was a little tiny kid, even when he first started walking. He would get mad and stay mad for hours. Still does. He's not a very friendly kid at all, really. Not a real turn off kid, but if there isn't something in it for him, just forget it. He's rather selfish, actually.

Does Bobby have any friends?

Funny you should mention it. I was just thinking of this one friend of his, a real holy terror, irritates everybody. The kid even makes Bobby feel so crazy he'll come running to me or his mother to control the kid because he just doesn't know what else to do. It's exasperating. The kid's got no boundaries and Bobby, well, he doesn't have the skills to set them. Does any kid?

Some do.

Well, not Bobby. Like this kid, Steven, will come over to our house whenever he feels like it and Bobby will just let him in, whether he wants to play or not. It's like he can't say,

"No," to the kid. I don't know if it's because he's afraid the kid won't be his friend anymore or if he's just apathetic or what. But it's horrible, because the kid will come in, Bobby won't even be paying attention to him half the time, and the kid ends up tearing everything apart, creating a real mess.

Do you or Bobby's mother ever get involved?

It's hard. I mean, I like Steven, too, but he is really hard to deal with. I don't mind telling you, I'm truly afraid to take them places, because Steven will cut up so bad. I get afraid that I'm going to lose my temper with him. You can lose your temper with your own kid, but you'd better not do it with someone else's. You know what I mean?

Tell me a little about this boy. You've known him how long now?

A couple of years.

And he goes in and out of your place?

Constantly, on the weekends and in the afternoons when school is out.

So you see him almost every day?

Five days out of the week, I see him.

And what is this child's activity level like?

Very high pitched. He is in a family where everybody is deaf. His brother's deaf, his mother's deaf, I forgot whether his father is deaf or not. So in order to get people's attention, he screeches, yells and hollers, because nobody hears him at home anyway. He's real fidgety. Two minutes with one thing, three minutes with another. He's also very demanding and manipulative. He gets on your nerves in about two minutes.

So back to Bobby. Would you call him a fearful child?

I would. I mean, he is kind of afraid to take even normal chances; afraid he might fall and get hurt.

Is he also shy?

Not shy, just not willing to take any chances, afraid to get hurt, afraid to do anything rough.

☙ • ❧

After Alan and I spoke a bit more, I gave him the *Magic Carpet* CD to try with Bobby. He returned about a month later to share his observations.

☙ • ❧

How did it go the first time you used **Magic Carpet** *with Bobby?*

The first time he tried it he took it in the family room, put on the headphones and listened to it for 20 minutes or so. Then he was out; he fell asleep.

Was this one of the times he had been acting up?

Yes, it was about 8:30 in the evening and we were hoping he might wind down some because he had been going from one activity to the next—driving everyone crazy. I said, *"Bobby, why don't you listen to this CD? It's a very special program that a friend of mine made."* So he listened to it for about 15 to 20 minutes lying on the couch and he was asleep. In fact, he slept the rest of the night.

And that's quite early for him to fall asleep, isn't it?

The earliest since I've known him, which is three years. After using the program a few times, he's started going to bed anywhere between 8:00 and 9:30.

Commonly, now that he's using the program?

Oh yes, he's started going to bed a lot earlier in general. Sure, he'll check the *TV Guide* to see what's on and he'll ask how long he can stay up. But now if I say he can watch one more program, but then he must go to bed at nine o'clock, then when that time comes he'll actually get up, say goodnight, do his thing in the bathroom and off to bed he goes.

Has he done that before? Has he ever gone to bed on his own?

I never saw him do it and his mother said he never did. And he's been doing this consistently now. I've also had him listen to the program when he was playing in his room and I felt like he needed to calm down. The first time I did it, I turned it down low so he could just barely hear it. I don't think he was paying any attention to it, the same way you would listen to background music.

He had been really active, but his playing mellowed out and he went to sleep early that night, around 8:15. A couple other times he has gotten the CD on his own to listen to on the couch, maybe when he wasn't feeling very good—agitated or upset about something. He figured it out after using it just a couple times that it made him feel better.

Does he also enjoy using it at night?

Yes, he will come look for it.

At this point, how would you rate the improvement in his sleep problem?

Well, 99% of the time he will go to bed on his own. When you absolutely have to ask Bobby to go to bed now, it's when he's not aware of what his schedule is the next day.

So it's a whole new attitude about going to bed?

He goes to bed very easily now; it's no problem any longer. He's so good about it; I just can't believe the difference. He's getting older, too, so normally, I would've thought that as time went on he'd want to stay up even later. So this is more than I even could've hoped for.

And that whole pattern changed over what period of time? How much time are we talking about?

Less than a week. It worked just like that. Pretty amazing. The other thing is he's not only going to bed, but staying in bed and falling asleep. Before when he would go to bed he'd always play for a while. Now he goes right to sleep.

Have you noticed any changes in his behavior during the day?

He's mellowed a lot these days. And now, when he does get mad, he doesn't stay mad as long as he used to.

And that pattern changed along with everything else?

Yes. And I also noticed that he's suddenly braver. He's now coming to me and asking if it's okay to go riding in the dirt field, where before he was only brave enough to go to the corner. Now he watches the traffic, walks his bike across the street and then rides like crazy.

So he seems more self-confident now?

Yeah, he even went out for soccer. At first he didn't like it and it seemed like his mind wouldn't stay on the game. But as he has continued using the CD and has gotten more relaxed, he seems to be getting a lot better at soccer. He was running all over the place and the coach said Bobby has really improved as a soccer player.

You think that happened at the same time as the other changes?

Yeah, when he got more relaxed, less irritable, more self-confident. It seemed to affect a lot of things. His grades even improved and now he's reading like crazy.

Really? Tell me about the reading.

Well, he decided to join a reading club, which is very competitive. Out of the 30 kids, he's now number four on the list; he reads a lot of books. That requires a lot of concentration and, as I think I mentioned last time, before he didn't want to be bothered with it. But now he loves to read.

You're saying that after he used the CD then all of a sudden he started reading all those books?

Well, it's not like it happened overnight. He kind of gradually got into it, but then it seemed to accelerate and he started gobbling up the books.

But for whatever reason, it happened shortly after he began listening to **Magic Carpet?**

Yeah, right after, he started concentrating better and being more relaxed in the evenings. Before, when he was irritable and anxious he wouldn't sit and read. He still likes TV, don't get me wrong, but he likes to read now, too.

What percent of his time is spent reading now?

As much time as people will allow him. Some books he wants you to read with him. So he'll go get you and sit you down and have you read with him. You read a page, he reads a page, until he gets through it. We've both spent time reading with him, but he also likes to read by himself. He's really into reading now and he'll tell you, "I read three books this week." You know he has to be relaxed to be able to read. You can't read or remember if you're all keyed up, and that's another extension of his mind being calmer now.

So, what percent of the time would you say he's reading versus watching TV?

Before he was looking at television about 90% of his free time and playing with toys about 10%. Now it's maybe 20% TV, 20% toys, and the other 60% reading. And when he does watch TV, he's watching particular TV programs rather than just sitting there turning channels and watching whatever is on. He'll look at choice things. He'll even turn the television off at night which, if you remember, before I couldn't get him to do. He's a very bright little boy. He just needed somebody to hang in there with him. I think somewhere in his little head there's been a storm going on, and I think the CD helped mellow it out. He doesn't feel the rage that used to be there. And he's more able to do a lot of things. He's got a heck of a memory.

So, do you think his memory has improved?

Yes. I think his memory has improved along with his concentration. He doesn't seem to forget anything now. Before when I asked him to do something, he was always saying "Oh I forgot," but now he remembers and just does it.

And that's a big change in him?

He's remarkably improved. And I don't think he is at a standstill. I think he's getting even better. He's much friendlier now, too.

And how about his selfishness? Any change in that?

Yeah, he seems less selfish. That and much more. You remember that friend of his I was telling you about last time?

The difficult one?

That's putting it nicely. Yes, him. Let me tell you about the way Bobby is with Steven now. Well, since you and I talked last, Bobby is now actually able to set rules so that Steven doesn't bug him so much. For instance, if Bobby is over at Steven's house playing and Steven gets bonkers, Bobby says *"Now, when you calm down in a while I'll play with you. I'm going to leave now."*

And then Bobby will come home. He'll do something around the house for awhile and then he'll get on the phone and call Steven up and say, *"Hi, Steven, how are you doing? Are you feeling better now? Okay, then we can go out and play a little bit more."* He won't just let this little kid steamroll him anymore. He won't let Steven come in our house anytime he wants to either. Now when Steven shows up, sometimes Bobby stops him at the door and says, *"Wait a minute, we'll play outside."* And nobody's telling him to do this.

Are you kind of amazed at all this?

Yes, probably even more so than his mother, because I am an observer. His mom is usually busy doing stuff and doesn't notice the subtle things as much as I do, but she's also been stunned. Now Bobby and Steven go outside and play for a while, and then Bobby will bring him in. He'll organize the game and tell Steven they are going to play in one room and not play all over the house. He keeps Steven relatively quiet.

And how is Steven responding to all this?

You know something? It's so strange, but he's been changing, too. I don't know whether Bobby is rubbing off on him, but I did bring him in recently and I played *Magic Carpet* while they were in the back room playing. This was about three weeks after Bobby started using it.

So Bobby was controlling him a bit better but Steven was still very hyper?

Yes.

So, the day you tried playing the CD, what was going on?

They were having an argument back in Bobby's room. Steven wanted all the toys, he wanted this and he wanted that. They were really going at it, so I put the CD on in the background. And he said, "What's that weird stuff and who's that talking?" I said, "That's a sleep CD." He said, "What's a sleep CD?" I said, "I don't want to explain it to you, Steven, just listen to it."

After a while, Steven got into playing with Bobby, and they were interacting in a more social and creative way, which was very different for Steven. I ended up going in the room and turning off the CD about two thirds of the way through. Steven started asking questions about what it was. They kept playing peacefully. There was no screaming or battering each other like usual. They played for another hour or so and then Bobby said, "I'm going to go do some reading, Steven, you have to go home now." When Steven visits now, you don't hear him screaming anymore. It really is quite amazing.

Did that happen all of a sudden, after he listened to the CD, or was it over a period of time as a result of your son taking better control the situation?

Probably a combination of the two. But it's interesting, Steven doesn't scream anymore, even outdoors. I also haven't seen Steven in a bad mood anymore.

When you played the CD for him, what was that playtime like compared to others you had witnessed?

There was a 100% turnaround. He was civil.

Okay, but have there been any other occasions when they played that well together?

Never before. Honestly. They had never been that calm or cooperative. Before, there would always be a fight with Bobby eventually stepping out of it to go get somebody to do something. They could never resolve it on their own. Five minutes of play and 20 minutes of fighting. But now they're getting along really good.

You have seen some nice changes with the children. It seems that in some way the CD has at least been a catalyst.

It really wasn't going on before we played the CD though. We've played it for both of them several times now and it really does relax them.

Thank you so much for sharing this information with me.

You're welcome.

❧ • ☙

RESISTANCE TO READING

Like Pamela in the previous interview, young Bobby was an avid TV watcher before listening to *Magic Carpet*. And as with Pamela, Bobby's TV habit probably fostered poor social skills and oppositional behavior. Bobby's oppositional behavior, however, was more severe, to the point of throwing temper tantrums. Reading was not only absent from his life, but it seemed anathema to him.

Fortunately, his use of the CD program appeared to turn him around. Many of the adults I interviewed after using the programs with their child reported either a spontaneously renewed or newly emergent interest in reading as a common thread.

HEARING STORIES VERSUS READING THEM

Although almost all children love stories, that passion doesn't always translate to reading. Many children grow up resisting reading. And the problem doesn't go away by itself.

THE LATER REPERCUSSIONS OF RESISTING READING

Resistance to reading breeds poor reading skills, and poor reading skills leads to further and deeper resistance to reading. Of significant long-term consequence, children rarely outgrow resistance to reading by themselves. In fact, as many studies have shown, left to their own devices, children who don't read grow into teens who don't read (a prevalent problem in today's world), who in turn grow into adults who don't read. Not only does this bode poorly for an individual's ability to find decent employment, but it vastly impedes one's ability to function adequately in everyday society.

WHAT'S A PARENT TO DO (AND NOT TO DO)?

A child might resist reading for any one reason or a combination of reasons; parents will consequently find it helpful to know what exactly it is about reading their child struggles with, for that knowledge may shine a bright light on the best solutions to the problem of resistance.

Before we get into that, however, let's take a moment to go over some methods to unequivocally *avoid* when trying to alleviate a child's resistance to reading. The following techniques will almost certainly *not* work in getting your child to read more (and enjoy it), and in fact may only lead to further and deeper resistance:

- bribery
- nagging
- judgment
- criticism
- unrealistic goal-setting

With this in mind, we can now proactively explore the predominant types of resistance to reading and identify appropriate ways of dealing with them.

APPROACHES TO THE COMMON REASONS CHILDREN RESIST READING

Typical reasons kids give for avoiding reading, along with practical suggestions on how you, as a caretaker, can handle them, include the following:

- *They find it boring.* This could be a response to the type of reading material they're facing, especially that which they're exposed to in school. Negate this complaint by making sure a child has enjoyable reading material at home, material that differs noticeably from the types of reading material she faces at school. Find out what types of stories, or information, your child likes, or finds interesting, and provide her with ample reading material of that kind.

- *They don't have the time for it.* Kids have busy lives, too. They may not have the kinds of responsibilities that you have, but that doesn't mean their lives aren't already filled with other demands on their time—school, friends, after-school activities, homework, chores, meals, shopping with mom or dad, and more. In these instances, help your child develop some time management skills, including scheduling in times for reading.

- *They find it too difficult.* Every child is different, and no two children develop at quite the same rate. Yet in our schools a child is typically expected to develop at the same pace as the rest of the class. If your child has trouble reading, perhaps you should discuss with your child's teacher some ways that your child can be taught to read at her own level, even if that means supplementing your child's academic coursework with at-home reading materials more suitable for her actual reading level. In extreme cases, a child may be dealing with a learning disability, such as dyslexia. Or, alternatively, a child could have vision problems in need of correction. In any of these instances, identify the source condition as the first step in identifying the appropriate course of action. Early testing for problems like these can spare your child years of unnecessary anguish and frustration. And once you provide the type of special attention your child needs, you might find blossoming within her a love of reading, not to mention learning in general.

- *They don't see the point.* Understandably, children don't realize how crucial reading is to their education, to their development, and to everyday living. They simply don't see it as important or relevant to their lives. A powerful approach to this problem is through reading material on subjects that matter to your child. Find out what interests her—animals, sports, astronomy, history, art, natural phenomena, etc.—and furnish her with material that excites those interests. Likewise, find reading material that broaches subjects your child may be confronting in life—moving, a new sibling, dog training, and so forth. Next time you and your child go to a bookstore or the library, let your child pick out her own books to read.

- ***They don't like it.*** Finally, whether a child reads well or not, the pressure exerted by parents, teachers, and others to read (and like it!) may be too much for her to handle. As such, children may resist reading purely in defense against the pressure put upon them to read. To alleviate this problem, find ways to take the pressure off. Help your child feel good about herself as she already is, and then find more subtle ways to make reading fun. For example, read comic books or the funny pages together. Get your child a subscription to a young person's magazine, or next time you're at the market pick her up a fan magazine she'll enjoy. Read the TV listings with her to find the show times for favorite programs. Read the instructions to her video games with her. Exchange letters together with loved ones living far away. Cook together from written recipes. Read riddles, jokes, *Mad Libs*, anything that may delight your child and make her momentarily forget she's even reading.

TEACHING BY EXAMPLE: DO YOU RESIST READING?

Best of all, teach by example. Make the enjoyment of reading an ever-present part of your household. Let your child see you and any other adults in the household reading and enjoying it. You don't have to make an issue of it or even point it out to them or in any way discuss it. Just make the pleasure you take in reading apparent to your child in a natural and unimposing way.

And if you yourself have a resistance to reading for enjoyment, then you have just hit on one possible influence in your child's own resistance. Remember, children always model their perspectives and behavior on what they see in their environment. And the number-one source for the perspectives and behavior they model is their caretakers.

HOW TO READ TO (OR WITH) YOUR CHILD TO ENCOURAGE READING

When you read to (or with) your child, be sure not to rush through the material. With bedtime stories, for example, a parent may wish to get to the end of the story so as to put the child to bed and move on with the evening. But this type of haste backfires in a combination of ways. First, it doesn't allow the child time to fully hear and absorb the material being read and, as a result, will likely lead to the child losing interest. And second, a child is sensitive to a parent's sense of hurriedness and is likely to interpret this as a disinterest in reading, one which the child is sure to model.

Take time to discuss what you read with your child. Ask your child questions about the material, such as what she thinks might happen next, why she thinks the character reacted the way he did, what she might do differently if put in the same situation, or what her favorite part of the story was and why. Another valuable purpose behind discussing what you read with your child is to identify any confusions or trouble spots your child may have had with the material. Many times a child won't voice her inability to understand something she read, for fear of derision or simple embarrassment, or for any number of other reasons. By opening up the subject for discussion, you make it safe for your child to bring up a part of the story she had a problem understanding.

By the same token, when you read to your child don't be blasé about it, even if you've read the same story 100 times. In fact, a young child commonly asks to hear the same story over and over again. When this happens, parents must essentially show patience with such seemingly outlandish taste for repetition, as a child's attraction to a particular story could have much to do with what the child is going through emotionally and developmentally at the time. Or the child might simply enjoy a sense of emotion the parent shows in their tone of voice.

When you read to your child, read with enthusiasm, with passion and verve, and your child is likely to find the same sort of excitement for the stories you read and, subsequently, with reading in general.

A Little Encouragement Goes a Long Way

As with any child development issue, positive reinforcement is paramount. Rather than scold or show disappointment with your child when she refuses to read, show enthusiasm and encouragement for even the slightest demonstration of interest in reading. A little praise goes a long way.

The DreamChild Adventures Programs and Reading

It would appear from the experiences of Alan and Bobby, Kenneth and Alicia and Pamela, and other families you'll meet in the interviews in this book, that children need to relax in order to concentrate and enjoy reading. But in terms of the *DreamChild Adventures* programs and their continued ability to somehow ignite children's interest in reading, I wonder if it's that simple—that the kids using these programs are reading more because they're more relaxed. Or perhaps there's more to it.

Might it be possible that the *DreamChild Adventures* programs actually stimulate these children's imaginations and "wake up" the visualization center of their brains?

In cooperation with the University of Arizona, we did some very sophisticated EEG brain imagery studies with mono, stereo and 3D sound, and sure enough, with the *3D Living Sound*, the visualization area of the brain showed greatly increased activity. Perhaps this forms the basis for an ongoing and lasting effect of these programs that makes reading more fun for kids.

A saving grace for you as a parent is reading is a self-perpetuating, self-feeding activity. In other words, the more a child reads, the better the child is able to read, the more pleasure the child gets from reading, and the more the child wants to read.

CHAPTER 4

IRIS/BEATRICE AND MELISSA

Interviewed:	Iris
Child:	**Beatrice, age 6**
Complaints:	*Difficulty falling asleep* *Yelling and whining in the morning*
Child:	**Melissa, age 8**
Complaints:	*Difficulty falling asleep* *Poor school performance* *Anger*

❧ • ☙

I*ris, do your children* sleep in the same room?

> Yes. They share a room.

And what kind of problems are you having around bedtime?

> The problem has been that they are up and down every night when it's bedtime, which is 9:00, playing, being silly, up for a drink, back down, up again. Kid stuff that usually goes on for about an hour and a half, every night.

It gets a little tiring?

> Yeah.

Do you ever lose your temper when you're trying to get them to settle down?

> Yes.

That's pretty typical for parents.

> Uh huh.

Let's talk about morning moods.

It's hard to say with my stepdaughter, because my husband gets her up earlier than my other one. Usually, the problem has been that they messed around so much at night that they didn't get that much sleep. Then he has to get her up at 6:00 in the morning, and she's tired and she just lays there and yells and I can hear her whining.

What about with your other child?

My stepdaughter, I think, has some adjustment problems.

Like what?

Well, she was abandoned by her mother when she was two-and-a-half. My husband has raised her since then. She had contact with her mother and spent last school year with her, and then she came back this summer and now she's back here to stay. I think that's been kind of tough on her.

Kind of a tough adjustment?

Yes. And she has quite a bit of difficulty in school. In fact, she failed, so she's going back and having to repeat the second grade.

So, is she sad at times?

Yes, sad and very angry.

❧ • ☙

After Iris and I spoke a bit more, I gave her the *Magic Carpet* CD and a couple weeks later I provided *Playhouse on the Beach* to try with her two girls. She returned three weeks after our first session to share her observations.

❧ • ☙

Last time you were here I gave you some programs to work with.

Yes, you gave me *Magic Carpet* and *Playhouse on the Beach*.

How long ago?

Magic Carpet, I got three weeks ago, and *Playhouse on the Beach*, I got about a week ago.

And what were your children's reactions?

They have their own [CD] player, and they're really proud of it. So we let them play it themselves.

With or without headphones?

Without. The first night I walked in and I was really surprised because I went to see if they were really listening and they were already asleep.

How long had it been?

About 30 minutes and it had been quiet the whole time, and they didn't get up once.

Had it been rare that they would go to sleep that quickly?

Very rare. Close to never.

What happened after that?

They kept doing it. We did it three more times that week with the same effect.

And what about in the mornings? Have you noticed any change in their moods?

Well, now that you mention it, I realize I haven't heard my daughter whining in the mornings lately.

How about that!

I didn't even think of that!

So, that seems to be different. What about your stepdaughter? Is she still waking up sad in the morning?

No, lately she's always pretty happy when she gets up.

What about the nights that you didn't do it?

Those were nights that we got home really late and they fell asleep in the car. And about a week ago we got *Playhouse on the Beach*. And they really liked it, too. They ask to listen to one of them every night when they go to bed, and they get into bed on their own now; it's become a ritual. They get the comforter, and then they lay down with their dolls and I let them put the program on by themselves and they're asleep within 20 to 30 minutes without getting up. It's very unusual for them and I don't see any other reason than the programs.

Thank you for your feedback.

Absolutely! And if you have any more children's programs we'd love to hear them.

I plan on having more, sometime in the future.

Great!

ACADEMIC PERFORMANCE

In my first conversation with Iris, we learned that her stepdaughter Melissa had failed the second grade and would have to repeat it, a harrowing experience for any child. Her trouble sleeping undoubtedly contributed to Melissa's poor academic performance. In this particular case, we don't know if her grades subsequently improved, but we can assume that there is an improved probability. Thanks to significant attention given the subject by the medical and scientific communities, there is no longer any doubt that—for better and for worse—duration and quality of sleep do affect academic performance.

The Connection Between Sleep and Academic Performance

It has been documented time and time again that improved academic performance ties in directly with sufficient sleep and good sleep habits, and by the same token, that impaired and deficient academic performance can result from sleep deprivation and poor sleep habits.

More specifically, medical research has found a definitive correlation between sleep deprivation and impaired alertness and performance, memory deficits, and delayed response times. A deficiency in REM (dream) sleep has been found to lead to increased irritability, anxiety, and even depression, not to mention impaired concentration, socialization skills, and the ability to execute complex and creative tasks. Sleep deprivation persistent throughout a child's young life and into adolescence has been explicitly associated with increased vulnerability to accidental self-harm and harm to others, and has significant potential for alcohol and drug use and abuse.

How did researchers figure all this out? In part, these discoveries were attributed to MRI scans that revealed a great deal about the differences between the way the brain processes information during the day and during the night. During the daytime, information is temporarily stored in particular areas of the brain until nighttime, and while we are asleep that information is then processed and transferred to the various parts of the brain where the information will be stored permanently; the more that children learn during the day, and the more complex the information, the more sleep they need at night. What's more, brain scans revealed that each stage of sleep has a distinct role to play in the process; therefore, a problem with any one stage of sleep almost invariably triggers a cascading problem for the entire process of absorbing, sorting, and storing information.

The Effects of Sleep Deprivation on Learning

The loss of plasticity of neurons in the brain caused by sleep deprivation leads to difficulties encoding memories. Translated, this is the biological explanation of how deficient sleep detrimentally affects a child's ability to remember what he's learned. The impaired ability of the body to extract glucose from the bloodstream, also caused by impaired sleep, explains how a child's alertness and attentiveness can be impaired. In addition, this deficiency of the energy necessary to fuel certain parts of the brain is directly related to detrimental effects on a child's ability to orchestrate thoughts in pursuit of a goal, predict outcomes, and perceive the consequences of their actions.

The Harm of Sleep Deprivation to Social Development

Tired students, moreover, have weakened impulse control and find it difficult to interact appropriately with their peers and teachers. Further, sleep-deprived children have trouble studying because they get distracted by more entertaining pursuits, and they have trouble taking tests because they tend to get stuck on an incorrect answer, failing to come up with creative alternative solutions to a given problem.

The Effect of Sleep Deprivation on the Brain

Children's brains continue to grow all the way up to age 21. Most of this growth occurs during sleep time. A reduction in or disruption of this imperative sleeping period, then, detrimentally affects vital brain growth, and naturally, a child's academic performance as well.

Why Children Need More Sleep, Not Less

Furthermore, a child experiencing a particularly challenging and exhausting day requires additional sleep in order to adequately process and store the same quantity of information that he could otherwise handle had the day been less taxing. It sounds like common sense (and probably is) and, yet, far too rarely do children compensate for those particularly tougher days with extra sleep.

Parental Perceptions on Their Children's Sleep

Interestingly, while, according to the National Sleep Foundation, 90% of parents believe that their children are getting enough sleep, 60% of children believe that they are not, and 25% of children surveyed believe that their grades have suffered as a result.

Statistics on Sleep and Academic Performance

It is now generally accepted that sleep-related difficulties are a key factor in poor academic performance. In one study that surveyed 1,000 students between grades 9 and 12, 90% of the students said they felt groggy during the school day from lack of sufficient sleep, and 25% of students reported having fallen asleep during class time at least once each week. Put that together with another frightening statistic from a related study, revealing that one hour of lost sleep can cause a child to function as though they had lost two full years of cognitive development, and you'll begin to realize the full scope of sleep deprivation.

Another of the studies, examining the sleep patterns of children in grades 3 through 5, found that 43% of the children experienced some sort of sleep difficulties lasting six months or longer. The same 43% were also more likely than their well-rested peers to fail at least one year of school.

Still another study compared 150 students with high GPAs to 150 students with low GPAs and found that the higher-ranking students went to bed earlier on school nights, woke up less frequently during the night, got out of bed later on school days, and displayed other indications of better sleep habits than did their poorer-performing peers. On standardized tests, students with a full night's sleep scored an average of seven points out of 100 higher than those of students who experienced deficient or disrupted sleep. Alarmingly, just 60 minutes less sleep than needed can make a sixth-grader perform like a fourth-grader.

Academic Subjects Most Adversely Affected by Poor Sleep Patterns

On an interesting and related side note, the academic subjects which seem most adversely affected by poor sleep patterns are math, reading, and writing.

How Much Sleep Does a School-Age Child Require?

To perform well in school, and in life in general, a school-aged child requires at least nine hours of sleep, with a more optimal level achieved at between 10 and 11 hours each night. Compare that to the actual data revealing that, on school nights, one-half of all adolescents sleep less than seven hours per night. And just a meager 5% of high-school seniors said they averaged as much as eight hours of sleep each school night.

Common Pitfall: "When I was Your Age..."

Now, parents might find it tempting to compare their children to themselves when they were young: *"I got less sleep than that and did just fine in school. Quit complaining, we're all tired."* But the bitter truth is today's kids get, on average, a full hour's less sleep than the kids of 30 years prior. Even children in kindergarten are getting an average of 30 minutes less sleep per night than kindergarteners of 30 years ago.

Common Misconception: Making Up for Lost Sleep

One cannot "make up" for lost sleep either. The harm caused by sleep deficiencies, including the actual damage to a child's cognitive development, cannot be reversed or compensated for by the child getting extra sleep at more convenient times. A more appropriate and healthier bedtime routine that includes the necessary time for adequate duration of sleep on a regular basis is clearly essential.

Does Snoring Affect a Child's Grades?

It also appears that children who snore at night, particularly those with sleep apnea (discussed in a later section) experience poorer grades and demonstrate lower functioning on psychology evaluations, as well as shorter attention spans, than their peers. Nearly 20% of children in the bottom 10th percentile of their class, according to one study, had breathing problems significant enough to disrupt their sleep.

Studies have also found that, of the children afflicted with sleep apnea and/or snoring, those who had their adenoids or tonsils removed tended to improve academically afterwards. Could it be because of improved breathing and a subsequent improvement in sleeping patterns? Many experts think so.

Bedtime Resistance and Poor Academic Performance

Bedtime resistance causes sleep problems significant enough to negatively impact academic performance. This makes sense when we consider bedtime resistance invariably leads to delayed onset of sleep, cutting down on the overall duration of sleep each night. And it doesn't help that, for whatever reason—guilt, laziness, resignation—today's parents tend toward being lax about enforcing bedtime schedules.

On the flip side, from now on when your children stay in bed until all hours on weekends and holidays, you can take heart that they are probably doing exactly what they need to take care of themselves and their still-developing brains. No longer, on such occasions, will you feel you should struggle to get them up and out of bed. That'll no doubt be at least one portion off your parenting plate. Getting your children to get to sleep at a decent time, however, is another story.

The Total Picture

This book explores in great depth many causes for sleeping difficulties, including both the schedules of the children and of the parents, interrupted sleep caused by obstructive sleep apnea or nightmares, and early school start times. Television and cell phones in children's bedrooms have also proven adverse to sleep patterns. Any of these alone can precipitate problems with academic achievement; taken in total, they can be devastating.

CHAPTER 5

ANGELA/COREY, ZOE, AND MOLLY

Interviewed:	Angela
Child:	**Corey, age 4**
Complaints:	*Difficulty unwinding at bedtime* *Bedtime resistance and not staying in bed* *Frequent nighttime wakings* *Nightmares* *Bouts of crying and screaming* *Bad moods* *Oppositional disposition* *Uncooperative behavior* *"A terror" in the morning*
Child:	**Zoe, age 10**
Complaints:	*Sleep-talking* *Restlessness* *Wake-up difficulty* *Lack of cooperation in the morning*
Child:	**Molly, age 2**
Complaints:	*Restless sleep* *Sleep-talking* *Nighttime wakings* *Crying spells in the morning*

✦ • ✦

First of all, what is your children's sleeping arrangement? Do they each have separate rooms or do some of them sleep in the same room?

All three of my children sleep in the same room.

Chapter 5   Angela / Corey, Zoe, and Molly

I see. And which of them have been having sleeping difficulties?

The oldest and the baby have had no major problems, but Corey has had a lot of problems settling down at night. Bedtime starts at 8:00 and they have to actually be in bed by 8:30. But then for half an hour to 45 minutes, it's back out for Corey, to see what Mom's doing, get a drink of water, on and on. Once in a while the baby will follow him, but it's basically Corey. Sometimes it will take an hour for him to go to sleep.

How long has he had this problem?

Since birth he had trouble falling asleep and couldn't sleep for long periods of time.

What is his behavior like at bedtime?

Basically, I say, "It's 8:30, your bedtime, let's go," and he'll fight at every step and ask if he can stay up and watch this or that on TV. Or he'll get to bed and I'll say, "Goodnight, it's time to go to sleep" and I'll go out and sit on the couch and two minutes later he's back up. "Mom, I have to talk to you about something," or, "I need a drink," or, "I have to go potty," or, "I can't sleep," and so on. Sometimes I actually have to lie down with him to get him to stay there and go to sleep, and half of the time I will fall asleep myself in his bed and wake up at 2:00 and then move into my bed.

Are nighttime wakings a problem?

Yeah, there's always been a problem with that. When he was a baby they were every hour or two. Until the age of 13 months, he was up and down all night. I would wonder if he was sick. It's been three years since his dad and I divorced, but Corey was quite close to him and one day Daddy said he was moving out and leaving. There was no warning for me, let alone the kids. He never explained anything to the kids and I think it's affected Corey the most. At bedtime and during the night there are bouts of crying, "I want my daddy," [or] "Why isn't my daddy here?"—especially when his dad first left. Often I'll hear him talking to his daddy in his sleep, and arguing with people, and then he wakes up.

Does he have nightmares?

About two or three times a week. Sometimes he won't wake up, so I'll have to wake him up before he works himself up, which bothers me and scares me a lot. Sometimes he will get up and walk out into the living room, if I'm sitting in the living room reading a book or watching TV. He'll walk down the hall, and I'll see him peeking around the corner. He'll say, "I can't sleep. Can I stay out here with you?" Sometimes he won't get to sleep until 11:30, sometimes 1:00 in the morning.

How often is he waking up, on average each night?

At least once, sometimes twice.

Will he get you up each time?

Yeah. I'll either have to go in his room and lie down with him in his bed or talk to him until he goes to sleep, or I'll have to let him get in bed with me. If I'm sitting up, he'll come out and lie down with me and eventually he'll go to sleep.

What is Corey like in the morning?

Corey is a terror in the morning. When I work day shift and have to get him up at 6:00 to get him dressed and fed, he fights me every step of the way while I'm attempting to get him dressed. He'll cry, scream and kick, and refuse to eat.

How often does that happen?

Every morning is like that. It's very hard on me and I know it's hard on him and I always feel really bad after I drop him off at school. I can never leave him at school with a good feeling, knowing he is okay. He'll be in a bad mood because we've fought all morning and then I'll have to resort to, "Corey, I'm going to have to spank you; you can't kick and yell at Mommy." And, "Corey would you please sit down and eat? You need to eat so we can go." He'll crawl off the chair and lie on the floor and say, "I'm tired, I'm too tired to eat—I don't want to eat." There is a lot of rebellion.

What about the other children? How have their sleep patterns been?

My oldest daughter is 10 and she never really had a sleep problem, but she talks in her sleep and turns over a lot. And in the morning her bed is a mess. You can tell she's had a restless night.

Tell me more about how she acts in the mornings?

There are days when she gets up and every movement is hard. I tell her to get ready because it's almost time for school and she yells back saying, "I know that!"

Do you have any idea what the source of this trouble may be?

When the kids' father left it affected all of them in different ways. I think it affected the baby the least, but it did affect Zoe in that her schoolwork suffered and she doesn't sleep as soundly at night.

Even though it's been a few years, you feel it's still a major issue?

When he first left, he was back and forth for a while. Slowly he just checked out of the situation. When he started checking out, it was harder for them to adjust, so it was kind of a prolonged thing because he kept things going.

How about your youngest? Any sleep troubles there?

Molly is more prone to lie there and talk and sing to herself. Bedtime is never really a problem, and she hasn't had a problem falling asleep, but she does toss and turn in her sleep a lot.

How old is she exactly?

She will be three in two months.

Is Molly kept awake by Corey?

Yeah. That's definitely part of it. They're kept awake because Corey is still awake and doing things. She is a very restless sleeper and her bed, just like her sister's, is always torn up in the morning. There are times when I can hear her talking in her sleep, but not as much as the other kids.

Does she have trouble sleeping through the night?

She does, yes. She usually gets up at least once and goes to the bathroom in the middle of the night.

How are the mornings for her?

Oh, it's awful. When she gets up, she'll immediately come into my room and sit on the edge of my bed and just cry.

And how often does she do that?

At least a couple times a week.

☙ • ❧

After we spoke a bit more, I gave Angela the *Magic Carpet* CD to try with Corey, primarily. She came back several weeks later to report on the progress of all three kids.

☙ • ❧

You started using **Magic Carpet** *with one of your children—Corey?*

Yeah, but since all three of my children sleep in the same room, the CD plays for all of them.

What happened in the first week of using the program?

The first night I told him that Dr. Jackson had made the program especially for him. I told him we were going to use it because he was having so many problems sleeping. The first night I set it up for him, but since then, he does it by himself and he wants to do it every night.

What happened the first night you used it?

He fell asleep in about a half hour. The next night he also fell asleep in about a half hour. He has requested it every night since then. He would say, "You know, I can't go to sleep without *Magic Carpet*." There have been times, very rare, when he has been someplace where the program was not available and it's been a problem. When we stay at my mother's house, if I forget it, we'll have a problem that night. The last time he hadn't gone to sleep by 10:30, and I had to go to work in the morning, so my mother stayed up with him until about midnight, trying to get him to go to sleep. He has started telling people, "I have a problem sleeping and Dr. Jackson made a CD for me and it helps me go to sleep." He doesn't take the program to his dad's house and I can tell the difference in his behavior the next day when he comes home because he hasn't used it that night. He didn't use it last night. He was at his father's house and we're having a harder time today.

Why didn't you send the program with him?

Because Daddy can't be counted on to send it back. That might sound selfish, but sometimes he won't return things and we just can't be without that program.

It sounds like you need a second program.

That would be great!

How hard is it to get him into bed now?

Not hard at all.

You mean he doesn't resist going to bed at all now?

He looks at the clock, and he's at the age where he can tell time now and he knows if its 8:30, and he'll say, "It's 8:30, Mom," and I'll tell him to turn off the TV.

Almost as though he's looking forward to bed?

Yep. He watches the clock.

How much has his resistance to going to bed improved?

Most of it—probably 90%. Every once in a while, depending on what's going on, there may be a problem. I go back to his father leaving because they were really close. He sees his father on a regular basis and I think Daddy is really indulgent with him. When he returns home and the rules are different, it's harder for him. So, I would say about 90% of the problem has ceased.

What's the average amount of time it takes him to go to sleep now?

Half an hour.

What about nighttime wakings?

Nighttime wakings—currently about twice a month. He rarely wakes up at night anymore. In the last month, I can remember two occasions. I work the night shift and he stays with my mother at night and he never gets my mother up now. On my nights off, Corey has had me up twice. I think it's just been a *"Mommy check"* to make sure I'm around.

Does he have a hard time going back to sleep?

No. I tell him I love him and it's okay, and he goes back to bed.

You haven't had to go to his room with him?

No. I just tell him it's okay and to go back to bed, and he goes and crawls into bed and that's the end of it. When I first started using the program and he would wake up in the middle of the night, I would restart it and use it to get him to go back to sleep and I don't have to do that anymore.

That worked?

Yeah. It would take him a while, but I wouldn't have to stay in the room.

So that was effective right from the beginning?

Yeah. I was able to go back to bed and not worry about it. I didn't have to stay in his room and lay down with him.

What's going on with his bad dreams?

He still has bad dreams, but only every once in a while, so that's a big improvement.

Has there been any change in his behavior in the mornings?

Yes, a very dramatic change. He wakes up in the morning, and if I'm up he comes to find me. If I'm not up he'll come into my room and stand next to the bed and say, "Good morning, Mommy," and come and give me a hug. And when I tell him it's time to eat breakfast he'll say, "Okay, what can I have?" It's a very dramatic change—he doesn't fight me at all. Every once in a while, which I think is normal for a four-year-old, I'll tell him he can watch cartoons after he is dressed and he wants to know why he can't watch cartoons now. But no acting out, screaming or crying or saying he's too tired for school.

How long was it before you saw that change?

It was a slow change. Slowly the mornings got easier. I can't say exactly when. I probably noticed it about five days after he started using the program.

Mornings are fairly easy now?

Yeah, mornings are real easy. Sometimes he has something he doesn't want to do, but it's not like it was before. It's not that he doesn't speak up for himself and let you know what his needs are. It's just that there's not the difficulty that there was before.

What about the rest of the day? What are the reports from school?

He's been in the same school for almost a year now. Shortly after I started using the program his teacher asked me what I was doing; if I was doing anything different with Corey at home. He's calmer at school; he sits for longer periods of time. His attention span is longer and they could see a change in his ability to memorize things and recognize letters and numbers. Attitude-wise, he has been calmer. He never had a problem with fighting, but it was kind of, "Let me show you how tough I am," and that is better. He's a lot calmer and his teacher did notice it. At nap time he used to tell the teacher he wasn't tired and didn't want to take a nap. At first, he was less resistant and would at least lie down and rest. But, gradually, he was relaxed enough to actually take naps, which he never did before.

And the other children? Has the program had any effect on them?

I can see some changes. Now when I stand in the doorway and watch, all three of them are asleep. It's a lot calmer. All three of them are sleeping more soundly.

Has your oldest daughter mentioned any difference in how she feels when she gets up? Have you noticed anything in the morning?

She acts a lot more refreshed. She's now easier to get along with. Now when I say it's almost time for school, she'll say, "Okay, Mom." She's a lot less cranky.

Is she more refreshed?

She looks a lot more refreshed. There's more color in her cheeks and she looks better.

And how about her schoolwork? Has that improved any?

Actually, her schoolwork *has* improved, as a matter of fact. I went in and talked with her teacher a few times and slowly, after listening to the program, her schoolwork began improving and she came back up to the level where she was before. I think it helped relieve the shock of Daddy leaving.

Okay. Now Molly, your youngest, was there any change in her?

Yeah, she goes to sleep faster. And she sleeps a lot sounder now.

Is she still talking in her sleep?

Not at all, honestly.

Is she still getting up in the middle of the night to go to the bathroom?

No, I haven't heard her doing that at all now.

Does she seem different when she gets up in the morning?

Yes. Instead of coming into my room crying, now she comes in my room with a smile and says, "Mommy, it's time to get up and have some cereal."

Is she ever coming into your room crying in the mornings?

No, now she never does that.

Okay, are there any other changes with Molly?

We've been using the program now for almost three months. She talks about it. She'll tell me about certain parts, "I like the part where you can hear the birds, Mom." She'll listen, and when your voice says something, she'll say the same thing. It's like she's got it memorized and sleepily she'll talk along with you.

It sounds like she's claimed it for her own.

> Yes. She'll close her eyes and be talking along with the program and pretty soon she'll say things like, "No, kitty, you can't go down there, because there's water down there." She's imagining she's taking her kitty with her, because she loves cats, and it's like she's talking to her cat while she's reciting the script. Yeah, it's helped her, though I've never seen any real behavior problems with her. Because she is so little, she hasn't had time to really develop many behavior problems. So the changes with her have been small. But she really likes it and it makes her bedtime more enjoyable.

Do the other children enjoy it too?

> All three of them do. It's kind of funny to listen in on them. If Zoe starts talking, Corey will say "You're talking too loud, I can't hear the CD." And it's cute how Zoe always makes sure that Corey has his CD. She's real good about reminding me to take it if we're going to Grandma's house to sleep. "Do we have Corey's CD?" It's been labeled Corey's CD. He'll rant and rave at me, if we forget it. "You *know* I can't sleep without my CD. You *know* I have problems sleeping, Mom." So I have to remember or I'm in deep trouble. So, it has actually helped all three of them, but I've seen the most changes with Corey.

Thank you very much.

୨ • ୧

CHILDREN OF DIVORCE

In Angela's interview, we learned that her middle child, Corey, had great trouble dealing with the sudden departure of his father from his life, even three years after the divorce. And while this is certainly understandable, understanding doesn't do much to help the boy sleep at night. Meanwhile, Angela's divorce from her husband also seemed to have negative effects on her oldest child's academic performance. Almost any adult who grew up a child of divorce will tell you that their parents' breakup presented a real challenge.

THE CRISIS OF DIVORCE

Divorce has become a prevalent part of our culture, so much so that now 50% of marriages in the United States end in divorce. Over one million children each year experience a family divorce firsthand. And although long-term difficulties are not a certainty for children of divorce, they are twice as likely as their peers from intact families to suffer mental and emotional struggles as a result of their parents' divorce that, if left unattended, could very well persist into and throughout adulthood.

On the surface, divorce changes much about a child's life: where she lives and goes to school, the family dynamics in the household, the family's financial situation. But even more changes occur beneath the surface, internally.

How Divorce Affects Children

Divorce affects a child's whole world view. It forces reexamination of the concepts of safety, stability, trust, and love. Common themes for children of divorce surface as problems in school and trouble relating with peers and authority figures. We commonly see aggression, regression, and other behavioral difficulties, as well as negative self-concepts.

Young children may not consciously process what they experience surrounding their parents' divorce; yet they often manifest their conflicted emotions as physical symptoms. One common category of these symptoms is sleep disturbance.

Common Childhood Sleep Disturbances Related to Divorce

Without much, if any, conscious awareness of what is happening around her, a child whose parents are considering, preparing for, or going through a divorce may experience bedtime resistance, bedwetting, nightmares, and night terrors (to name just a few)—even if no such symptoms have ever occurred before. Some other possible symptoms, not directly related to sleep, include thumb-sucking, headaches, tummy aches, tearfulness, and oppositional behavior.

Approaching the Challenge of Divorce with Your Child

There is little doubt that divorce often has traumatic effects on children, and that trauma of any sort can lead ultimately to anxiety and depression. How you and your children navigate this difficult period, however, will help determine whether these effects are short-lived or long-lasting.

The shock brought on by divorce often triggers a child's fight-or-flight response. And if the child doesn't have adequate means of appropriately expressing her feelings about these changes—such as a common feeling of powerlessness—she may very well withdraw, freezing up and closing down from you and the outside world.

If, however, you find ways to proactively confront the challenges of divorce with your child, you create opportunities for you both to build greater inner strength, improve relational skills, and develop a better overall ability to cope with change and adversity. For it is not the act of divorce itself that has the potential to cause trauma, but the child's experience of the act of divorce as molded and modeled by the divorcing parents' words and deeds. Every challenge, including the divorce of one's parents, introduces an opportunity to develop new and better mechanisms for managing all of life's challenges.

How to Have Open, Honest, and Clear Communication with Your Child Around Your Divorce

Most importantly as a parent, be open and honest with your children about the divorce and all that it brings up for them. Keep the lines of communication open between you and your children to minimize the trauma that all of you go through around the experience.

Encourage Your Child to Express Her Feelings

Make it okay for your child to openly and honestly express her feelings of fear, anger, sadness, and any other emotions, positive as well as negative; you will automatically pave the way for your child to resume feeling safe, secure, and cared for again. Do not assume that your child feels the same about the relationship and its dissolution as you. Rather, ask. And be prepared to accept and allow whatever emotions come up, however surprising, or even threatening, they may feel to you. Judging your child for her reactions to your divorce, and challenging or invalidating those feelings is quite counterproductive at this point; your child needs acceptance and patience.

And, for your own peace of mind, don't fear your child's negative emotions. Sadness and disappointment are natural, healthy responses to trauma. If unexpressed and invalidated, however, they may join with more harmful emotions like hopelessness and despair in a downward spiral, which can then lead to more serious problems like the aforementioned anxiety and depression.

Give Them Time to Adjust on the Inside Before Life Changes on the Outside

Don't, consequently, wait until the last minute to broach with your children the subject of your impending divorce. Don't wait until actual lifestyle changes occur before you begin discussing the situation with them. If at all possible, plan a time to sit down with your children and your spouse all together, so that you are both present to convey to your children that what is happening is a reflection on the two of you and not on them. It may seem obvious to you that your divorce is not their fault, but it isn't so obvious to them. In actuality, children often find all sorts of ways to put the onus for the divorce upon themselves.

Be clear and up front with them about the changes to come, and make space for them to ask whatever questions they may have; then follow through with the answers to the best of your ability. Ask them about their fears concerning the divorce, and address those fears. Your children need to know you understand how big an impact this divorce will have on their lives; you may not even know yourself until you try to put into words your answers to their questions. And you can best demonstrate this by listening to everything they have to say on the subject and by providing answers instead of rebuttals.

Addressing Your Child's Needs

Assure your children that you and your spouse will still meet all of their needs. The format will change, yes, but their being taken care of will absolutely not. Most of all, remind your children that you and your spouse both love them dearly, even though the bond between you and your spouse may be irreparably damaged.

Expect Many Conversations

One conversation will probably not suffice, either. Helping your children cope with your divorce will be an ongoing process, one in which you will probably have to repeat yourself frequently, reminding them as often as needed that the divorce is not their fault and that both you and your spouse will always love them.

Be Gentle but Honest...

Tailor the language you use to the age of your child, but don't sugar-coat the situation. Don't speak down to the child. And don't lie to her. If you and your future ex-spouse do not plan to remain friends after the divorce, for example, then don't pretend that you will. Likewise, don't give your children false hopes that you and your spouse may someday get back together. They must understand your decision to divorce is final, or they will never find the kind of closure they need to begin the process of healing.

...And Keep Your Marital Troubles Out of Your Child's Life

Equally imperative, don't expose your children to your marital strife. Some studies have found, in fact, exposure to the parents' discord impacts children more than the actual divorce itself. Therefore, do your best to shield your children from your arguments. Worse, don't involve your children in any sort of power-struggle between you and your spouse or ex. When you use your children as bartering or negotiation tools, that's exactly how they feel—like helpless pawns held hostage to the vicious battle between the two people they love most.

After the separation is final, try your best to maintain some modicum of civility between you and your ex-spouse in front of the children. And when your ex-spouse isn't around, keep the gloves off. Badmouthing your ex-spouse to your child is in no way the same as being open and honest with your child. Avoid at all costs telling your children how they should feel about the other parent.

Refrain, as well, from quizzing your children or pumping them for information about your ex. Don't use your child to send messages to your ex. And certainly don't ask your children to take sides. Instead, find alternative venues for dealing with your feelings rather than dumping them onto your children's already laden shoulders. In the plainest terms—just don't put them in the middle.

Full Disclosure-For Your Child's Sake

Be sure also to inform the adults instrumental in your child's daily life—teachers, doctors, babysitters, etc.—of the divorce to help foster the network of support your child needs (not to mention to help prevent awkward moments).

Taking Care of Your Child Means Taking Care of Yourself

And speaking of finding other venues of support, you shouldn't, and don't have to, go through any of this alone any more than do your children. Importantly, in fact, set a good example for your children about drawing on your existing support network. That's what it's there for. This includes relatives, friends, teachers, counselors, civic and religious leaders, mental health experts, and trained professionals. Seeking support from outside sources and encouraging your child to do the same will help restore the community and family foundation the divorce may very well have crumbled.

In particular, seek out avenues for expressing and processing your more negative emotions about your divorce so you can better guide your child through the experience in a positive, healthy, and proactive manner, so that, in other words, you don't project your guidance for your child through a veil of bitterness. For you will not be much good at caring for your child's needs during this trying time if you aren't taking care of yourself. Children are extremely sensitive to the emotions of their parents, and if you feel guilt, blame, shame, or resentment about the rift in the relationship, your child will model those feelings herself.

Now more than ever you need to stay on top of your mental, emotional, physical, and spiritual health. Eat right, sleep well, socialize, exercise, pray or meditate—maintain a healthy lifestyle in every way possible as you go through a divorce and throughout its aftermath so that you are best poised to help your child go through it in as healthy a manner as she can, too.

Furthermore, if you were a child of divorce yourself, your own divorce may bring up unresolved issues you must be careful not to project onto your children. Just as everyone handles death differently, you cannot assume your children will manage the divorce and navigate its aftermath the same as you did the divorce of your parents.

You're Still the Parent, She's Still the Child

Beware, too, of letting your child parent you while you go through your divorce. It may sound absurd, but in truth many children, upon witnessing one or both of their parents going through severe distress, may try a bit of role reversal, taking on the position of parent as their actual parent heals. While this is admirable (and even adorable) it is not healthy—not for you and not for your child. Likewise, avoid telling the child, "Now you are the man/woman of the house."

The experience of a divorce is difficult enough for a child without the added burden of the role of a grownup and the consequent burden of grownup responsibilities. That's your job, not hers—no matter how hard you may find it at the time. Further, such role transference sets a precedent for dysfunctional patterns of future parent-child interactions you'll find difficult to break.

Nip the Matchmaker Syndrome in the Bud

It is also not a child's job to fix their parents' relationship or get them back together. And while this may seem obvious to you, you very well may need to spell it out for your children. Again, you may need to make it perfectly clear to your child that your decision to divorce is final. You couldn't fix your relationship and neither can they, no matter how hard they try, no matter how often they watch movies like *Parent Trap*. And they need to understand this implicitly so they don't put themselves through unnecessary heartache.

Compensate for Choices Lost with Choices Gained

Children of divorce naturally (and justifiably) feel like victims of their parents' breakup, especially when issues like custody, visitation rights, and child support come into play. Sadly but simply, your child has little say in what happens between you and your ex- (or soon to be ex-) spouse. But you can help establish a sense of empowerment within your child by allowing her as much choice as possible in areas where such freedom of choice is appropriate. For example, give your child the freedom to choose what clothes she's going to wear or what food she's going to eat; control over such basic choices help her feel she hasn't lost all control over her environment, but that there are indeed many areas of her life where her will is still honored.

COMPENSATE FOR STRUCTURE LOST WITH STRUCTURE GAINED

Divorce also threatens to destroy children's vital sense of continuity. To a child, continuity equals stability and security, and they need it from you to build necessary feelings of safety and trust in you, in themselves, in others, in their environment, and in life itself. A loss of this sense of continuity introduces chaos and fosters a breakdown in your child's feelings of safety and trust.

To help nurture those feelings of safety and trust, then, establish or maintain structure in your child's life wherever you can. Mealtimes, bedtimes, rituals like church or afterschool activities—all of these offer valuable opportunities for children to understand that just because one element of their lives has changed drastically, doesn't mean that the rest of their lives will follow suit.

A child of divorce must also understand that the impending changes will be no excuse for unacceptable behavior. Household rules must still stand. And if new living conditions demand new rules, responsibilities, and limitations, then so be it. Rules, responsibilities, and limits promote structure in a child's life as much as routines and rituals do, and structure is integral to a healthy upbringing.

COMMON PITFALL: COMPENSATING WITH GIFTS AND LIBERTIES

Along the same lines, showering a child with gifts or giving her added liberties does nothing to help her recover from the pain of her parents' divorce. It only assuages your own guilt in the short term and, in the long term, promotes a dangerous sense of self-righteous entitlement in the child that grows increasingly difficult to break. Santa Claus need only come once a year; but a child needs proper parenting 365 days a year, divorce or no divorce.

JUST BECAUSE THEY'RE NO LONGER YOUR FAMILY . . .

For kids of divorce of any age (and quite likely for you as well), weekends, birthdays, and holidays can be especially tenuous times, and require particularly conscientious attention. Likewise, a child must be allowed to maintain her relationship with both sides of her extended family. All of this will no doubt take some careful coordinating on your part but it is, after all, your duty as a responsible and loving parent to do so.

SIGNS OF MORE SERIOUS TRAUMA TO WATCH FOR

Finally, be alert to the following warning signs of more serious trauma associated with divorce that may require more intensive, and possibly professional, attention:

- sudden absence of spontaneity
- decreased self-esteem

- apathy
- deep sadness
- irascible moodiness
- irrational fearfulness
- excessive clinginess
- inappropriate displays of anger
- poor hygiene and self-care
- sleep disturbances
- difficulty concentrating
- alcohol or drug abuse
- sexual promiscuity
- self-abuse
- allusions to suicidal thoughts

THE GOLDEN PROMISE: I'LL NEVER DIVORCE YOU

Helping your kids deal with your divorce takes a careful combination of sensitivity and self-control. Let your behavior show you're there for them in whatever ways they need you to be. And most importantly, show them you may divorce your spouse, but you can never, nor would you ever wish to, divorce your children.

CHAPTER 6

JANICE/TIMOTHY

Interviewed:	Janice
Child:	Timothy, age 7
Complaints:	*Aggression toward his sisters*
	Fear about moving
	Fear around separation from his biological father
	Mouthiness
	Disrespect

ଛ • ଏ

Hi, Janice. Please tell me *a little bit about your children.*

I have three wonderful children. The oldest one is 13 and she's a gem in her own way, and Timothy, he is seven and Gina, a little girl, is five. About a month ago we made a decision to leave the state. We are going to move to Oregon where the kids will have woods to play in; they can go fishing and things like that. And it seemed like a good decision to everyone, except that my son is really attached to his dad. He lives here in Seal Beach and, even though he's close by, his daddy has been really distant and not wanting to spend a lot of time doing things with him. So I think we've made a good decision, because he's going to have a good father figure there who will do a lot with him and I think it will be good. But because of this decision, he developed some anxiety about leaving his dad.

Have you been having any behavior problems with him?

They're all real good kids. They all go to private Christian schools. They're all real intelligent kids and Timothy has been at the top of his class the last two years. And he wasn't having any behavior problems, but recently, Timothy has become real mouthy, real hard to deal with. He acts like, "Well, you don't love me; you don't like me," and picking on his sisters; that sort of thing. He hasn't had any sleep problems and he hasn't been doing bad things except for being mouthy. And I'm getting real concerned. He's getting more and more disrespectful towards me and towards his teachers and picking on his sisters. In quiet moments he'll tell me, "Mama, I don't like to be mean." And at other times he'll just be hell on wheels. So I'm getting worried. I don't want my son to grow up being a disrespectful little guy that nobody likes. I'm concerned, and I decided I needed to do something.

So he isn't very good at expressing his feelings?

It seems like he isn't able to put into words how he's really feeling. Instead he'll just rant and rave and get mean and say "You don't like me," and so on.

❧ • ☙

After we spoke a bit more, I gave Janice the *Magic Carpet* and *Playhouse on the Beach* CDs. Several weeks later she returned to tell me how it went.

❧ • ☙

Have the programs had any effect on Timothy's behavior?

Magic Carpet and *Playhouse on the Beach* have been real effective for Timothy. He likes the programs a lot.

Tell me what happened.

Okay. He listened to them. All three of the kids listened to them when I first received them. We were in the kitchen getting dinner and cleaning up and so forth. And Timothy stood in front of the player listening and he said, "I really like how Dr. Jackson's voice sounds," and they all enjoyed the music and the sound effects, and they had lots of questions about where the sound effects came from. Your voice and the others on the CD seemed very real to them and made them feel that somebody loved and cared about them.

So it doesn't require any effort on your part to get them to listen?

They want to use them all the time. "Mama, where's my CD so I can go to bed," type of thing.

So it's actually entertaining?

Very. They like the imagery and all the interesting things they can see happening in their mind. When they're on the *Magic Carpet*, they're flying and they get to visit all those places and then they get to shrink down into tiny people, and all the other things that happen. The first time we listened to it we were all together and it was interesting to watch them; they got really quiet and then I could see them imagining what they were hearing.

So Timothy has been listening regularly. Have you noticed any change in his behavior?

He's calmer. He's easier to deal with. Now, when we're sitting and watching TV, he won't say, "Well, you like her better than me." He'll come and crawl up on my lap and say, "Can I come and sit with you, Mama?" It's much easier to hug him and play with him when he acts loving and I'm not feeling hateful toward him.

So when he's acting nicer it's easier to be nice to him?

Yes. And he's not picking on his sisters nearly as much. He's a little boy, so I guess he'll always be picking on his sisters, but he's not doing it anything like he was. Yesterday he was picking on them, and I talked to him and told him to go get the program and listen to it and when he finished I said, "Now do you feel better?" And he said, "Yes. I feel better." I said, "Do you feel nicer?" And he said, "Yes. I feel like I love my sisters more." And at times he has said, "Mama, I feel mean towards my family sometimes and I don't want to feel mean." So this is helping him express that; he's putting more words to how he feels about things.

There is a significant change in the area of him actually expressing his feelings?

Yes. He never said things before, like, "Sometimes I get these feelings in my head, and they make me hate people, and I don't want to hate people." He just couldn't tell me that before.

So it was a sudden change?

Over the last week or so.

How long has he been listening to **Magic Carpet***?*

For about a week.

Thank you so much for sharing. That was an interesting story. So you'll be moving soon?

Yes, it will be about a month before we move because there's a court thing going on. I think Timothy feels the pressure of that, plus the stress. He's going to leave all his friends and everybody's uprooting. He hasn't actually talked about leaving his friends, but he does talk about not being able to see his daddy. And he's also voicing his concerns about where he's going to be and where he will be going to school. Before he would just say, "Yeah, I want to go," but he wouldn't talk about any of the parts that might scare him.

So he's giving you the opportunity to discuss these issues.

Yeah. We're able to talk about it and say, "Yes, you're going to have your toys and new friends, and it's going to be a big change. And some of the changes will probably hurt for a little while, but it's going to get better." So we can talk about things a little bit easier. And Gina wants to go because she's going to get a kitty.

Hey, that's a good enough reason. Well, thank you very much for talking to me.

You're welcome.

SIBLING RIVALRY

In my interview with Janice, she explained how, after her divorce from her husband, her son, Timothy, started acting out, in particular by lashing out at his sisters and competing with them jealously for Janice's attention. Child experts commonly hold that some degree of animosity and an element of competition between siblings are inevitable. And whether that is true or not, sibling rivalry is certainly a prevalent issue faced by children growing up in the same household.

INFLUENCES AFFECTING SIBLING RELATIONSHIPS

A number of influences, including the following, affect the relationship between siblings:

- birth order—who was born first, second, third . . .
- age—sibling dynamics tend to change as siblings age
- age difference—how far apart in age the siblings are
- gender—relationships between brothers, sisters, and brothers and sisters are all considerably different from one another
- individual personalities—such as when one child is particularly shy or particularly aggressive
- number of siblings—rivalry increases when there are more children than one per adult in the home
- parental treatment—including influencing factors like favoritism

HOW AGE AFFECTS SIBLING RELATIONSHIPS

One child psychologist, Dr. Sylvia Rimm, suggests sibling rivalry is strongest in siblings of the same gender who are close to one another in age. When children are close in age (and especially when they're of the same gender) they feel a deeper need to establish their own individual identities and a strong delineation of the differences between them and their sibling. They, in essence, compete to define themselves—to find their own unique talents, skills, interests, and abilities as distinct from those of their sibling(s).

On the other hand, siblings more divergent in age develop rivalries, too, though for altogether different reasons. It's a positional type of conflict that arises between siblings of different ages. The younger child wants to be treated as an equal; the older child wants to be recognized for being older. Thus we see the common behavior in which a younger sibling mimics everything the older sibling does (much to the older sibling's vexation). Age divergence also helps explain why older siblings tease and bully their younger siblings in order to demonstrate supremacy.

Both, of course, occupy difficult positions, and neither one holds the ideal position. First, the older sibling has to share the parent. Then as the younger sibling ages, the older one has to share his play space, toys, and so on. And later still, when the younger one is finally old enough to be allowed to go outside to play, the older one feels his turf is being infringed upon once again. On the other hand, the younger sibling has to watch as the older one continually gets all the privileges first, including those which the older sibling perceives as a chore (such as taking out the trash). And when the older sibling is asked to take care of the younger one (as in feeding, bathing, or babysitting), neither child is happy with the arrangement.

It is also between siblings of divergent ages that this positional rivalry has a greater potential of turning dangerous. An older sibling typically knows how to manipulate and bully more effectively than does a younger sibling. And a younger sibling may have fewer developed skills for behaving appropriately under stress than does an older one.

A New Baby's Arrival

Even the arrival (or impending arrival) of a new baby in and of itself can initiate sibling rivalry, as most children feel threatened by the baby's demands on the parents' attention. Often, in fact, this sense of threat begins as anticipation before the new baby is even born. Include the child in the process of welcoming the newborn into the household to help defuse these fears, but don't expect to allay the fears altogether. The anticipatory fear is natural; you simply want to keep the lines of communication open and prevent the fear from developing into anxiety.

How Individuality Creates Sibling Rivalry

Positional rivalry aside, the personal characteristics of each individual sibling, regardless of differences in age and gender, also play a huge role in the nature of their relationship with one another. Sibling rivalry is therefore also common, in families where one of the children is particularly gifted, or anxious, or temperamental, or easily bored or flustered, and so on. Likewise, a child with learning disabilities or developmental difficulties (such as with attention span, language, and socialization), may also be more prone to engage in contentious behavior with his siblings.

How to Handle Sibling Rivalry

So what is a parent to do? Surprisingly, in many cases, nothing.

In the best-selling book she co-authored, *Siblings Without Rivalry,* Adele Faber explains, "Our relationships with our siblings prepare us to interact with people in the larger world." Many of life's lessons we first learn in our relationship with our siblings. Children learn valuable skills like sharing and compromise, assertiveness, self-control over aggressive impulses, acceptance of people's differences, and valuing of other people's perspectives.

Common Pitfall: Refereeing Your Children's Relationships

Furthermore, playing referee to your children's infighting often has the opposite of the desired effect. Rather than dissipating the animosity, it often gives the siblings more to fight about. More significantly, though, it also subverts children's development of vital life skills, like the ability to negotiate peaceful solutions on their own. Verbal arguments between your children may get on your nerves, but they are not necessarily harmful, and in fact can help both children develop useful problem-solving skills. So conflict between siblings is actually a valuable tool for them, a training ground where they establish their individual identities, practice their skills of self-reliance, and vent negative emotions in a safe and familiar arena.

You can inadvertently exacerbate problems between siblings by taking sides, including trying to figure out "who started it." It doesn't matter "who started it"; what matters is that the children both find a positive way to finish it peacefully. The less you get involved in minor disputes, the sooner your children will develop the skills to manage those conflicts themselves, and the better they will become at conflict resolution. These skills they take with them throughout their lives to help them navigate all kinds of adversity.

THE CRITICAL CAVEAT: VIOLENCE

If physical or emotional violence of any sort comes into play, however, a parent has no choice but to intervene. And while staying out of your children's conflicts as much as possible, it is also incumbent upon you as a parent to monitor those contentious interactions to make sure that neither child's safety is threatened.

If a verbal argument between siblings becomes physical the parent must help the siblings understand that they may have whatever feelings they have, but also understand the limits between acceptable behaviors and unacceptable behaviors as a means of expressing their feelings. You can honor your child's right to his feelings, in other words, while still teaching him to be responsible in his actions. Validate your child's emotions, and even help him understand the root causes of those emotions, but at the same time train him in appropriate ways to deal with and express them. As you monitor sibling rivalry, by the way, be sure siblings know the boundaries of personal space and that the destruction of each other's personal property is completely unacceptable behavior.

Most times, however, violence will not be a part of your children's contentious interactions. And of course, besides stepping back from it all to let them work it out between themselves, you'll see ways to help transform these conflicts into mutual opportunities for growth.

COMMON PITFALL: WHO STARTED IT?

First, hold both children accountable for the conflict. Again, it doesn't matter "who started it." It only matters that both of them engaged each other in "it." For all intents and purposes, both of them started it. If children know it takes two people to make an argument but only one to keep it from happening, then they may feel empowered to walk away if an interaction with their sibling becomes too uncomfortable. Gradually, they can learn to ignore their sibling's attempts to draw them into a conflict.

EQUALLY ACCOUNTABLE BUT NOT EQUAL ACCOUNTABILITY

Second, be aware that holding both children accountable for the conflict does not mean that both children have equal accountability for their behavior in the conflict. In other words, while both children are responsible for fighting with one another, each child is uniquely responsible for his specific conduct. Clarifying this will better help children recognize their responsibility for the matter and begin to examine alternative ways of responding to the same types of stimuli.

The One Exception: "Separate Corners!"

Third, while mediating your children's arguments is a bad idea, separating them from one another can be a splendid idea. Instruct them to use their "alone" time to think about what happened, about their responsibility for it, and about how they might be able to resolve their dispute peacefully. Even if one or both of them fails to come up with a suggestion for a positive resolution of their differences, the time spent alone will, at the very least, help each child calm down some and regain his composure.

You Can't Force Love, but You Can Enforce Civility

You can't force siblings to love each other or express love for one another. That must come from within themselves, lest your efforts have the opposite effect and breed bitterness and resentment. Keep in mind the big difference between being friends with one another and being civil to one another. You cannot insist that your children be friends with each other—and in fact you may want to inform your children they do not even have to be friends—but, regardless, your children must be aware that you insist on their being civil to each other.

Give Them Nothing to Prove

Equally important, express praise for who your children are inside, as people, and not just for how they behave on the outside. When a child feels appreciated simply for being who he is, that child is less likely to feel the need to prove himself through negative actions. Let your children know what you love about each of them and you'll thereby promote the growth, development, and enhancement of those qualities to the point where they begin to infuse all of your children's behaviors and actions.

Common Pitfall: Showing Favoritism

Beware especially of any favoritism, coming from you or other caretakers. You can unwittingly provoke rivalry between your children by treating one of them better than the other(s). "Why can't you be more like your brother/sister?" Eliminate that criticism from your own behavior, for it only breeds jealousy, bitterness, and resentment—a guarantee of further sibling rivalry. Such comparisons not only weaken sibling relationships, but also hinder their growth and personal development as individuals.

What's Fair?

"**It's not fair!!**" How many families with siblings haven't heard that accusation? But fairness is a double-edged sword when it comes to raising children. Consider the following:

> A teenaged child thinks that because he's older he should have special privileges not granted to his younger sibling. And if he doesn't get what he believes he has coming then *it's not fair*. The younger sibling, however, thinks that both children should be treated equally or *it's not fair*.

Who's right?

In a sense, both of them are. That wedges you squarely between the proverbial rock and a hard place. But treating people equally is only one quality of fairness; treating each appropriately according to his unique personality and needs is another aspect of fairness. Fairness honors both commonality and individuality; that leaves parents at a total disadvantage in any rational argument of fairness. Many parents therefore, when stuck in this messy quagmire, will often resort in frustration to irrational outbursts like, "Life isn't fair," or "Just do what I tell you."

Find ways to give each child the time and attention that each needs, separately and independently from one another. Parenting siblings is not so much about giving of yourself equally to each child but rather giving each child what he needs as an individual. Different kids have different needs, and when a child feels his needs are met, he is much less prone to feel the time and attention you give his sibling is "not fair." More on the concept of fairness shortly.

But for now, let's remember each child needs to know the time and energy you expend showing love and affection for his sibling doesn't take away from the time and energy you expend showing love and affection for him; your love for your children must not be a zero-sum game. In other words, one child does not have to "lose" in order for the other to "win." It's up to you to get this message across, through your words and through your actions, not just now and then, but every single day of their lives.

Get to Know Them as Individuals . . .

When you spend alone time with each child, inquire as to what each one likes best and least about his sibling. This information will be extremely useful in helping you keep a keener eye on their interactions as they develop. This time alone with each child individually reminds them they are special—even simply seeing it in your eyes makes them special. And all children need to feel special; secure in that feeling, a child may be less inclined to compete with his sibling. Plus, you'll find celebrating the positive uniqueness of each child quite easy, and you'll find that in turn an utter joy for you, for whom most other parenting tasks might not be so simple.

In addition to spending quality time individually with each sibling, separate from the other, further opportunities to support your children in having independent identities may include promoting:

- separate social circles
- separate toys
- separate spaces in which to be alone
- separate extra-curricular activities
- separate goals
- separate schools

. . . While Facilitating Positive Siblinghood Scenarios

On the flip side, joint activities the siblings (as well as the whole family unit) can enjoy participating in together help strengthen the bond between them and in turn, help counter the tendencies toward friction between siblings. This in turn homes in on another significant point about sibling rivalry: such rivalry

rivalry often acts as a mirror or gauge of the general level of harmony or discord in the household as a whole. Working together on your overall family dynamics, then, carries powerful potential to reduce the propensity among your children to squabble.

Don't Take the Bait!

Do your best to avoid being drawn into no-win arguments over fairness, and instead express genuine empathy for what your child is going through. "I understand that this doesn't feel fair to you. That must be terribly frustrating for you." Your child will very likely reply, "Yeah, it is." But feeling understood goes a long way toward helping a child overcome frustration. It's okay to validate your child's negative emotions. In fact, it's more than okay; it's healthy. And honoring your children's emotions helps them to find ways to reconcile how things are with how they want things to be.

Positive Reinforcement Is Your Friend

Remember, too, good behavior must be praised at least as diligently as poor behavior is pointed out. Children learn a great deal from positive reinforcement—more in fact, many experts believe, than they do from punishment. All children crave attention, and prefer even negative attention to no attention at all. To combat this potential for adversity, then, be sure to outwardly express your appreciation for appropriate behavior. Don't ignore good behavior under the premise you don't need to reward your child for behaving as he's supposed to. A child needs to experience how good behavior produces desirable responses just as much as (if not more than) he needs to experience how bad behavior produces undesirable responses.

Help Them to Help You Help Them

And you can help, additionally, by educating your children in ways to solicit positive attention from you, from each other, and from the outside world. For example, teach your children how to appropriately invite siblings to play, and by the same token, teach them how to handle rejection in a positive and productive manner when the other child does not respond as they had anticipated.

Teaching by Example: How Do You and Your Siblings Relate?

Do you yourself have siblings? What is your relationship with them like? Are your children aware of this? How do they see you behave in relation to your own siblings? Remember, children model what they see from the adults who are close to them, especially from their parents. If you have a contentious relationship with your siblings, your children will probably imitate this. Teach, then, by example. Let your children see you interacting appropriately with your siblings and they'll start modeling those behaviors instead.

Examine all the dynamics in your household, as your children will tend to model all of them. If angry screaming and yelling occurs frequently, for example, then you can only expect your children to model that behavior. It's in their nature to model after you. If a heavy blanket of stress overshadows the joy in your home on a regular basis, then it would be only natural for your children to emulate that stressfulness in their relationships.

Working on developing better ways of dealing with anger and stress yourself, therefore, you'll give your children better examples to model. You can actually help your children learn to work out their differences, then, by working on your own personal challenges. A household that's filled with fun and lightheartedness, mutual respect and appreciation, and calm, peaceful communication will promote all those same energies in the dynamics amongst your children.

Indications that Professional Help may be Called For

Finally, in certain circumstances, you may want to consider seeking professional help for handling your children's sibling rivalry, particularly if you observe any of the following:

- their conflict starts to take a toll on your relationship with your spouse or partner
- you perceive a serious and present danger of one causing physical harm to the other
- the mental/emotional well-being of one or more of the children (or other family members) seems severely affected by the conflict
- you suspect more serious psychiatric conditions may be at play in the conflict (such as depression or substance abuse)

If you're wondering whether professional assistance is appropriate for your particular situation, discuss your concerns with your child's doctor and get his opinion on the matter. If he does agree that some sort of professional aid is in order, he will probably be able to recommend a qualified expert with a practice near you.

CHAPTER 7

PRISCILLA/HARRY AND CHLOE

Interviewed:	**Priscilla**
Child:	**Harry, age 6**
Complaints:	*Nighttime wakings*
	Nightmares
	Exhaustion in the morning
	Waking parents at night
	Whining in the morning
	Bedtime resistance
	Lack of confidence
Child:	**Chloe, age 9**
Complaints:	*Nightmares*
	Whining
	Feelings easily hurt

❧ • ☙

Please tell me a little *about your children's sleep problems.*

My son continually has trouble sleeping through the night. He'll come into our room. "What's the matter, why are you here?" "I had a bad dream." So he'll come and sleep with us.

How often?

Very frequently for the past six to eight months and then last night he fell out of his bunk bed while he was sleeping, and he was traumatized by that. He had a lot of trouble last night relaxing and going back to sleep. It was very frightening and it took me almost three hours to calm him down.

Tell me about his mood during the day. What is his mood like, generally?

Well, he drags. It's like he's exhausted. His dreams either keep him up or keep him from relaxing or sleeping. He doesn't want to get up in the mornings. He's always whining and I have to go to his room three or four times to tell him he has to get up because we have to go. I tried giving him some responsibilities in the morning to do, and I would give him a quarter, but it still wasn't getting him out of bed.

Have you ever had problems getting him to go to bed?

Nothing out of the ordinary. But yes, he'll want to stay up and watch a movie or he'll want to play a game.

So there's a little bit of resistance going to bed.

Yeah, I wouldn't say out of the norm, though.

How about his older sister? Does she have a sleep problem?

She's has nightmares.

How consistent have her nightmares been?

Well, last Friday, she had a nightmare. She spent the night with the babysitter and she woke up about two or three in the morning and then could not sleep for the rest of the night. She dreamed she was out in the front of the house and her father was sitting on the porch where he could see her and someone was trying to take her away and her father wasn't doing anything about it. She got anxious and didn't want to go to sleep because she was afraid she would have the same nightmare.

How often has she had bad dreams?

Not as often as my son, but two or three times a month.

Does she have any problems with daytime behavior or attitudes?

When she has a nightmare she tends to be much whinier, much more flighty. And at the drop of a hat, she can get her feelings hurt by something you said and she'll cry, where normally she doesn't do that.

❧ • ☙

After Priscilla and I spoke a bit more, I gave her the *Magic Carpet* and *Playhouse on the Beach* CDs to try with both of her children. She returned several weeks later to tell me how it went.

❧ • ☙

So you first started using the programs with your son?

Yes I did. It was the day after he fell out of his bunk bed that I decided some sort of action needed to be taken. Then I met with you and got the program for him and started to use it with him.

And which program did you use?

> First I tried the *Magic Carpet,* and he really enjoyed it but it seemed almost too animated for him because he got so involved in the story that he wasn't falling asleep. So I then played *Playhouse on the Beach* for him. The first night, I had to play *Playhouse* twice before he actually fell asleep. Again, I think he was enjoying the story so much that he wanted to stay up and listen; he was concentrating on the program. The second night, I played *Magic Carpet* and then *Playhouse* in that order. The third and fourth times I probably played them the same. Then the fifth night, he said, "I like *Playhouse* better." Now, he consistently wants to hear *Playhouse on the Beach.*

I gave you both the male and female voice versions of **Playhouse.** *Does he have a preference for either?*

> He enjoys the male voice of it because he can relate better to the male voice. The female voice seems a little more animated. So I think he relaxes better to the male voice.

Is there any change in his willingness to go to bed at night?

> Actually, there is. He's not resisting at all. When I ask him to get ready to go to bed, he'll take 10 minutes to get his teeth brushed and get washed up, but he doesn't fight or argue. He will go ahead and get ready to go to sleep.

So going to bed is a more pleasant experience for him if he knows he has the program to listen to?

> It seems to be. There are nights that I have not gotten ready to put the program on, and he'll say, "Mom, aren't you going to put the CD on?" So I'll put it on. He seems to enjoy the program and wants to hear it. Once, he wanted me to turn it up, and I said, "If I put it any louder it's going to keep you awake," and he said, "No, I want to do that." So I turned it up so loud that the whole house could hear it, but he still fell asleep.

Okay. So what has happened in terms of him coming into your room?

> He has not been coming in. Since the start of the program he hasn't done it.

How long has he been using it now?

> Approximately two weeks.

And he hasn't come in one time?

> Not once.

And the quality of his sleep is better?

> Yeah. It's like he's getting that non-interrupted sleep, where he's feeling more relaxed when he wakes up.

Has he talked at all about his bad dreams?

> He hasn't had any bad dreams. Absolutely none. And he wakes up in a different mood. Since he started using the program, he's been getting a better night's sleep and he wakes up ready to do some chores. I think it's because he's getting more sleep and better sleep.

How much more sleep has he been getting?

Actually, most of the time he's sleeping more, but not always. The last two weekends he stayed up longer than usual, but yet, he still woke up in a much better mood. He's not dragging, he's not sluggish, and he's not moody when he wakes up now.

So he just seems to be generally in a better mood in the morning?

Yes.

Have you noticed any changes in how he seems during the day and evening?

During the day, I don't know, because I work. But in the evening there has been a change. Whereas before he would tend to stay close to me, want to play things with me, or want me to sit and watch TV with him. Now he will go on his own and play, or even with his sister or with kids in the neighborhood.

A little more confident in his interaction with others?

Yes. He's separating a little more and feeling more confident.

That seemed to come about right when he started listening?

Yeah. It all started to happen right at that time. He was starting to get to know other kids in the neighborhood, but he still wanted me to be outside with him. He's more confident now. He can go out and play without me being there.

Any other changes that you can identify?

I don't think so, but it's still early. I'll be looking.

Now, his older sister. Did she listen to the programs?

Yes, I didn't have headphones so both of them would listen at the same time. She seems to like *Magic Carpet*. She liked it because of the music in it, so she wants to hear that one, but she can fall asleep to either one. She really likes the song. Both of them will run around the house singing "Magic Carpet, floating up, up, and away." They like the things that happen in *Magic Carpet*.

How many nightmares has she had since she started listening to the programs?

Just one that I know of.

Being so infrequent to begin with, though, it would be hard to say if they've improved, since she's only listened a short time.

That's right, but she really enjoys them.

Okay, so it would be hard at this point to know if there's been a change in that.

Well, before she had the programs, she'd play a little game before bed and she'd say, "Give me good thoughts, give me gum drops," hoping she could ward off the nightmares, and recently she hasn't been doing that, so maybe that's a good sign.

Does she seem different in the morning?

Not too different, but she was able to verbalize her feeling about her bad dream and that was different. She actually talked about it and then seemed to feel okay.

Thank you very much for sharing this with me.

You're welcome.

❧ • ☙

Nightmares

Both of Priscilla's children were losing considerable sleep because of nightmares. In addition, both the lost sleep and the nightmares themselves had enduring effects on their days, too.

What Causes Nightmares?

Nightmares—deeply upsetting or terrifying dreams—are often caused by the ordinary conflicts and struggles that are all part of normal development. The emotional anxieties that create nightmares vary and can originate in fears of many different kinds. Almost anything a child finds frightening during the day can set the stage for nightmares. But they can also originate in a wide range of psychological, developmental, organic, and genetic factors.

For example, nightmares can be spurred by a particularly traumatic event or a physical/medical condition like a fever. Nightmares triggered by a stressful mental, emotional, or physical event can persist up to six months after the inciting event took place. In some extreme cases, regular nightmares can result from some sort of severe trauma and may be an indication of PTSD (post-traumatic stress disorder), in which case they may persist for much longer than six months.

Nightmares can also arise from nothing more than the typically active imagination most children have, and in fact some nightmares can occur for no apparent reason at all; they do occur in almost all children at one time or another. They do not discriminate according to gender, race, or cultural upbringing.

Statistics on Nightmares in Children

Scary dreams have been known to occur in children as young as two years old. Though variations in diagnostic criteria make it difficult to calculate an exact figure, several studies report that more than 50% of children between ages 3 and 6 experience nightmares disturbing enough to cause disruptions in both their sleeping patterns and those of their parents. About one in every four children has nightmares more than once per week.

When Are Nightmares Age-Appropriate?

Young children have a hard time understanding that dreams aren't real. As such, nightmares tend to be most problematic in children between ages 4 and 6. By age 7, nightmares usually become less of a problem, as most children of that age finally understand that dreams, although frightening, are not real.

Effects of Nightmares on Waking Life

A Canadian study published in the journal *Sleep* revealed that children prone to nightmares tend also to be more anxious and restless during the day and develop a more difficult temperament as well. Whether the nightmares are the effect of such personality traits or their cause is still subject to much debate.

The Time Nightmares Are Prone to Occur

It does appear clear, though, that nightmares typically occur in the middle of the night and in the early morning, the two periods of time when dreaming (REM sleep) is most prevalent.

What Distinguishes a Nightmare Disorder?

A nightmare disorder occurs when frequent and repeated nightmares continually disrupt a child's sleep. If your child experiences frequent nightmares (several a month), you may want to work with her during the day to try to determine what underlying fears may be causing them and then to try to resolve the trouble on that level. If the nightmares continue, I suggest you discuss your concern with your child's doctor.

The Stuff of Children's Nightmares

Generally, a child's nightmare involves some sort of clear and present danger, whether a physical threat such as being chased or a psychological threat such as being taunted. Children's nightmares might involve monsters or ghosts, dangerous animals, or threatening people. But commonly in most children's nightmare scenarios, the child experiences a lack of control over the scene taking place and fears imminent injury.

Upon Waking From a Nightmare

When a child awakens from a nightmare, she usually reorients to her surroundings quickly and is usually quite receptive to efforts of calming and consolation as well. Also, a child upon waking from a nightmare ordinarily recalls much of the content of the dream.

Now although a child waking from a nightmare typically becomes quickly aware of her familiar surroundings, the effects of the sleep disturbance leak into her day, and may cause impairment and distress in daily functioning. In addition, quite often a child who experiences a nightmare will awaken one or both parents, causing a disruption in *their* sleep patterns which can, in turn, lead to the parents' experiencing impairment and distress in their daily functioning.

The Best Cure Is Prevention

Prevention is the challenge, but also the best solution. Make bedtime a comfortable and safe experience for the child. Spend time with the child at bedtime, reading and otherwise helping her to relax. A soothing bedtime ritual might also include a relaxing bath, a gentle massage, a warm mug of herbal (caffeine-free) tea, or even something as simple as being tucked in with regular hugs and kisses.

Or, if your child seems to need a sense of company at bedtime, instead of remaining in the room until she falls asleep, you might have her listen to *Magic Carpet*, *Playhouse on the Beach*, or *Country Friends*. You could also use these programs directly after a nightmare occurs as a way to help her get back to sleep and to prevent recurrence of nightmares that night. This change in mental focus draws attention away from the upsetting event and leads her into a state of feeling safe. And keep in mind that listening to the *DreamChild Adventures* programs has been helpful in eliminating nightmares for many children.

OTHER WAYS TO HELP PREVENT YOUR CHILD FROM HAVING NIGHTMARES

Although it is unrealistic to expect to stop your child from having nightmares altogether, there are a number of other ways to try to decrease their frequency.

MONITOR TELEVISION AND VIDEO GAMES

For one, be sure to monitor the television programs and movies your child watches and the video games your child plays so as to avoid those that might be too scary, violent, or otherwise disturbing.

DISCUSS DAILY STRESSORS

In addition to discussing the content of your child's bad dreams in an effort to uncover their cause, it may also be worthwhile to examine your child's daily routine. Might there be something happening at home or school or elsewhere in your child's daily life that could be causing enough distress to possibly lead to bad dreams?

For example, might another child be bullying your child at school? Could a close friend be moving? Is there any current strife in the home that could be upsetting her, such as an impending separation or divorce?

ENCOURAGE EXPRESSION

By age 3, your child can begin to talk directly with you about any concerns and worries that could be triggering nightmares; then you can offer reassurance and guidance for dealing with those causes. Allow your child, at any age, to express feelings in appropriate ways. Try to assure your child that her feelings are understandable and normal. It is important to maintain open communication with your child by expressing your willingness to discuss any concerns she may have, no matter how difficult or touchy the issue may be.

If your child has difficulty expressing either the content of the nightmares or the concerns in waking life that could be causing them, consider exploring these issues in more creative and less explicit ways, for example by drawing or playacting.

How to Deal With a Child's Nightmare in the Moment of Crisis

At this point, let's say you're on the back side of prevention and are trying to cope with the crisis of the moment—a nightmare. You need to take an appropriate action to help your child move beyond the fright of the dream. Whatever you do to help your child deal with nightmares, do not ignore her cries in the middle of the night and try not to get angry, frustrated, or impatient with her (such as for waking you up). Let's look, then, at proactive courses of action.

You can employ any number of additional other strategies for dealing with your child's nightmares as they occur. Most importantly, simply stay alert to frightened wakings in the middle of the night (easiest to do if your bedroom is close to your child's, but if not, consider installing a baby monitor). As soon as you hear your child waking up frightened (screaming, crying, whimpering, etc.), go to her immediately and reassure her with comforting words, soothing her just as you would if she became frightened by an event during the day.

Remember, however, as you sleepily grope for the right thing to say, telling a very young child, *"It's only a dream,"* is unlikely to help since young children don't yet understand that dreams aren't real. With children who are at least three or four years old, though, it may be helpful to remind them that they were dreaming, although they, too, may still have difficulty understanding the nature of dreams.

Cuddle with your child. Gently stroke her head or back. And listen to your child's fears with empathy, understanding that her fears are perfectly real, and should not be discounted under any circumstances. If your child wishes to discuss the nightmare, by all means encourage it. Then offer reassurance and comfort until your child has calmed down sufficiently to return to sleep. Keep in mind that if your child is afraid to go back to sleep, this may require your staying in the room until that time comes. If she is very frightened you will need to do whatever is required to help her calm down, possibly by reading a story or enjoying a simple, distracting, and—above all—relaxing activity together. Or perhaps lie down with your child or even let her join you in your bed. You may find it helpful to provide a nightlight in your child's room, but make sure it isn't casting scary shadows or you'll defeat the purpose of its being there.

Remind your child that she can think comforting thoughts to soothe herself as well. Suggest, for example, that she imagine the nightmare scenario ending in a happy manner. Don't underestimate this method, for it helps teach your child to conquer her nightmares by actively imagining taking charge of the scene. This activity may also help her develop confidence, self-esteem, and a sense of proactive control over her responses to issues in daily life. As in waking conflict, unpleasant dreamtime scenarios typically include stages of threat and struggle. Whatever methods you follow, look at the nightmares as opportunity to help your child learn to use the innate tools she has for achieving resolution of her fears and confidence in her ability to face up to the frightening events of her life—both sleeping and waking.

What Distinguishes Night Terrors from Nightmares?

Night terrors, sometimes called "sleep terrors," differ from nightmares in significant ways. For starters, night terrors occur during deep sleep, as opposed to REM sleep, and are therefore not remembered.

When a child awakens from a night terror, she does not have any recollection of having experienced a particularly disturbing dream or, for that matter, of having any of the symptoms of night terrors so apparent to anyone observing the event.

Night terrors are most common in children from age 3 to 6. They can be associated with stress, changes in routine, sleep deprivation or a new environment. Fortunately, as a child gets older, night terrors tend to go away on their own. When they do happen, however, just let the episode pass naturally, without intervening. Don't try to awaken the child because they will just be confused and disoriented.

How to Handle a Child's Night Terror While It's Happening

Although night terrors don't appear to consciously disturb the child, they often quite alarm the parents, as they are generally characterized by the child uncontrollably screaming, crying, and thrashing around in bed. A child experiencing a night terror may also be sweating and breathing rapidly.

If you try to talk to your child during one of these episodes, she will not respond because she is asleep. It is, in fact, quite difficult to awaken a child in the midst of experiencing a night terror, this characteristic alone can be extremely disconcerting to parents. Some children will even open their eyes, appearing to have awoken from the night terror, but in actuality turn out to still be asleep.

Are Night Terrors Dangerous to a Child?

A night terror poses no danger unless the child is thrashing around in a manner that may cause harm, in which case it is advisable to clear the surrounding area but not to restrain her. If your child's night terrors are also marked by incidents of sleepwalking, then it is doubly important to create an environment that would protect your child from injuring herself in such instances.

Handling Nightmares and Night Terrors—In a Nutshell

Most children generally outgrow nightmares and night terrors eventually. Until that time comes, your role as a parent is simply to make sleep as safe, comforting, and relaxing for your child as it can possibly be. If your child experiences recurring nightmares, if the nightmares end up causing your child difficulty in everyday living, or if they persist even as your child ages, then consider talking to your child's doctor or consulting a therapist.

Chapter 8

Kevin/Kelly

Interviewed: Kevin

Child: Kelly, age 10

Complaints: *Trouble falling asleep*
Insecurity
Death of her grandfather
Nervousness
Over-sensitivity to feelings of rejection
Fear of separation from parents
"Worry about everything"

☙ • ❧

Tell me a little about the problems Kelly's been having.

She's been going through tough times and is having problems with sleep and feeling fearful and worrying a lot. She's been more nervous than usual and acting really insecure. She has really wanted to be the focus of our attention. And that's okay up to a point, but she has been clingy and seems to need to be right there with my wife and me, but we just can't be there all the time for her.

So when did this all start?

Actually, the sleep problem first showed up at the beginning of summer. My wife and I are both working, so we arranged to have Kelly's aunt watch her over the summer while she was out of school. But her aunt is only 20 and my daughter doesn't view her as a "real" adult. She was fretting so much she started having problems falling asleep. That eventually eased off once she got used to her aunt, but then her sleep got a lot worse in October, five weeks ago.

What was going on at the time?

Both Kelly and her sister, who is 6, were out one evening at Shakey's Pizza with their mom and their grandfather. You need to understand that Kelly has been very close to her grandfather, who we call *Grampi*. He's been a super Grandfather. Really loving toward the kids and just a great guy. He owns a roller skating rink across town and they've spent a lot of time with him there. It's been really fun for them, especially with him being the head honcho and all.

So, they're out with him the night before, and then the next day my wife gets a telephone call, and Kelly is standing there watching while her mom starts screaming and crying, and then Kelly starts crying and she's begging her mom to tell her what has happened and mom finally says, "Grampi is dead." He was only 59, and he died of a massive heart attack.

This has been a hard time for my wife, too. Her dad seemed young and healthy and we had never really thought about the possibility of him dying. So it was a shock. I'm afraid that my wife still hasn't had time to really deal with her own loss. She's been so busy taking care of everyone else, handling paperwork as executor of the will, and selling the rink. So she's been trying to hold it together emotionally, but as soon as she slows down I think it's going to hit her harder. Anyway, we're all handling it in our own way.

And how has Kelly been handling it?

Not very well. But it's her first experience with death and this whole thing has been hard. To start with they didn't even have the funeral for ten days. There were so many things that needed to be arranged. It was just pandemonium and tears. We let Kelly go to a viewing of the body. She wanted to, and she even touched Grampi. She said he felt stiff. I know some people might think you should shelter a little girl from death, but that's not how we feel, so we let her do what she wanted. The hardest part of the viewing was probably seeing Grandma break down over the casket; it was heart-wrenching.

I couldn't tell you, for sure, what effect all of this has had on Kelly, but her sleep has gotten a lot worse and she is a lot more nervous than usual. Kelly has been with my wife the past four weeks, and my wife needed to be with Grandma, so the girls spent most of the past four weeks at her house, around all of the things that remind them of Grampi. They've been helping Grandma with all the company, and there's been a lot—almost a constant flow—of family and close friends coming through. People flying in from all over the country to stay for a few days, and each time someone would leave, someone else would come.

And each time someone new arrived, everything would get emotional again and there'd be lots of crying. And then they'd leave and more company would come, and everyone would go through it again. Over and over, and Kelly has been in the middle of it.

So how has Kelly been affected by losing her grandpa?

Well, she started having problems falling asleep again, even worse than before, and she's having problems staying asleep, too. And it seems she's getting more and more insecure. She started wanting to be with us all the time. She wants to know exactly what we are doing at all times. She's been much more fearful. I got a cold and she got really worried about it—like I might get really sick and die. She also started feeling overly sensitive and was getting her feelings hurt very easily. Like, "So-and-so didn't want to play with me today. No one likes me." Kelly has always been a little nervous but, right after Grampi died, you could just see the anxiety all over her, especially when she flew with Grandma to Colorado. She was just panicked. She couldn't think about anything else. The questions were endless. I think she convinced herself she was going to die before she got on the airplane. Anyway, when she got back that's when I decided she needed some help, something to help her relax. So that's when I called you. I have to say she's a bit more nervous than the average child. That's just her personality. She's just wound tight. At the beginning of summer, she had been having stomach aches, frequently. We took her to the pediatrician and he ran a bunch of tests and couldn't find anything physical. Her anxiety was just affecting her stomach.

And how are you doing through all of this?

Well, I've been going through my own grief. You know we all have our own way of going through something like this. That became really clear to me when I went to grief groups after my mom died a couple years ago. The groups help you to see that everyone feels the same sense of pain and loss, but we all handle it in different ways. Some people are very emotional and others may hold it in, but we're all feeling pretty much the same thing. Everybody's so unique and at the same time we're all the same. It's become easier to just accept that, "*Oh, this is how I handle these feelings*." How you do it doesn't seem as important; there's no right or wrong way to handle your pain. Grandma has been going to a grief group and I think it's really helped her. Anyway, I'm doing fine, but it really seems to be taking a toll on Kelly.

༄ • ༄

After we spoke a while longer, I gave Kevin the *Country Friends* and *Magic Carpet* CDs to try with Kelly. Several weeks later, he came back to report on her progress.

༄ • ༄

What did Kelly think of the programs?

She had already heard the adult one and liked how it made her feel, so she was quite happy to have others to listen to. But she's really only using *Country Friends*. She listened to *Magic Carpet* once, but she really likes *Country Friends*. In fact, the first day she got it she listened to it for about five hours straight. She just loved it. The 3D sound was such a new experience. The program allowed her to go off into this other world where she felt safe and comfortable. I think it reassured her that she could feel good and not have to depend on us to feel that way. It was her first experience listening with headphones. Until then, she had only used the ear buds that came with her iPod.

How did she react to using headphones?

She liked them. I think they kind of gave her a feeling of being able to go into her own world; a place where she could get away, without really going anywhere. It allowed her to be close to us and far away at the same time. She knew she could just open her eyes and we'd be close by, but the story took her far away and gave her an experience that was independent of us, but enjoyable. I think it helped her feel like she could do something on her own and still be okay. Before using the program she was getting really anxious every time she thought about leaving us. But when she started listening, you could see her begin to unwind. The anxiety and fear just started melting away, and her sleep suddenly got better. Now she's really not having any problems sleeping at all.

How often has she been listening lately? Does she listen at bedtime?

She has listened to it at various times; sometimes in the evening, but not really right before bed. At the beginning she listened daily, and then every second day, or so, and now maybe every three days. Sometimes she does it on her own and sometimes I see that she needs to relax, so I'll suggest that she listen and she always does. And it makes her feel better. At this point, she's pretty much back to her normal self.

How is she doing in general?

She's no longer questioning where we're going and what we're doing and how long we're going to be. She's much more relaxed—not so worried about everything. I'm really glad that she is doing so much better. And I think she's even been a little more sensitive to others' feelings.

What do you mean?

Let me give you an example. She has always been pretty self-centered. I think that's normal for kids her age. My wife works as a nurse, and she does private duty, so she may be with a particular patient for four or five years. Well, one of her long-term patients just died, and when Kelly found out, her first reaction was, "Oh, that's the guy who used to give us chocolate chip cookies, isn't it?"

But then she starting saying, "Oh, his wife is going to miss him, isn't she?" And then she said, "He probably has grandchildren, too, and they're also going to miss him." So her initial thought was, *"No more chocolate chip cookies,"* but then she pretty quickly got around to the feelings of all the people involved. I guess that's what going through it yourself helps to give you—empathy for others.

Gaining empathy is a process for children. It doesn't happen overnight and it doesn't happen without real life experience. I guess that's part of why I don't think kids should be sheltered from death. If we pretend that it doesn't exist and kids don't experience it, they are cut off from an important part of human experience. And how else are they to develop real empathy for others who are experiencing it?

Well, I really appreciate the feedback on **Country Friends** *and everything you have shared.*

You are very welcome.

DEATH AND DYING

In this interview, Kevin described the terrible impact Kelly's grandfather's death had on her. This experience illustrates a common issue that all of us face at some point or another in our lives, and that most of us feel totally unprepared to deal with: the death of a loved one.

Then again, how can anyone actually be "prepared" for such an event. There's not much that can be done beforehand. It's something that you simply have to go "through" when it happens.

HOW A CHILD PERCEIVES DEATH

Death is one of the most difficult concepts for children to understand. Think of it this way: we learn about the concept, for example, of *"hot"* first, in reality, when we touch something someone has told us is hot; once we experience *"hot,"* we form the concept of "hotness," the degrees, so to speak, by which we expand on as our experience with *"hot"* grows. But the first time a child experiences the death of a loved one, there is no previous experience on which to base the concept.

So when Kelly touched her grandfather, her senses told her he was "stiff." Probably much more traumatic, she witnessed firsthand her mother's "screaming and crying" and her grandmother's "breakdown over the casket." Kelly's senses gave her some tactile and emotional information. Do those add up to the same concept of death we form in our own adulthood? Probably not. But Kelly, at the time of her grandfather's death, didn't have much more to go on. So she formed a concept of death limited to her own experiences including her observations of the adults close to her, which resulted in some unrealistic fears.

And this isn't particularly surprising since most adults have trouble coming to terms with death. Our first childhood experience of death is often the loss of someone old, like a grandparent. Studies in the United States show that one out of every six children experience the death of a grandparent, parent, sibling, or friend by the age of 10.

Preschoolers usually view death as temporary; after all, they play games in which someone is "dead" and then gets back up again. By age 5, however, children generally view death as permanent, final, and universal. Even so, children age 10 and older may resist talking about their feelings about death. Being young, they tend to believe that death is a long way off and rarely think about it as something that will happen to them.

EXPLAINING THE DEATH OF A LOVED ONE TO A CHILD

Explaining the death of a grandparent, or anyone for that matter, presents quite a challenge. And while in all likelihood the death of a grandparent will deeply affect your child, you and your spouse will also be mourning, and you will have your own feelings to deal with. How you explain the death of a grandparent depends somewhat on the age of the child and the closeness of the relationship.

If your child is a preschooler, you must be sure you use language that can be understood. Provide short and simple answers to questions and put the concept into real terms they can understand. For example, if the grandparent used to take the toddler to the park, you can explain that the grandparent won't be taking him to the park anymore, but he'll still be able to go there with you. If your child is older, you still don't want to make your answers too complex, but you can present more detail.

Even if a child wasn't especially close with a particular grandparent, it can still be a struggle to explain the death to the child. But it is less likely that the child will be as deeply affected if he didn't see the grandparent very often. If the grandparent saw the child on a regular basis, you can expect the child to take it a lot harder.

When you explain the death of a grandparent, you may wish to communicate your religious or spiritual beliefs to your child as well. You won't want to get into a long theological discussion, but you might just say that you know that she misses her grandparent, and that the grandparent is okay and is in heaven.

Common Pitfall: Sheltering Them from the Truth

While parents naturally want to "protect" their children from loss and pain, even the youngest child knows that something is very wrong and wants to know why everyone is crying. Attempts to shelter them from the truth only serve to rob the child of the opportunity to develop coping skills that will be necessary later on in life. And at some point there will be no parent around to protect him from grief because it is the parent who has died.

How to Have Open, Honest, and Clear Communication with Your Child on the Subject of Death

To help a child deal with a death, try to stay open to his questions and answer them as truthfully and as completely as possible, given the age of the child. Don't go into more detail than is necessary and if you don't know the answer to something, just say so.

When talking about the deceased, avoid euphemisms. Don't say that the person "passed away" . . . he *died*. Don't equate death with a journey because the child may become fearful when a parent goes away on a trip, thinking they may never return. Don't equate death with sleep. You shouldn't say, "He just went to sleep and now he's with God." Your child may fear falling asleep and be angry with God for taking someone he loves away. And, as the preceding interview illustrates, you might want to explain the difference between a minor illness and a fatal one. The child may think someone will die the next time that person catches a cold.

Try to accept all forms of emotional expression without criticism. Some children may try to use humor to help them deal with the situation. At times, we all react to stressful situations with laughter. Even if their attempt at humor feels inappropriate, let it pass. This is a time when your child needs to feel cared for and accepted whatever his reaction.

Everyone Grieves in Their Own Way . . . Children Included

It is advisable to let children decide what they will take part in. If they want to attend the funeral, then let them. If they want to view the body with the rest of the family, let them, but explain beforehand what will happen and what they will see. It's important for them to feel they are part of the family, but don't force them to participate in things if they don't want to.

Every person, including children, must grieve in their own way. The grieving process is long and doesn't follow a fixed pattern. When we refer to the pain of grief, that pain is very real. In fact we may experience it very much like physical pain. When someone says he feels "heart broken" his chest may actually hurt. And "gut-wrenching sorrow" describes well the physical sensation that may accompany grief. And just as one must heal from a physical wound, a healing process must take place for emotional and psychological wounds as well. We all heal in our own way and in our own time.

Emotions Happen: Let Them

Death precipitates a huge range of emotions—panic, guilt, anger, sorrow—all of which are normal. Try to accept your own emotions and the emotions of those around you. There is no "right" or "wrong" way to feel. Generally, the best way to get "through" this process is by allowing emotions to be expressed. It's okay to cry, scream or beat on a pillow.

As time passes, the waves of emotions will come less frequently and less intensely. But don't be surprised if just when you or your child seems to be "getting over it," suddenly another wave of emotion washes over you. It's just the nature of the process and it may go on for some time. Grief can last for one to two years or even longer. Don't get down on yourself, or your child, because someone else thinks the grief should end in six months.

Taking Care of Your Child Means Taking Care of Yourself

Adults who find themselves having a very difficult time dealing with a death might want to seek out others by joining a support group. Grief groups can help, as the above case also illustrated. Such groups are also available for those suffering a particular type of loss such as the death of a child or death by suicide. No one can know exactly how you feel, but others who are going through similar experiences can be of great comfort and support. In the case of children, if a child's mood doesn't improve at least some after several months, or if their grief is interfering with their ability to function, I suggest seeking the assistance of a therapist.

Chapter 9

Vivian/Georgia

Interviewed:	**Vivian**
Child:	**Georgia, age 4**
Complaints:	*Fear of abandonment*
	Difficulty falling asleep
	Regressive behavior
	Fear of monsters in her bedroom—crying and screaming
	Behavioral reactions to marital discord and separation
	Oppositional behavior
	Anger

Vivian, please tell me about the problems you mentioned on the phone that you're having with Georgia.

> She's a wonderful girl but she has been having some really bad issues. The big one is going to bed at night. She's always saying, "I don't want to go to sleep, I'm afraid that you'll leave me." And she'll stay up late, she'll get up and say she has to go to the bathroom, she whines—mounds and mounds of excuses to get up, and won't go to sleep at night.

How long has this been going on?

> I'd say it's slowly evolved over the last six months that her behavior has really started to change. And it's gotten to a crisis in the last month or so.

You say it's changed. What were her sleeping patterns like before?

> Georgia was always hard to get to sleep as a baby; we took a lot of time with her. We would hold her and walk with her until she nodded off. We read to her. We spent lots and lots of time with her as a baby. I rocked her in a rocking chair until she was two.

And did all that work?

> Oh yes. It used to work great. She'd be sound asleep in 20 minutes or less.

But that doesn't work anymore?

I wouldn't know. We just don't have the time or energy for it anymore. What with Willow being born and . . . oh, it's a mess. And, now, when she gets up in the morning, she's really whiny and irritable.

What was Georgia like when she got up in the morning before the problems started?

Before she had a sister, she was real bright and happy. She used to get up when she was really little and come into our bedroom and say, "The sun is up," which meant "Mom and Dad, get out of bed, it's time to start life again."

How long does it usually take you to get her into bed now?

Her bedtime is 8:30, and sometimes she's still awake at 10:00.

What's the average amount of time after you put her down to get her to go to sleep?

About an hour.

What are her behaviors like at bedtime?

She'll get up and say she has to go to the bathroom. She'll get up and say there are monsters in her room. She'll start crying and screaming. We'll run in, frantic, saying, "What's going on? What's happening?" and she'll say, "I'm afraid you're going to leave me." And so we talk to her and explain to her that we'd never leave her and ask her if there was some reason she thought we were going to leave her. We really can't figure out if there was one particular instance that may have caused her to feel this way.

Were you having any other problems with her before then?

No. She was always pretty compliant, but she was always the center of attention before.

And now?

Georgia is the first grandchild on both sides, and she's been everybody's little darling since birth. Now, suddenly, this strange little person comes into her life—her sister.

So you think her problems seem to be closely associated with the birth of her sister?

Oh, yes, her sister is at a stage now, she just started walking and talking a little, so everyone's saying, "Oh, what a cute baby, isn't she a darling?" This is a rough period for Georgia. Her sister's a very happy child, and she's getting a lot of attention. But Georgia is used to being the center of our attention. She used to act like she was on stage a lot—we'd call her our "ham bone" because she loved to perform so much.

Great entertainment?

Oh, yes! No batteries required. And we've always been an attentive audience. At least we used to be. But since Willow was born, we've had our hands full. We haven't been able to give Georgia the same sort of undivided attention we used to.

How has her behavior changed as a result?

Georgia has regressed, like mimicking the baby's behavior. Whatever the baby does that gets her attention, Georgia will mimic that. So it's been pretty clear that she feels left out. Before Willow was born, when Jim and I were talking at dinner and Georgia would interrupt, we would stop talking just to hear what she had to say. Now she's almost four and she needs to know that it's important not to interrupt. Plus Dad and I have a lot of things we need to talk about, so she has to be silenced sometimes. And she's not very happy about that. She seems to feel like, *"Maybe I'm not so cute anymore since everyone around me is not paying much attention to me."* A lot of things changed in our home since we had another baby.

What else has changed?

Since I've been on day shift, back from maternity leave, Georgia is with the babysitter more than she has been, and now she has a sister to compete with. Plus my husband and I started having some problems, too. He was actually out of the home for a while. Georgia is very attached to her dad, and it was very hard for her. She just sobbed when her daddy was gone. When he came back, he and I had to work on a lot of issues. We've always been pretty good about not talking about things in front of her, but I'm sure she felt our distress. It was certainly in the air.

Have you talked with her about how all this is affecting her?

I try, but she won't tell me anything. That's part of why I'm here. It's so frustrating being a therapist and feeling like you can't help your own child. I feel like there are things going on with her but when I try to get her to tell me about them, she clams up. So her dad and I are left having to try and guess what's going on with her.

And what guesses have you come up with?

The abandonment issue is really big with her where she is just terrified that we are going to leave her. In her own way, it seems like she is telling us that we have emotionally abandoned her already. We brought in a sister, we're having problems of our own, we're spending less time talking to her, I'm working more, she's at the babysitter more, and she's not getting the quality time and attention that she used to. I think her fear that we would leave her is based on the fact that, in a way, we have already left her during the day.

One day I was angry, and she came up to me and said, "Mom, you're not mad at me, are you?" I said, "No, I'm not mad at you," and I explained to her what had me angry. She seems to feel like she has a responsibility for everything that's going on in the world, including Dad being out of the house.

Kids crave attention, good or bad, which can cause "emotional snowballs" to build and go off in all sorts of directions.

Yeah, she is doing a lot of aggressive things, little things, you know, when she's angry. Like when I get home and play with her she plays rough, and *"accidentally"* kicks me. It's kind of obvious that she's angry with me. And she won't talk about what's bothering her. She is just really angry.

Does she get mad at the baby at all?

She doesn't express much anger at the baby. It's more towards Mom and Dad.

Besides not paying as much attention to her are there other reasons that you think she might be angry with you?

Occasionally, we spank her for not going to bed at night. I think that's just making her angry and not helping at all.

Do you spank her for anything else?

You know, we don't spank her a lot. Occasionally, we spank and, whenever we do, we always feel afterwards that it was not something that was a useful tool with her. It just causes her to have angry feelings. It doesn't work. She responds a lot better to positive reinforcement than to spanking.

What other methods have you tried using to get Georgia to sleep so far?

We started using stickers with her. We gave her a calendar and we bought some cute little stickers and we called it a bedtime calendar. We explained to her what she needed to do to earn a sticker.

And what did she earn with her stickers?

Initially, it was just stickers. And that was great. We were a little weak with it though. We found ourselves giving in to her. She's got us pretty well manipulated. And we would give her a sticker anyway, and then we realized we weren't doing her any favors with that.

It's natural to want to make your child feel good, but that's not always what's best for them.

Yeah. So we finally made it a little more stringent, and made it clear what she needed to do for her stickers. And then we added in that if she got 12 out of 14 stickers in two weeks she would get an outing with her dad.

Something special.

Yes, a one-to-one thing without her little sister.

Did the stickers help?

They seemed to help with her compliance; not so much with her attitude and feelings.

Was it helpful for getting her to sleep?

Not really.

Well, it was a good idea to try the stickers, which can be effective for some children, but they just weren't particularly effective for her.

She was in bed, she was compliant, but she wasn't happy.

Let's talk a little more about spanking.

It bothers us to spank her and we do it out of frustration. And you do see that it does great harm. You're angry, you've hurt them; it violates a trust between parent and child. Kids just don't buy the line, "We're doing this for your own good." They interpret it as angry feelings. It puts space between parent and child. In essence you're saying, "I'm going to force you to do something you don't want to do," instead of a loving approach saying, "This is something you need to do; it's important for you to do it." That kind of attitude, instead of, "I'm your parent and I'm a lot bigger than you are, and I'm going to force you to do this whether you like it or not, and I don't care about your feelings."

And that, to me, is what spanking says to a child and what forceful kinds of actions do. You take choice away from them. You humiliate them and take away the option of them complying on their own. We were at a point with her that we were so frustrated with what was going on that we just wanted to beat this kid and throw her in bed. It was a feeling of total frustration. We've got this kid that doesn't want to do what we want her to do. She's obviously manipulative; she's obviously doing things on purpose. We know something is going on with her, but we can't figure out what the hell it is. She, by her behavior, is obviously telling us something, but we can't really put our finger on what has triggered what is going on.

So you know there are some obvious issues, like Dad being out of the house, but you don't know for sure what is causing her behavior?

We never know whether we're reading something more into it or if it's maybe something so small we aren't aware of it. Our feeling is that it isn't something small, but something is genuinely going on with her. She has a lot of issues to deal with for a three-and-a-half-year-old; she has to go to the baby sitter, Dad was out of house, Mom and Dad are both working. And we aren't focusing the majority of our attention on her during the week. So there is a lot for her to deal with and feel angry about. What'll we do with this kid? She won't go to bed, she won't do what we ask her to do, and she's got a smart mouth. And you end up smacking them. But it just doesn't work.

It's important to keep the perspective that you can be unhappy with her behavior, but still love her.

Love her to death! We say, "We love you very much and we will always love you," but that's a hard one for her to understand. And that's such a big issue. We tried to explain to her, "You didn't get a sticker because of your behavior, not because you are a bad person." It's really a hard concept for children, but a really important one for them to learn. If she doesn't get it she might go on thinking her behavior makes her a bad person.

She might think that if she doesn't live up to others' expectations or, for that matter, her own, she's bad.

> When you feel like your kid is out of control, the parent is out of control, too, because the parent is feeling like, "*What the heck am I going to do now? I've tried sweet-talking her, I've tried manipulating her, I've tried tricking her, I've tried bribing her, I've tried beating her . . . and nothing is working.*"

You start to feel like you're failing as a parent.

> Yeah. Feeling like, "*This problem is uncontrollable and what am I going to do?*" The kid has nothing to count on when they don't have that security of "If I do this, I can expect that to happen."

Well, thank you for sharing what's going on. I'm sure a lot of parents could relate to your frustrations.

> We're letting her manipulate the heck out of us, on the one hand, and then being unrealistic with our demands, on the other. We're trying to force things. "You're going to do it, like it or not." I'm not saying that there'll never be times that I don't have to put my foot down because she's kicking and screaming.

Yeah, dealing effectively with the overflow of emotion is an important parenting skill. It's really unhealthy when you require kids to cut themselves off from their feelings and their emotions; and their expression needs to be allowed, up to a point.

> Yeah, and we do. We tell her we understand how she is feeling, but we ask her to go into the other room to kick and scream. "We know you're upset although we'd rather not listen to that right now, but you're free to do it. You're welcome to go kick and scream down the hall."

※ • ※

After Vivian and I spoke some more, I gave her the *Magic Carpet* and *Playhouse on the Beach* CDs to try with Georgia. Several weeks later, she returned and reported on her findings.

※ • ※

How long has Georgia been using the **Magic Carpet** *program?*

> For about two weeks now. That and *Playhouse on the Beach*.

And have you noticed any effects?

> She's started sleeping better.

That's wonderful. I'm so happy to hear it. Has it had any effect on her behavior?

> Her behavior has changed a lot; she's much happier.

What's going to bed like now?

It's much smoother now. She happily goes to bed. There is not the resistance, there's not the angry feelings coming up, there's not the emotionality, that's all gone now. It's much more like the way she used to go to bed, very happily, "Goodnight, I love you." I guess she's feeling much more secure. She's into a routine of saying, "Good night. Can I listen to the program?" She listens to it every night. Initially she could stay awake when she listened. When the talking stopped she'd be up and say, "It's over now, you can have it back." More recently she's begun to fall asleep with it on. One night, I went in to speak to her and in taking the headphones off she started crying and said, "No, it's not over, don't take it Mom." So I reassured her and gave it back and moments later she was out.

How long does she average before going to sleep?

She's usually falling asleep within 20 minutes or so.

If she does take the headphones off before it's over, does she go to sleep right afterwards?

Yeah, she's not staying awake. She's falling asleep right away. If she brings us the player she's tired, she's droopy eyed, she's going right back to bed and going to sleep.

What is she like when she gets up in the morning now?

When she wakes up in the morning, she's delighted. She comes up and says, "Do I get my sticker?" And she's smiling and she's happy. Now it's that same kind of joyful attitude as before the problems started.

What about during the day?

Yeah, yeah. Much more compliant and much happier. And I think we are more willing to give out positive strokes to her, so it's just been a more positive attitude all the way around.

How about her manipulative behavior? Has that changed at all?

It sure has. She no longer tries to manipulate us like she was doing before. That has all stopped. We've done a lot of talking with her about what manipulation is, what tricking people is, and that it's better just to tell us what she wants. We'd say, "Don't try to manipulate us out of something, because that's kind of like lying." So she'll occasionally ask, "Is this manipulation?"

How has her anger been lately?

The last week or so she's been less angry.

And has she been talking about her feelings?

Yeah. She's finally telling me about what's going on at the babysitter. She hasn't been happy there, and she'd say, "Mom, I didn't like it there today. I wish all those kids would stop beating on me." And I felt so bad. "What's happening?" "Well, so-and-so hit me because of this, and this other kid was mean to me." Suddenly she seems to feel that it's okay to tell me what's happening with her.

Do you feel, generally, that she's verbalizing her feelings better?

Yeah, she is. She's talking about things more than she used to. In the past, she wouldn't even tell me what happened at the babysitter that day. She'd be angry, but she wouldn't talk about it. But she's finally starting to talk about things now. And she's made it clear that she's just not happy at the sitter's. She's not getting along with some of the kids there and she normally gets along with children, so it's not working well, and she's talking about that more now, so we're working on getting some kind of resolution there.

We've been trying to explain to her that if somebody hits her, she doesn't have to take it. She shouldn't hit anybody else, but it's good to talk about it. It's okay to say, "Hey, I don't like it when you treat me that way." And so we're talking about it, and we may eventually end up taking her out from the sitter, if it doesn't get better soon. But, we're going to give her a chance to work things out with our help.

Have you seen any change regarding her abandonment fears?

Yes. Generally, she's much less fearful. So we've been trying to talk with her, give her more individual, quality time, and reassure her that we love her and will always take care of her. And she's getting more positive. We're really trying to get away from the negative stuff with her, because that just seems to snowball in a direction we don't want to go. The CD has been really helpful—it's part of our more positive approach, and she's feeling much better about herself.

And what has happened with the spanking lately?

Well, when you put in the positive stuff, we've seen with Georgia that she really wants to work to get that special outing with Dad. She really wants to do it, not just to get something, but because she wants to please us. She wants to be compliant, and she wants to make us happy. She's at an age where she's very susceptible to guilt and shame about all sorts of things. She truly feels bad when she doesn't please us, and by spanking her we cause her to feel guilty. So we're much happier when we can get her to do what we want in a positive way.

There's just such a difference in her and the way she feels about herself. It's been extremely dramatic. She's delighted that we're pleased with her and we're now responding to her better. I think her feeling abandoned really heightened everything. And of course she felt abandoned when her parents were doing something hostile to her. How else is a child supposed to interpret an assault like spanking? But sometimes you get so frustrated you don't act rationally.

It's all part of being a parent, isn't it?

Right.

Can we continue this later?

Sure.

Two Weeks Later

Well it's been a couple weeks now since we last talked about Georgia.

Yeah. And she is still doing well. She's still my wonderful kid again. Behaviorally, she's a lot nicer to deal with. We've set more limits with her, but the limits are more loving.

When you say the limits you are setting are more loving, are you saying that your reaction to her is different now?

Oh, sure.

So things are still moving in a more positive direction?

Yes. Now she's expressing her feelings, but they're not so hostile. Even if she gets a little mad she's better at following directions and we're more loving, because we're not so frustrated. And we, as parents, are saying, "This is not a monster, this is a three-and-a-half-year-old, and though we are bigger than her, that doesn't mean we have a right to push her around." The whole atmosphere is changing. It's turned into a much more positive situation.

She's had two special outings, since we started her sticker thing around going to bed. She's had some days when she didn't get a sticker and she really took that well. We've been working on trying to separate her behavior from who she is. Like many children, it's hard for her to see the difference between her behavior and who she is. It's easy for children to feel like, *"I'm a bad girl because I did something bad,"* not, *"I did something wrong, but that doesn't mean I'm a bad person."*

That same concept is a real challenge for parents, too.

Yeah, and that's our focus right now with her and I think she's starting to understand. But if she's feeling bad about herself, listening to the program seems to help. She listens to it every night. She asks for it and she loves it. And then she's just easier to deal with. She's easier to reason with, just nicer and much more pleasant. I'm really enjoying her a lot more.

If you were to put your enjoyment on a scale of 1 to 10, where were you before she used the programs and where are you now?

I was probably rating a 3, and now I'm a 9 or 10. I think a parent, as well as a kid, often doesn't separate the child from the behavior that you don't like. And it's easy to forget how much you really love your child. You always love your kid, whether they're going to bed at night or not. It's easy to label a kid as bad, and make black-and-white judgments when you're really frustrated. It's much easier for me to differentiate now instead of feeling like, *"I'm just going to write this kid off because she's such a pain in the ass."*

Easier to keep your whole child in mind?

> Oh yeah, and to remember she's just three and a half, and it's really hard for her verbalize what's going on. But she's a heck of a lot more open now. She's more grounded. That's the best way to describe it.

So you're saying you have continued to see more positive changes?

> She has made progress in other areas, but more subtle than what we saw initially. The immediate response we noticed was that she was more cooperative. The power struggle was eased between us and she was more willing and happier to go along with things and she has maintained her cooperativeness. But now, as far as working with feelings, a little something will come up here or there, and she'll reveal something that's important. She talked last week about how she felt at the babysitter when this child wouldn't play with her.

So, she seems to be expressing her feelings more openly?

> Oh yeah, she's much more able talk about them.

Is this something new for her? Of course, she's so young, just developmentally she may be hitting that point.

> She seems to be getting in touch with what her feelings are. And we've always encouraged that, but being able to verbalize it is a first for her.

That's interesting in a sense because the programs talk about feelings quite a bit, but really only positive feelings.

> And she's now able to share her negative feelings, too.

What about her expression of positive feelings?

> Oh, yeah. Earlier we had talked about how she's rough with her play. And now she's been much gentler and saying things like, "Mom, I need a hug, can I sit on your lap for a while?" which is what she was like before all this started happening. She's more open and loving.

A little clearer about what she needs in terms of how she's feeling and asking for it?

> Absolutely.

And you said she's happier, too?

> Sure, she's happier. And so am I. The little girl I love is back again.

Thank you for sharing your story.

> You're welcome.

SPANKING

At their wit's end with their unruly daughter, Georgia, and her mounting problems, Vivian and her husband, Jim, resorted to spanking Georgia in an attempt to gain some compliance. Each time afterward, they would feel guilty and wonder if their actions might have any negative effects on their daughter. The answer is, it appears, almost certainly, "Yes."

TEACHING BY EXAMPLE: YOU'RE THE MODEL

Few people would deny that parents are their children's primary models for acceptable behavior. Everything gets modeled: "This is how you hold a baby." "This is how you hold a football." "This is how you wash your hands." "This is how you wash a car." "This is how you hit a baseball." "This is how you hit your sister." *What's that?*—you ask. *How you hit your sister? I would never say that!*
No doubt you wouldn't. Not in words, at least. But if you spank little sister, that is exactly what you are modeling. You can say, "Do as I say, not as I do," until you're blue in the face, but that's hardly ever how it works out. Children will almost always do as their parents do, *not* as their parents say.

WHAT SPANKING TEACHES

By spanking, parents unintentionally teach a number of problematic behaviors at once. They teach that it is okay to control another person's unwanted behavior by using force and inflicting pain. They teach that it is okay to strike out when you are frustrated. And they teach that it is okay to accomplish what you want with violence toward others.

A BRIEF HISTORY OF SPANKING

In earlier generations, spanking a child was commonplace, and considered a natural part of responsible parenting with many subscribing to the belief, *"Spare the rod and spoil the child."* This phrase is often incorrectly attributed to the Christian Bible, but it first appeared in a poem by Samuel Butler in 1664. In more recent times we've seen a widespread shift in attitude, primarily because of our more informed awareness of the long-term consequences of our actions towards children.

A CAVEAT ON SPANKING AND CHILD ABUSE

Before we go too much farther, just to dispel any myths or alleviate any misgivings about the material to follow, I need to emphasize that by no means is *all* spanking child abuse. That is simply absurd! Each incidence of spanking varies in frequency, intensity, and circumstance. Nonetheless, one cannot ignore the definitive, and largely concordant, conclusions reached in the abundant research on the subject of spanking.

IS SPANKING EFFECTIVE?

In his book, *Beating the Devil Out of Them: Corporal Punishment in American Families and Its Effect on Children*, University of New Hampshire sociology professor Murray A. Strauss writes that corporal punishment is not as effective a form of punishment or behavior modification as the alternative methods—like time-outs, verbal corrections, and logical consequences; in fact, he writes, corporal punishment produces dangerous side effects that may include depression, domestic abuse, and juvenile delinquency. One of Strauss' contemporaries, psychologist H. Stephen Glenn, takes it even further, asserting that corporal punishment is the least effective of all forms of discipline in that it "reinforces a failure identity." What's more, he points out, compliance resulting from spanking is typically short-lived.

Hitting versus Discipline

Dawn Walker, of Canada's Institute of Child Health, draws a distinction between discipline and hitting, asserting that while hitting may be detrimental, discipline is a necessary part of responsible, proactive, and effective child-rearing. This can be incredibly helpful to parents worried that, without spanking, their child might get "out of control" or who believe that the sole alternative to spanking a child is imposing no discipline whatsoever.

Potential Consequences in Adulthood

In his book, Strauss cites a study which found that people who were spanked as children have greater difficulty with interpersonal relationships and a greater likelihood of antisocial behavior than those who weren't spanked as children. And one among many consequences of these two traits, he notes, is difficulty obtaining and maintaining decent employment. In the shorter term, these effects might show up as problems with academic performance. According to Straus, "Not all children who are spanked will develop negative social behaviors, just as not all heavy smokers will develop lung cancer."

But that in no way discounts the exhaustive evidence that there are indeed significant potential long-term negative consequences of spanking children, not least of which is that spanking can teach children, especially boys, to rely on physical aggression to solve the problems they face, promote lower self-esteem, poorer interpersonal skills, and depression, and condition them, especially girls, toward immediate, unquestioning obedience to any domineering force.

Ms. Walker also comments, "We know that children who are under the threat of violence or aggression develop a fight-or-flight response system that has an impact on creativity and imagination, both of which could influence their IQ."

Anti-spanking advocate John Benjamin Guthrow (1994, United States Department of Education, *Elementary and Secondary School Civil Rights Compliance Report*) found that the ten states listed as having the greatest incidence of corporal punishment in their schools also had disproportionately higher murder, incarceration, and poverty rates, as well as poorer overall physical and mental health of their citizenry and fewer of their students acquiring high school diplomas than did students in the rest of the country.

Spanking's Sexual Component

A 2001 survey of developmental experts that revealed spanking in childhood leads to problems in adult life also revealed that women, in particular, who were spanked as girls tended to continue to experience violence in their adult lives. An increasing number of experts agree that boys spanked as children are more likely to depend on violence as a means to certain ends, whereas girls who were spanked as children have a propensity to accept and submit to violence.

This brings up the question of a possible sexual component of spanking. Anatomically, the nerve endings that travel to the genitalia also travel to the buttocks, giving any action done to one area definite implications for the other. Striking the buttocks with the intention to cause pain—especially when done by a male authority figure, parent or otherwise—can lead girls to form negative associations about their genitalia.

POTENTIAL PHYSICAL DAMAGE

Perhaps even more frightening, and too-infrequently discussed, spanking can potentially cause unexpected long-term physical harm as well. Boxing the ears can burst an eardrum. Shaking can cause concussions, whiplash, brain damage, blindness, and even death. Smacking the buttocks can injure the tailbone, pelvis, sciatic nerve, and spine. Even smacking a child's hands can cause physical damage (some irreparable), including burst blood vessels, broken bones, torn joints and ligaments, and early onset of osteoarthritis. Not to mention that when a child is hit, he could accidentally fall down and suffer all sorts of injuries.

IS IT TOO LATE TO CHANGE?

Now, all this may convince some parents who've already spanked their children that it's too late, the damage is done and there is nothing they can do now to "fix it." Nothing, however, could be further from the truth.

When you change your behavior and the relational dynamics between you and your child, you change his view of the world—plain and simple. It's never too late to give a child a new and improved perspective on the world. As reported in the *Canadian Medical Association Journal* in 1995, "There appears to be a linear association between the frequency of slapping and spanking during childhood and a lifetime prevalence of anxiety disorder, alcohol abuse or dependence and externalizing problems." Ceasing to spank your child now and shifting towards more proactive disciplinary methods will go leaps and bounds towards healing any wounds you feel you may have caused, and conditioning your child to have a more positive and healthy attitude about life.

WHAT THE U.N. CONVENTION ON THE RIGHTS OF THE CHILD SAYS

Article 19 of the United Nations Convention on the Rights of the Child (signed by every federal government belonging to the UN . . . except the United States), states:

> Parties shall take all appropriate legislative, administrative, social and education measures to protect the child from all forms of physical or mental violence, injury or abuse, neglect or negligent treatment, maltreatment or exploitation, including sexual abuse, while in the care of parent(s), legal guardian(s) or any other person who has the care of the child.

A BETTER WAY?

Quite possibly the best conclusion parents can reach from all this evidence is that, when they think, "There's got to be a better way than this"—'*this*' being spanking as a means of modifying their child's behavior—they are absolutely right.

CHAPTER 10

LIA/ANA

Interviewed:	Lia
Child:	Ana, age 10
Complaints:	*Difficulty falling asleep*
	Overexcitement
	Oppositional behavior
	Bedwetting
	Low self-esteem
	Anger
	Unhappiness
	Crankiness, especially in the morning
	Restless sleep
	Temper tantrums, often lasting hours
	Demanding behavior
	Obesity
	Frequent stealing

❧ • ☙

Lia, *please tell me, what are Ana's sleep problems?*

Going to sleep, she's overexcited, wants to stay awake, lots of requests, you know, those kinds of things.

Okay. What's the average time it takes for her fall asleep?

Between 30 minutes and an hour-and-a-half.

From the time you get her in bed until she falls asleep?

From her bedtime—her bedtime is 8:30. Until about six months ago she would usually be asleep in 30 minutes. But lately it's been around an hour and a half.

What are bedtimes like?

I have at least been able to get her into bed on time, but she plays around, dawdles, and then tries to sneak in some television watching. She plays, you know, and just does all kinds of things to keep from going to sleep.

How is she sleeping at night once she gets to sleep?

She is sleeping very restlessly. She's all over the bed, starting at one end at night, and in the morning she's at the other end. The covers are all messed up. I have to remake the bed every day. She also has a bedwetting problem.

Have you been doing anything for that?

We have her on Tofranil, 25 mg, at bedtime for her bedwetting.

What's the longest time she's gone in the past without medicine that she didn't wet?

Only one night.

One night is all she's ever gone?

Yeah. Maybe once in a while it's been two nights, but that would be the maximum. I don't remember for sure if there was ever two nights, but I don't think so.

Does she usually wet her bed once at night or more often than that?

Well, we change her and change the sheets, but if it happens more than once, we often get lazy and put a towel under her and move her to the other side of the bed.

Does she frequently wet more than once?

Yes, often. In the hospital they were keeping records of how many times she would wet during the night, and it was usually five, six, or seven times.

Really?

She would go minimal amounts, but they were keeping exact records. That's how I know. My husband has told me that he changes her, puts her back to bed, wakes up a little later and gets her to the bathroom, and she is already wet again. That happens pretty often.

After she wets herself and is uncomfortable, does she wake you up to change her?

No. She doesn't wake us up. She never wakes us up. We go in there and find out, but sometimes she'll pull the sheets off the bed herself.

Do you set an alarm? I mean, how do you deal with that?

Whenever we wake up in the middle of the night, we check on her. We have it down to a routine where we are waking up every morning at 2:00 just to get her up. We set alarms in the beginning, but we've been doing it so long, it's just become second nature. Now, I always wake up around 2:00 in the morning.

What is she like in the morning?

Well, our home is by the beach, so it's very cold in the morning. She wakes up ice cold. I guess that's probably how our little morning routine got started.

And what is that?

Every morning she comes into my room and we cuddle together before we start the day. But then, as soon as she gets out of bed she becomes a little terror. She's usually very oppositional, especially in the morning. She is cranky, nasty—you'd have to be a saint not to fight with her.

So in addition to her sleep problems, she has some behavior problems as well?

Where do I start? There's so much. At the school she is in, she is classified as an SED kid, *seriously emotionally disturbed*. And she is in the most structured school environment they have. I think it all stems from the fact that she has excessively low self-esteem; she's a very angry, unhappy little girl. Ana was hospitalized recently for approximately two and a half months. She was hospitalized for self-destructive kinds of behavior . . . temper tantrums so out of control that they could not be stopped for hours at a time. When she was released from the hospital, her out-of-control behavior was much better but still not what I'd consider normal or healthy.

Has she been going to any follow-up therapy since then?

Oh yes, every week.

Does she mind having to go?

She doesn't have any control over that. She does much better in therapy when Frank and I are not there.

Does she mind going to those sessions?

When we're there, she doesn't like it because we're talking about the things she's done wrong and she doesn't want to hear it. When she's going alone she's more willing. The therapy is pretty unstructured, so she gets to do play therapy and they do artwork. Ana just loves to be involved in anything that she can do herself.

She likes doing things independently. She doesn't want me to choose what she's going to wear. She doesn't want me dressing her. She doesn't want me making her breakfast; she wants to make it herself, which is a problem because of how she eats.

Oh, and how does she eat?

Non-stop.

Is she overweight?

She would be considered obese. She is about 30 pounds overweight. She's nine years old and weighs about 100 pounds.

That must be tough for her.

Chapter 10   Lia / Ana

Oh yes, children pick on her, say things that make her cry, call her fat. Things like that have been very, very hurtful to her.

Have you ever tried to encourage her to limit her eating?

We've been doing that since day one, since she started getting overweight. She started having a problem about the time she was a year and a half old, when she was able to get into things and get food for herself. We tried to stop it. Our kitchen is now to the point where there is no food in it. It is bought on a daily basis, so there's nothing extra for Ana to get into. She has never been motivated and never wanted to comply with a diet. She is always sneaking food, going off with a friend, buying candy, or even stealing it.

Really?

Oh, let me tell you about her "shopping trip" to the mall.

Please do.

She came home from Galleria North with two shopping bags full of merchandise. We totaled up the tags and it was over $500. I mean two huge bags!

So how long has she been stealing?

She has been "light fingered" forever—even as a small child in preschool. When she saw something she wanted, she picked it up and walked off with it.

Other children's things?

It doesn't matter. And she always tears them apart to see how they work.

So this is a problem in her daycare?

She's had this problem in every environment she's ever been in.

❦ • ❧

After Lia and I talked a while more, I gave her the *Magic Carpet* CD to try using with Ana. We met again in two weeks to discuss their experiences.

❦ • ❧

You received a children's program recently.

Yes, *Magic Carpet*, two weeks ago. I started my daughter on it the first night. She was very excited that she would get to listen to the program and go to sleep with her headphones on.

Special treat?

Yeah, very special. She stayed awake through the first listening. But by the middle of the second listening, she was asleep, so it was still earlier than normal for her. I didn't notice any major difference in her daytime behavior the first two or three days. What I did notice was she'd ask me every night, "Can I have the CD to go to sleep, Mommy?" Over the weekend she shared it with every little friend she could drag into the house.

How long would it take her to go to sleep?

By the second night, she never made it through the first listening. In fact, last night she didn't make it through five minutes.

Have you noticed anything else?

We are having other changes as well.

Okay. Please describe them.

We stopped the Tofranil four nights ago and she hasn't wet yet. This has not been the pattern in the past. We've gone through about six trials off medication, and within two days of stopping the medication she has always wet again. She has done that and it's been four days, now, that she's been dry.

That's excellent. I'm so happy to hear it. Anything else?

Oh, yes! A big change is that her oppositional behavior, in particular, has improved. For the last nine days she has not awakened cranky. She has been more pleasant; we've got a decrease in intensity and duration of outbursts, of oppositional kinds of behaviors. She's just a nicer kid. She's calmer. She's happier. She's not a normal child altogether, but we do see a very significant decrease in this type of behavior. She's just a nicer kid to be with.

I mean, she's not—she hasn't completely reversed. I mean, it's not a major, major change, but it's certainly enough for me to notice, and it's enough for me to note because I do a behavior chart on her every day for her therapist. I've shared *Magic Carpet* with her therapist, and she thinks it's the greatest thing since peanut butter. She would also like to use it. I advised her to get in touch with you because it's your stuff. Anyway, her therapist really likes it.

Very interesting.

And I'm overjoyed. Absolutely overjoyed!

And what does this mean for you?

I wake up happy in the morning.

Have you been listening to the program?

Not since that first time. I listened to it with her the first night. You know, last night was the first time I had to remind her listen to it so it might be losing some of its novelty now.

Well, I'm giving you **Playhouse on the Beach** *today so she'll have a little variety.*

Great, I'll start *Playhouse* tonight. But, like I said, it's not a miracle, it's not a huge change, but it certainly is a significant one. We intend to continue using it.

How about the restlessness in bed? Have you noticed any difference in how the bedding appears in the morning?

It's no longer all messed up.

So she's sleeping differently?

She's less restless and sleeping more deeply, which is why I think she's being friendlier in the morning.

So is her daytime mood different now?

Yes. For example, when she came out of that two-and-a-half-month stint in the hospital I told you about, she was somewhat better, but not nearly as happy and calm as she is now. And she still needs to get calmer, but she didn't return from the hospital as contented as she appears now, after listening to *Magic Carpet* for two weeks.

I would like some continuing progress reports.

No problem. I'll be happy to give them to you.

Thank you.

ಜ • ಜ

ONE WEEK LATER

ಜ • ಜ

Okay, another week has passed.

Yes, I've had *Magic Carpet* for two weeks, and *Playhouse on the Beach* for one week, so we've got a total time of three weeks.

Tell me what has changed.

We're basically seeing the same changes, but to a greater degree. They're getting more positive. There was an incident this week, which a short time ago would have destroyed her. Her one and only friend in the neighborhood is moving away and Ana responded appropriately. She was very tearful, very upset, feeling like she was being rejected. What normally would have happened is it would have turned into anger, and that would have been taken out on every person in her life for an extended period of time.

How long would that kind of incident have triggered behavioral problems before?

Sometimes it went on for days, sometimes it went on for weeks before we figured out what it was that she was angry about and we intervened. And sometimes with Ana, it was very subtle, those things she'd be angry about, and sometimes it would take us a long time to figure out what they were.

And this time you felt it was different?

Yeah. To give you an example, Ana thought this same friend was moving three months ago. She became inconsolable. There was no talking to her for a week and a half. She would cry, she would yell, she wouldn't respond appropriately. You couldn't engage her in a normal conversation. She was very oppositional, very angry, and very sad. That went on for 11 days.

So she didn't think her friend was going to move, but then she found out her friend really was moving after all. And then what happened?

Ana was told that she was going to move. Then the family decided to move out of state. Before she was just moving to a different city, which was close by. Now they're moving to a different state, so she'll definitely be gone and Ana won't even be able to visit her. Ana came home very tearful, tears running down her face, crying so hard she was hiccupping, telling me that her best friend was moving away and she was never coming back and she would never have a best friend again, and she'd be all alone.

We did a lot of comforting and soothing, and I spent about 45 minutes with her just talking to her calmly, which she listened to this time. And after consoling her and telling her I understood why she felt so bad, I was able to take her mind off of it and engage her in a game that we got involved in playing. Last time that would never have worked. Not only did she have a shorter duration of hysteria, it was much less intense. Maybe a maximum of an hour and a half, and no tantrums since. There's been some sadness. "I'm sorry Deanne's going away, I feel sad because she's going." But that's the extent of it. It didn't go beyond that into all the anger and acting out. And for me, that's like a different child.

How many days has it been since she found out?

It's happened on Sunday morning and this is now Thursday, and I've spoken about it with her every night. She would be looking sad and I would say something like, "You're sad because Deanne is moving away now, aren't you?" And she'd say, "Yes, Mommy, I am," and that would pretty much take care of it.

Are you and she still sharing the morning cuddling ritual together?

Yes, and I'm glad you asked, because that's changed significantly, too. Now, when we're done cuddling, she gets out of bed, smiling, and offers to make toast for me or something. She's very nice now, most of the time. This nice little girl is who we see the majority of the time, as opposed to rarely, which was before.

Last week you said you weren't willing to call the changes major.

Now I am. That's what I was just going to tell you. I would qualify this as a major change in behavior for her. I have acquainted her therapist with the programs; she is just as excited as can be. Because all the work we have been doing with therapy, trying to do behavior modification and all of that, had some effect, but not as dramatic as this has had. Now I don't know if it will hold, but it certainly is there. Time will tell.

But it did withstand the first challenge.

It certainly did. Brilliantly! I mean, my stomach didn't hurt all day. I usually get an attack of ulcers when Ana goes through something like that. Now, I mean, we're *all* feeling a lot better. As I told you about the programs, she really likes them; one day will be *Magic Carpet*, and one day will be *Playhouse on the Beach*.

She seems to stay awake longer when listening to *Playhouse* than she does with *Magic Carpet*. She may get through most of the CD before she goes to sleep. At least, when I monitored her the last couple nights that's what happened. Last night was not fair because we have broken headphones and she couldn't listen to it. She was quite upset. We're getting a new headset tonight.

How long did it take her go to sleep without being able listen?

I put her to bed at 8:30. I went to sleep about 9:15. About 9:10, I could still hear her in there playing. The last time I yelled at her to go to sleep was at 9:10. So she didn't go to sleep as quickly without the program.

What's it like at bedtime now? Do you still have to struggle with her to get her to go to bed?

Nope. Since she started listening, we don't see that happening anymore. She goes right to bed, puts on her headphones, fiddles around until she gets everything just right and then I can kiss her goodnight. She really likes the fact that she's in charge of listening to the program.

Okay. What about the bedwetting? What has happened with that?

She's not wetting. She's been off medication for 18 days now. And we've had no occurrence of bedwetting, and that's the first time this has ever happened.

Indeed. Until now you'd said she could only go one day without the medication before wetting the bed.

Exactly.

Has she said anything about it?

She hasn't talked about it specifically. She's more self-confident now. Perhaps she's feeling more in control of herself and that's translating into better self-esteem. She's just so much happier now and it's so much easier not having to deal with the bedwetting.

She probably feels better not having to sleep in a wet bed.

Exactly. She's not waking up all yucky and cold, you know, and smelling bad, and being all chilly.

That's probably about it for this week. Can we continue this later?

Yes.

Thank you very much.

THREE WEEKS LATER

It's now been about three weeks since we last talked. How is Ana doing?

Ana is remaining stable. We've had a couple of incidents. Last night she had an episode of bedwetting after some severe anxiety over the welfare of her brother.

What happened?

He was supposed to come back to us by plane from South Carolina. We waited all day long and all night long. He never showed up. She was aware that he was supposed to come, so she had a rough night.

Was that the first time she had bed wet recently?

Since she started listing to the programs six weeks ago. A new change in Ana is she is now self-motivated to start a diet, which she started two days ago. She is being very methodical about it, incorporating all of her friends into it—a double support system.

Has she ever been on a diet before?

No, never wanted to. Never was interested in it. The stimulus for dieting isn't new. It's been there forever, but it never motivated her to do anything about it.

It sounds like she's finally developing some internal control.

Yeah. She's still a disturbed child, but she's coming along well.

Have there been any changes in her stealing?

As a matter of fact, I'm getting reports from her daycare that she's much easier to manage, including the fact that the incidence of stealing is down.

Down? What does that mean exactly?

She's not doing it anymore. We used to check all of her belongings before she left home in the morning to make sure she didn't take something to school that she wasn't supposed to. And we'd check her belongings before we brought her home to make sure she wasn't bringing something home.

When did that change? Since she's been listening to the programs?

We had one incident, the first week. The big stealing thing happened about a week and a half before we started the programs. And we had one after that, about a week into it. We had instituted some behavioral consequences for that. She had to write a letter of apology, take it to the person she stole from, and apologize to the person.

Did she ever have to do that in the past?

Not all of that. We increased that consequence, because she had to write a letter to the individual *and* at the same time go and apologize to the person.

So that may have had some bearing on it, too, but she's also not taking things in the house?

Not taking things from me anymore. She was *"light-fingered Louie"* for my makeup and things like that. She doesn't even do that anymore. She asks now.

Any other changes reported at her daycare?

They are reporting that she's a happier little girl, easier to manage. They feel that they can control her better than they ever could before. They don't know about the programs so they are attributing it all to what wonderful therapy she is getting. I doubt they'd even believe it if I told them it's your programs, so I haven't. And we're thinking about pulling her out of there because she's doing so much better. She's leaps and bounds above the other kids now. I think her teacher is only hanging on to her because she likes her now.

Has this change happened over a long period of time or just recently?

Some of these changes have been happening for a while, but they were pretty subtle. We didn't see the rapid movement in them, the dramatic differences, until she started listening to the CDs. Her therapist can verify that.

Okay. Thank you very much for the update. Can we continue this later?

Anytime you want. No problem.

ॐ • ॐ

ONE WEEK LATER

ॐ • ॐ

It's been another week now since we discussed Ana. How is she doing?

Okay. The first thing I want to share with you is that this morning, before I left for work, Ana asked me, "Are you going to see Dr. Tom?" And I told her yes, I was going to see you, and she wanted me to give you a message: "Thank you for making me a good girl." She really said that.

Wow!

It made me tear up, too. Of course, I gave her all the credit. I gave it back to her. You know, "The CDs have helped you Ana, but you are the one who has done it. They only helped." I, of course, want to build her self-esteem.

She's seeing herself in a different light.

She's giving you credit for it right now, but I'm trying to get it so that she takes at least some of the credit.

She's now viewing herself as a good girl. I imagine that's quite different for her.

Yes, she's always been "a bad girl" and now she's "a good girl." Even when she's angry or hollers she knows she's a good girl.

That's wonderful.

Yes it is. And here's something that's interesting. Her CD player broke about five days ago. She has not been able to listen, and we have seen the same good behavior. There's been no regression to past behavior. And the bedwetting is still stable with no medication at all. She's bitching, of course; she wants her CD player back, and we'll have it back for her probably tonight or tomorrow.

Is she still going to sleep okay?

She's still going to sleep fine. No mood problems. I've learned with Ana—I'm able to understand her better now—when she gets upset about something. For example, she came last night and told me she didn't want to take a bath at her regular time. She argued with me; that wasn't what she was upset about though. She was upset because I had tripped outside the house and I'd fallen and skinned my knee, and that's what I guessed she was really upset about. So I was able to talk to her about it. I said, "Ana, I know you're not upset about your bath, and I know you're not angry with me, and I know you're not angry with Daddy. I think you're upset because Mommy got hurt." And she looked at me, and tears welled up and she said, "Yes, Mommy, that's it." I was able to talk to her about it, and she went in and took her bath five minutes later.

On her own?

On her own.

So, you're gaining in your insights?

She's a little less complicated to understand now, because there's less going on. It's now easier to have a clear picture of what's happening with her.

You have a chance to keep up with her.

Absolutely.

So it was just too overwhelming in the past to understand her behaviors?

We were dealing with problem behaviors all the time. They weren't specific to a time frame. Now, when she's upset, it is in reaction to something that just happened, so it gives us a chance to figure out what it is that is bothering her. She's still not able to identify exactly what she's upset about, we have to help her with that, but it's not so chaotic that we can't see what's going on. So it's now much easier to help her. I would consider her much more like a normal 9-year-old now.

Have the changes you have seen simply held or do you feel there have been any further improvements?

They've not only held; they've increased further. Now they're holding even when she doesn't listen to the programs, which I think is a big step.

Well, this is truly exciting.

I want to thank you for not only making Ana a good girl, but a much happier girl.

You are more than welcome, and thank you for all of the wonderful feedback.

It's been my pleasure.

∽ • ∾

CHILDHOOD OBESITY

Ana experienced many unexpected benefits from her program use, but I thought the weight issue was of particular interest, especially in the light of the current epidemic of obesity in children. This issue, perhaps more than any other, may negatively impact the future health of a whole generation. Being an overweight child can create a number of health problems, including ones that were once confined to adults, such as diabetes, high blood pressure, and high cholesterol.

STATISTICS ON CHILDHOOD OBESITY TODAY

In just the last two decades, the incidence of being overweight doubled for children ages six to eleven, and tripled for American teenagers. A recent *National Health and Nutrition Examination Survey* conducted by the Centers for Disease Control and Prevention found that about one-third of the children in the U.S. are overweight or at risk of becoming overweight; in total, about 25 million children and adolescents are overweight or nearly overweight. This epidemic is not confined to the U.S. but is seen in all industrialized societies, where many people live sedentary lives and eat lots of convenience foods. A recent report, in fact, has revealed that there are currently more obese people in the world than there are undernourished people.

IS MY CHILD AT RISK? SIGNS AND SYMPTOMS OF CHILDHOOD OBESITY

You may not know if your child is at risk by just looking at her. Children carry different amounts of body fat at different stages of development, and some children have larger-than-average body frames. If you're worried that your child is becoming overweight, talk with her doctor or other health care provider. A complete weight assessment will take into account your child's history of growth and development, family history, and your child's position on growth charts. A thorough evaluation will help determine if your child's weight is in an unhealthy range.

CAUSES OF CHILDHOOD OBESITY

Although there are certainly some genetic and hormonal causes of childhood obesity, most excess weight is caused by poor eating habits and lack of exercise. If children consume more calories than they burn, they gain weight.

Other factors that can influence a child's likelihood of becoming overweight include the following:

- **Diet**—Regular consumption of high-calorie, low nutrition foods, such as fast foods, baked goods and vending-machine snacks, contribute to weight gain. Soft drinks, candy and desserts, which are high in sugar and calories, can also cause weight gain.
- **Inactivity**—Studies have shown a direct correlation between the number of hours that children watch television or play video games and obesity. In addition to being sedentary and not burning calories, children tend to consume large amounts of high-calorie snacks during these activities, so it's double jeopardy.
- **Genetics**—In a family of overweight people, children may be genetically predisposed to put on excess weight, especially if high-calorie food is always available and physical activity isn't encouraged.
- **Psychological factors**—Some children overeat to comfort themselves when they experience stress or anxiety, which, in some cases, is a behavior modeled by parents.
- **Family/social factors**—Children imitate their parents, who have the most influence on their lives. If parents are headed down the road to obesity, their children will follow them. Ultimately, parents are responsible for providing healthy food and encouraging an active lifestyle. Further, obesity can cause or exacerbate many social and emotional issues.
- **Low self-esteem**—Children can be very insensitive to the feelings of others and often tease or bully their overweight peers, resulting in low self-esteem and sometimes depression.
- **Behavior problems**—Overweight children tend to experience more anxiety and to have poorer social skills than normal-weight children; this anxiety may lead to social withdrawal or to increased interpersonal conflict and disruptive school behavior. Children who have behavior problems are nearly three times as likely to be overweight. And children who have behavior problems are as much as five times more likely to become overweight as they grow up.
- **Academic problems**—Overweight children experience increased levels of stress and anxiety which often have tremendous negative impact on academic performance.
- **Unhappiness**—Overweight children often feel socially isolated and have low self-esteem and subsequent feelings of unhappiness leading to a significantly higher incidence of depression in this population. If your child loses interest in normal activities, appears sad, emotionally distant, or cries a lot, or perhaps experiences a change in sleep habits, and you are suspecting depression, take action. Talk to her about her struggles and feelings and try to determine the extent of the problems, and share your concerns with her doctor.

THE EFFECTS OF SLEEP ON CHILDHOOD OBESITY

Many factors increase a child's risk of becoming overweight, including lack of sleep, as more and more research demonstrates a link between sleep and obesity. A recent study in the journal *Pediatrics* demonstrated that every additional hour per night that a third-grader spends sleeping reduces the child's chances of being obese when they get to the sixth grade by 40 percent. In this study, of the children who slept 10 to 12 hours a night, about 12 percent were obese by sixth grade. In the group of children who slept fewer than nine hours a day, 22 percent were obese in sixth grade.

A number of possible reasons underlie this correlation. Sleep-deprived people, for example, produce greater amounts of a hormone called *ghrelin*, which promotes hunger, and less of a hormone called *leptin*, which signals fullness. And children who receive adequate sleep are more energetic and more likely to get involved in the kind of activities that burn more calories.

How to Deal With an Obese Child

Never isolate a child from the rest of the family. One of the best strategies to combat excess weight in your child is to improve the diet and exercise levels of your entire family. If a child is identified as having a "problem" and is treated differently from other members of the family, her anxiety levels may simply increase which can, in turn, cause an increase in emotionally-based eating. Health is a family affair — every member should participate.

But try to be patient if you are attempting to introduce a variety of new foods or activities. Children need to encounter a new food an average of ten times before they readily accept it, and it may take nearly as long for children to start enjoying new sports and activities, especially if they aren't very athletic.

Weight Loss versus Weight Maintenance

For children under age seven, the goal will often be weight maintenance rather than weight loss. This strategy allows the child to add height and "grow into" a more appropriate weight. But keep in mind that for an obese child, such a strategy may be as difficult as losing weight for adults.

For children over age seven, or for younger children who have pressing weight-related health concerns, weight loss may be the goal, which should be slow and steady, in the range of one pound a week to one pound a month, depending on factors like the existence of any health conditions that might either require urgent weight loss or preclude certain weight loss methods (*i.e.,* specific exercises or dietary changes).

If the goal is maintaining weight or losing weight, the methods are the same: increased activity and a healthier diet. And any success achieved will be primarily a result of your determination to help your child with these changes.

Common Pitfalls: Over Fixing

But try to avoid focusing too intently on your child's eating habits and weight. This can easily backfire, and sometimes cause a child to overeat even more, or possibly make her more prone to developing an eating disorder. In addition, avoid getting into food-related power struggles with your child, such as providing or withholding foods such as sweets as rewards or punishment. This sets up food as a potential weapon for control, another proven link to the development of eating disorders.

Ideally, avoid criticism or judgment. Emphasize the positives—the fun of the activities, the healthfulness of the food, the benefits of exercise (apart from controlling weight) like stronger muscles or improved endurance. If you can make exercise enjoyable, and establish healthier eating, the weight issue will tend to take care of itself.

Healthy Eating Basics

Keep in mind, parents control what food is purchased, how it's cooked, and where and when it's eaten:

- Purchase more fruits and vegetables and less convenience foods, which are high in sugar and fat. And make healthy snacks available all the time.
- Limit sweetened beverages, including those that contain fruit juice, because they provide little nutritional value and are high in calories.
- Avoid artificially sweetened sodas, which recent research has shown to cause sugar cravings, and increase cholesterol and blood sugar levels.
- Cook meals in healthier ways, using methods lower in fat. Avoid fried foods whenever possible.
- Colorful foods are generally more nutritious. Eat more green and yellow vegetables, and fruits. Substitute whole-wheat bread for white bread and brown rice for white rice. Avoid sugar and high-calorie desserts as much as possible.
- Avoid eating in front of the TV or computer. When the mind focuses elsewhere, people tend to eat fast and enjoy it less not realizing how much they eat.
- Limit eating out, especially fast-foods. Eating away from home has been linked to higher caloric intake and weight gain. In the year 2000, Americans spent 47% of their food budget on foods consumed away from home, and this percentage continues to grow. When consumers eat out, they are offered a large variety of low-cost, energy-dense foods in large portions. In fact, portion size has been increasing for the past 25 years, and people do tend to eat what is put in front of them.

Exercise and Activity Basics

A critical component of any weight loss program, and one that's particularly important for children, is physical activity. Such activity not only burns calories, but is healthful for growing bodies and improves sleep and daytime alertness.

To encourage greater activity levels, consider the following:

- **Limit sedentary activities**—Children who watch more than three hours of TV per day are 50 percent more likely to be obese than those who watch fewer than two hours. Make it a priority, therefore, to limit the time your child sits in front of a screen (computer or TV) or talks on the phone to fewer than two hours a day. In one notable exception, some video games such as Nintendo Wii *Sports*, the *Dance Dance Revolution* and the *EyeToy* actually require physical exercise. Recently I played Wii *Tennis* and was surprised when I broke a sweat in about ten minutes. In addition, the Wii *Fit* game, introduced in 2008, uses a balance board that measures players' weight and body mass index, and has a controller with a suite of games that focus on aerobics, yoga, balance and muscle conditioning. Although playing real sports burns more calories than these video games, they certainly rank higher than playing regular video games and can also help improve kids' confidence and hand-eye coordination.

- **Emphasize activities that involve body movement**—Children often resist structured exercise programs, and really, you simply want to get them moving. Outdoor activities such as basketball, jump rope, hide-and-seek, or roller skating burn lots of calories and improve fitness. And of course encourage your child to get involved in team sports like soccer.

- **Incorporate activities that your child enjoys**—If your child likes being in nature, drive to the countryside and hike together. If she likes to fly kites, walk or bicycle to the park for such an activity. If she enjoys your family dog, why not offer the job of walking the dog as a way of earning an allowance? If your child goes to the movies regularly for entertainment, alternate this with activities like bowling or miniature golf.

- **Create an active lifestyle for the whole family**—Identify healthful activities that everyone in the family enjoys, and engage in them together as part of your normal routine.

- **Make small, gradual changes**

Slow and Steady Wins the Race: Making Small, Gradual Changes

We've been discussing lifestyle change, not just a new diet. Time and again, diets only help people lose weight in the short term, only to gain the weight back, and usually more, in the long run. Thus, well over 90 percent of weight lost by traditional dieting comes right back; only by fundamental lifestyle change does one lose weight permanently. So be realistic. Introduce changes gradually, one at a time. Establish each change as routine before moving on to new ones. You'll more likely find success this way rather than by trying to make many large changes that last only a short time. Set achievable goals and stick with them.

Teaching by Example: Watch Your Own Weight

Whether or not your child is currently overweight, the suggestions in this discussion of obesity will help to protect you and your child from becoming overweight and will contribute to your overall health. You will have a much easier time helping your children to live a healthy lifestyle if you set a good example. Remember, children often translate "Do what I say, not what I do" into action as "Do what I do, not what I say." Invite your children to join you in diet and activity levels consistent with good health. Make this your formula for long-term success.

The Best Support You Can Give

One of the most critical roles a parent plays in helping an obese child is to aid in the process of building self-esteem and making her feel accepted and loved. Our society places far too much emphasis on slimness as opposed to health and fitness. Talk instead about health and fitness, but be sensitive that a child may view your concern as personal criticism and rejection. Do your best to accept your child as she is without being critical or judgmental. Express your appreciation for her, and praise her whenever possible. And as always, encourage your child to talk about feelings; listen with patience and understanding, so you create an emotionally supportive atmosphere that will sustain her through the inevitable trials and tribulations of growing up.

CHAPTER 11

ANDREW/DARREN

Interviewed:	Andrew
Child:	Darren, age 14, maturational age 9
Complaints:	*Hyperactivity*
	Learning disability
	Poor attention span
	Emotional problems
	Anxiety
	Oppositional behavior
	Behavior problems—violent threats, violence toward others
	Destruction of property
	Insomnia
	Bedwetting
	Poor self-esteem
	No regard for rules and limits

 •

Tell *me a little about Darren* and his difficulties.

His main problem is that he is hyperactive—he has difficulty keeping his mind on one thing.

How long has this been a problem?

Since he was four or five, so about 10 years.

Was he ever diagnosed as having Attention Deficit Hyperactivity Disorder?

He was never officially diagnosed as having ADHD, but he has some other learning disability—I don't know the name offhand.

Did they ever use medication?

Chapter 11   Andrew / Darren

They've been using antipsychotic medication to modify his behavior because he is so oppositional. He's on Seroquel, 150mg twice a day.

Has he ever been psychotic?

No.

So, they are using the medication just to tranquilize him?

Right. In school, his attention is zero. He was in special education classes and even in those classes he wouldn't pay attention or sit still. He wouldn't pay attention long enough to figure out a basic math problem. He's 14, but he only functions at about fourth-grade level.

So he probably has a lot of emotional problems?

I'll say. I'll give you another example. He goes out with friends at night and stays out 'til all hours with no regard whatsoever for how it affects those around him.

Does he ask for permission before leaving the house?

No, he'll just tell you what he's going to do and that's that.

Does he experience a lot of anxiety?

Yes, a lot of anxiety. By watching him you can tell that he struggles with it. He has told me that he feels inadequate and embarrassed that he can't measure up to other people. And he really wants to try to please people, but he can't. He doesn't know why, he just can't.

Has he had therapy?

He's been in therapy at a county mental health clinic for the past four years.

How has he responded to that?

He's very oppositional in the area of treatment for himself. He doesn't want to feel like there is anything wrong with him. Up until the last six months, the therapy has done nothing positive for him. In fact the last few months there has been talk about placing him in a locked residential treatment facility.

Have his behavior problems been so severe that the family doesn't feel like they can handle him?

Right. He has a lot of emotional outbursts; he's threatening, and sometimes violent.

Oh, he's actually been violent?

He's been threatening at school and violent at home and there have been occasions when he has assaulted kids at school.

Has he hurt people at home?

No. He broke out a window a couple of times, but he hasn't attacked anyone. But he has been threatened with residential placement and he knows that we are actively pursuing that. He's been trying to keep it together because he doesn't want to be taken out of the home and placed in a facility. It's the only thing that has worked so far—that has made a dent in his behavior—the threat of placing him in a residential facility. But that hasn't changed anything with regard to school or his outlook about himself or his sleeping at night. It's just stopped him from acting out physically. The only thing that has changed in the past six months is the fact that he has been less violent.

You alluded to trouble sleeping at night. Let's talk about that for a moment. Has he had problems both getting to sleep and waking up at night?

He has a lot of difficulty falling asleep and waking up in the middle of the night. And when he wakes up in the morning he's in a really bad mood. He'll have nightmares pretty often, and when he does it will take him a whole day just to get in a better mood.

Does he have any other sleep-related troubles that you know of?

He has a history of chronic bedwetting.

And I'd imagine that has a considerable effect on his self-esteem.

Absolutely. He already has a really poor body image. He draws a lot and often draws a picture of a person. If you ask him what the pictures are, he will say, "Me." They usually show a real distorted body with an extremely large abdomen and small head. He is overweight for his age, but he is not obese. He draws those pictures constantly throughout the day.

Do you see him on a daily basis?

Almost.

༄ • ༅

After speaking with Andrew, I gave him the *Magic Carpet* CD to try with Darren. Five days later, we met again to discuss the effects.

༄ • ༅

What was his reaction when you first gave him the **Magic Carpet** *program to listen to?*

He didn't like the idea. Again, he was oppositional about it. He felt like it was another form of treatment. Another person telling him, especially his uncle who works in mental health, that he needs this. I made a contract with him that he would listen to it at night, just for me, and he agreed to do that.

And how long has he been using it now?

Let's see . . . wow, it's only been five days. It's hard to believe because the changes are so drastic.

Really? What feedback have you received at this point?

He called and said that he is getting to sleep much earlier. He just called me right up, with no prompting on my part or by his parents, and told me that he's been able to sleep without getting up at night.

Have you heard of any changes in his bedwetting behavior?

In the five-day period he hasn't had any difficulty with that at all.

Did he report that as a difference?

Yes, that's what he told me, and he is sleeping like he's never slept before.

How are his mornings now?

In the past five days, he's waking up all smiles, in a good mood, right when he gets up. I think he's starting to feel better about himself. He's even showing a different attitude about how he looks.

So what is going on with the pictures?

He's still drawing but he hasn't been drawing those distorted pictures of himself. Basically, he seems to have a better body image now.

Has he mentioned anything that might be relevant to his level of anxiety?

I didn't get a chance to question him. He's not very in touch with his feelings. The only thing he said is that he feels rested. But his mom mentioned that he is calmer.

Did she know he was using the program?

Yeah, I told her I wanted to try it with him.

Did she notice other differences since the program has been used?

Yep, she confirms all the same observations I have. This is just after using the program for five days.

So you're saying, this is the first thing that has really made a big difference?

Yes, more difference than all of therapy and medications combined. He's a good candidate because he has a lot of underlying emotional problems and if we can get him to be able to sleep at night and to develop a better perspective of himself, the other modes of therapy that they are using may start having more effect. Up to now, the therapy hasn't done a thing for him though.

But as you mentioned, he's been very oppositional.

Right, and that is beginning to change—he's been more cooperative.

In terms of what?

In terms of staying out, doing what he wants with his friends and not coming home when he should. He's been coming home and asking for permission to go out, which is given to him as long as he's back by a certain time, and now he's back by that time.

Thank you for sharing your experience.

You're welcome.

ಞ • ೞ

BEDWETTING

According to Andrew, the program had a profound effect on young Darren, not the least of which was the cessation of his bedwetting. As you've no doubt noticed while reading this book, many of the children discussed in these interviews wet their bed.

THE PROBLEM OF BEDWETTING

That should come as no surprise. *"Nocturnal enuresis,"* as it's officially called, affects approximately five to seven million American children age 6 and older and, if left unchecked, can very easily persist well into a child's teens or, sometimes, even beyond, into adulthood. According to researchers at Canada's University of Quebec, in line with the slow maturation of the bedwetting child's nervous system, is the concurrent possibility of delays in his achievement of certain motor skills, language skills and behavioral development.

CAUSES OF BEDWETTING

The medical community remains uncertain as to the exact causes of bedwetting. It was once thought that it was an intentional behavior that children used to get attention, but that is no longer considered true. It is, in fact, widely considered untrue that bedwetting has its root causes in emotional dysfunctions, as currently no scientific or medical evidence supports this belief. Nevertheless, emotional upset does seem to exacerbate the problem.

More recent research on the subject of bedwetting suggests that the major cause is rooted in a delay in nervous-system maturation and an imbalance between nighttime production of urine and the bladder's capacity to hold it. The brain of the bedwetting child has difficulty in recognizing the messages sent by a full bladder to the sleep arousal centers that would normally awaken the child to appropriately take care of the need to urinate. Also, bedwetting children commonly have smaller bladders as well as smaller stature than their non-bedwetting peers.

Some evidence supports the theory that heredity plays at least a part in bedwetting, for often one or both parents of many children who suffer from the condition wet the bed as children themselves. In fact, a parent who wet the bed as a child has a 45% chance of producing a child who wets the bed, too. The odds increase to 80% if both parents were bedwetters as children.

Other proposed causes of and/or contributors to bedwetting include:
- anxiety and stress (as previously mentioned, not considered causative but often play a role)
- urinary tract infection

- allergies
- constipation
- metabolic disorders
- hormone deficiencies
- neurological disorders involving the spinal cord
- diabetes
- kidney failure
- side effects of medications the child may be taking

In stark reality, however, rarely does just one single cause lie behind a child's regularly wetting the bed. Keep in mind, incidentally, that only about 2% to 3% of bedwetting cases result from medical conditions.

STATISTICS ON BEDWETTING

Bedwetting is actually a prevalent behavior among children up to age 3, the typical age at which most children are completely toilet trained, because the functions of nighttime urine production and bladder control take time to develop. But bedwetting thus remains a relatively common problem in children even up to age 8. Statistically, bedwetting is far more common in boys than girls (while daytime "accidents," incidentally, are more common in girls). About 20% of 5-year-olds wet the bed; by age 6, this number decreases to only 10% (again, predominantly among boys). For this reason, medical treatment for bedwetting rarely commences before a child reaches age 6. The percentage of bedwetting continues to decrease at a rate of about 15% per year from age 6 onward, with just 2% to 3% of adolescents and young adults continuing to wet the bed.

SIGNS AND SYMPTOMS ASSOCIATED WITH BEDWETTING

Although psychological causes of bedwetting remain in debate, there is little question that several prevalent psychological symptoms typically accompany bedwetting. Any child who wets the bed likely feels ashamed about the behavior. He may also feel "dirty." Complicating matters, parents of a child who wets the bed often feel at fault for the condition, as though they did something wrong in raising the child.

EFFECTS OF BEDWETTING

Bedwetting can lead to a host of other emotional and environmental concerns for the whole household, for bedwetting disturbs more than just the child's sleep: it leads, for example, to a constant excess of laundry and places pressure on both the parents and the child to identify the source of the problem and resolve it. The situation often results in significant frustration and guilt for parents who feel at a loss for a solution and, in turn, lash out at the child.

LONG-TERM PSYCHOLOGICAL CONSEQUENCES OF BEDWETTING

Long-term psychological consequences of childhood bedwetting may include difficulty forming and maintaining healthy relationships, obtaining and holding down employment, taking trips away from home and, most typically, low self-esteem and even depression. In fact, as most cases of nocturnal enuresis dissipate naturally in time, a parent's concern for their bedwetting child should really focus on managing these psychological symptoms.

Won't Children Outgrow Bedwetting?

The consolation for most parents is that their children usually outgrow bedwetting. Sadly, however, this is not always the case. And even when a child does eventually outgrow nocturnal enuresis, much of the psychological damage from the problem until that point has already occurred.

Common Pitfall: Anger and Frustration

By all means, don't get angry with him, blame him, put him down, embarrass him, punish him, or—heaven forbid—spank him.

What to Do if Your Child Wets the Bed

If bedwetting seems a chronic problem for your child, consult your child's pediatrician in order to rule out any underlying medical causes that can be appropriately treated. If a child's bedwetting is accompanied by poor daytime bladder control more serious medical concerns are more likely involved. So, too, may be the case if your child's bedwetting is accompanied by pain in the urinary tract while urinating, or by back pain, abdominal pain, or fever. If the urine has a strong, unpleasant odor or if the child awakens regularly in the middle of the night intensely thirsty, a pediatrician's counsel is also wise.

If your child wets the bed, first and foremost reassure him that the problem is common and not his fault. Assure him you know he's not wetting the bed on purpose. And above all emphasize the behavior doesn't make him a bad person. Encourage your child to communicate openly with you about his bedwetting, while at the same time supporting discretion and protecting his privacy regarding the matter. Remain watchful that siblings don't tease, embarrass, or humiliate him for having the problem. A convenient side benefit of giving your child compassionate support is that doing so tends to decrease recurrences of bedwetting.

In establishing the steps to employ to curb, and ultimately prevent, bedwetting, allow the child an element of choice in which of these methods, if any, he will attempt, as it helps diminish the negative effects of bedwetting on his self-esteem and may even help improve his self-confidence. Likewise, having choices helps support the child in taking responsibility for dealing with a wet bed when nighttime enuresis does happen.

Prevention is the Best Cure

For starters, consider these proactive measures:

- Remove caffeinated beverages (and foods, like chocolate) from the child's diet, especially at nighttime
- Encourage the child to drink more fluids (especially plain water) during the day so that they are less inclined to feel thirsty and drink more at night

- Have the child urinate twice immediately prior to going to bed, the second time just five or ten minutes after the first
- Enforce scheduled bedtimes and even consider earlier bedtimes; sticking to a routine, and longer, regular durations of sleep have been reported to help control bedwetting
- Make it easy for your child to get up in the middle of the night to go to the bathroom, such as by putting a nightlight in your child's bedroom or giving him a flashlight by his bed should he need it
- Encourage calmness and relaxation immediately preceding bedtimes, avoiding roughhousing and other activities that may produce excessive excitement (such as playing video games before bed)

As a practical stopgap, try a waterproof sheet on the child's bed to help alleviate some of the secondary stressors associated with bedwetting. Other similar strategies include PODS (Potty On Discreet Strips), absorbent underpants, protective diapers, and pull-ups. Just remember these stopgap measures are just that: they'll relieve some of the stress you and the child feel over bedwetting while you and the child home in on permanent solutions.

How Better Hydration Helps Prevent Bedwetting

Proper hydration, ironically, actually plays a major role in preventing bedwetting. Many children avoid drinking fluids all day, only to guzzle down large quantities at night. Additionally, many children wait to drink anything until they're parched, at which point they drink sugary, caffeinated beverages to squelch their thirst, only making the problem worse, for caffeine and sugar act as diuretics; rather than increase the body's fluid levels, they actually inhibit fluid retention and conversely promote increased urination rather than less.

Aggravating the problem, when a body suffers from an imbalance of fluid intake, it demands replenishment of fluids at the most inconvenient time of day possible, namely in the early evenings. Proper hydration, supportive of the ability to sleep through the night without wetting the bed, is best achieved by consuming smaller quantities of water at a time, consistently and frequently throughout the day. Think ahead. Encourage proper hydration, for example, by including a bottle of water in your child's backpack before he leaves for school each day.

Exercises to Prevent Bedwetting

A physician may also recommend certain exercises for stretching the bladder and developing muscle strength in the bladder area, thereby making the bladder capable of containing larger quantities of urine before requiring elimination, as well as increasing a child's control over where and when that elimination occurs. In one such exercise, the child, when he feels the need to urinate, holds off for as long as possible before going to the bathroom. In another, he intentionally interrupts the stream of urine when he does urinate, thereby developing better strength and control over the sphincter of the bladder.

Medications to Treat Bedwetting

Occasionally, a pediatrician might also prescribe certain medications, including *desmopressin*, the currently preferred agent, and, in the past, tricyclic antidepressants, to temporarily eliminate nocturnal enuresis, but these medications do not "cure" the problem, and therefore must not be used with that intention in mind. Children have died from overdoses of tricyclic antidepressants and most authorities agree that they now have no place in the management of childhood enuresis. Medication may be indicated if a child is going through cognitive behavioral therapy, or other types of therapy, at the same time as he is experiencing bedwetting. Additionally, physicians may prescribe medication to a child who will not be sleeping at home for a period of time, such as at a friend's sleepover or at sleepaway camp. Treatment with *desmopressin* offers a number of advantages including rapid onset, lack of side effects, and safety, but after treatment is stopped only about 30% of children experience lasting improvement.

The Latest Word on Bedwetting: Alarms

The current consensus is that enuresis alarms are the preferred method of treating childhood enuresis, according to the results of an evidence-based review of research in the Cochrane Library, as reported in the June, 2006 issue of *Evidence-Based Child Health*. Such alarms are triggered by urination, waking the child up during these events, and this treatment eventually results in successful control of bedwetting 80 to 90% of the time. Several months after these alarms are removed from an affected child's bed, two out of three are able to maintain the benefits they have achieved.

Being Realistic About Timelines for Results

Keep in mind that while chronic bedwetting typically goes away by itself in time, it doesn't go away all at once. Generally, the process starts with the child having fewer instances of bedwetting each night, followed by a decrease in the number of nights that it occurs each week until the problem ultimately goes away altogether. There may, however, be considerable fluctuation in the progression of this process before the problem completely disappears, taking perhaps even several years.

Secondary Enuresis

All of the material in this commentary so far regards what is known as "primary enuresis"—or enuresis that has persisted regularly since infancy—but there is another type of bedwetting parents should also be aware of called "secondary enuresis." This is bedwetting that occurs after a period of at least six months in which no instances of bedwetting occur at all.

The reason why this distinction is so important is that primary enuresis is developmental—or to put it another way, completely natural. Secondary enuresis, however, might merit more concern. If your child is 5 years old before he starts wetting the bed, then it could be due to a medical reason and should be brought to the attention of the child's doctor as soon as possible.

If Bedwetting Persists

In the final analysis, if your child's chronic bedwetting persists, especially if the concern is secondary enuresis, seek guidance from a pediatrician who has given your child a complete exam, including a full urinalysis.

CHAPTER 12

SUSAN/HEATHER AND TAMARA

Interviewed:	Susan
Child:	**Heather, age 5**
Complaints:	*Malignant brain tumor*
	Brain surgery
	Insomnia
	Pain
	Anxiety
	Fear
	Stress of radiation therapy
	Morning crankiness
	Nightmares
Child:	**Tamara, age 13**
Complaints:	*Anxiety*
	Over activity
	Short attention span
	Insomnia
	Bleeding ulcers
	Diarrhea
	Stomach cramps
	Nightmares
	Headaches

꙳ • ꙳

Susan, *would you please tell me about Heather.*

Yes. She seems to have a lot of fear at night. We still don't know why it's going on, if it's something she's going through or someone has scared her.

How do you know she's frightened?

The screaming. We'll put her to bed and everything is fine, but in no less than five minutes she'll scream at the top of her lungs. Everything in the room bothers her. We had a hanging lamp that we had to take down. We took pictures down. We moved rugs away. We moved her bed, we left the lights on. So far, nothing has helped.

How long does it usually take her to calm down and fall asleep?

Sometimes three or four hours.

Frequently that long?

Oh, yeah. Or she'll fall asleep and wake up a half hour later and be up for three or four hours screaming and crying.

Does she complain of nightmares?

Yes. She says she has nightmares.

How many times does she usually wake up during the night?

Sometimes three or four times a night and it's always very hard to get her to go back to sleep. I'll have to sit in the hallway or in her room every night.

Have you asked her what's scaring her so much?

She actually doesn't know what's scaring her. Her pediatrician doesn't know what's wrong. There's no explanation as to why. This happens during the day, too. During the day she won't even go in her room and play. There doesn't seem to be anything that will help her.

Shifting gears a little, you have another child, Tamara, who is 13. Please tell me a little about her.

Poor girl, she's just so overactive. She can't relax. Everything will be going through her mind.

What is her attention span currently?

About three minutes.

Are you serious?

Definitely. You can ask the school. Even in school, maybe five minutes and then she'll be bored. She just can't stay focused on anything. She has had this trouble in school ever since kindergarten. Even so, her doctor doesn't think she has attention deficit disorder and only suggested that she get involved in some sort of activity.

How long is she able stay focused on something that interests her, though? Like television, for example?

It depends on what's on. If there is something on that she really likes, maybe 15 minutes. But that's not really what's had me worried lately.

What has?

Well, recently she's started having really severe diarrhea, before going to school. And sometimes it will happen in school.

How long has that been going on?

She's had it off and on for three or four months, and then it got worse so we took her to the doctors and they said they couldn't find anything wrong except that she's very nervous.

Has Tamara had any other problems?

Yes, she has headaches, too.

How often is she having headaches?

Almost every day. And often at the same time that she's having diarrhea. She was taking Tylenol with codeine for it, and it would take some of it away, but it made her sleepier than I would want. I still have the prescription, but she's no longer taking it.

Does she have problems with nightmares or crabbiness in the morning?

Terrible. The nightmares are on and off. And, yeah, crabbiness is also a problem, because she knows what will happen in the morning, so she wakes up in a bad mood because she doesn't want to go to school.

After speaking with Susan, I gave her the adult *Natural Sleep* and *Natural Relaxation I* programs to try with her daughters, since I had not created the children's programs yet. She returned two months later to tell me how it went.

So let's start with Heather. How has she been doing with the sleep program?

When we started using it, it was like she had a companion in the room. It took effect almost immediately. Right now, she does not get up at all. This has been for a while now.

What about toward the beginning, say after a month's use?

After a week she slept through the whole night with the exception of one time when she woke up screaming and wanted to know if we were there. As soon as I said, "Yes," everything was fine, she turned on the CD again and she went right back to sleep. After a week, she wasn't getting up in the middle of the night at all.

Was she having any kind of sleep problem after one week?

Maybe once every nine or ten days she'd wake up, but she doesn't wake up screaming anymore.

At this point does she have any anxiety around being in her room by herself?

No. Many times I have to go upstairs to find her, because not only will she play upstairs now, but she'll play with the door shut. She never had the door shut before.

And what about going to sleep at night?

Before, she insisted on having all the lights on in her room. She does have a night light in her room now, but it's mainly so she doesn't fall when she goes to the bathroom. She actually doesn't care if it's dark now and she sleeps with the door closed.

Did you notice any change in her behavior upon arising in the morning?

Oh, yes. When she was scared during the night she would wake up cranky, and she felt like she never had enough rest. After using the sleep program, she's waking happy, more contented.

She seems more relaxed?

Much more relaxed. It's like a different child; we are really amazed. We're surprised that the change had come so quickly for her.

Have you ever had to push her to use the programs?

No, definitely not.

What's her attitude about the sleep program?

She's fascinated. She's fascinated by the voice. It makes her relax and sleep. It stimulates her imagination. It's also made it so she isn't alone. She has developed an amazing imagination. She adds things to the program.

Really?

Oh, yeah. I know she does. It's like she makes it her own story book. She takes various toys with her and will bring a friend along. She is very creative. Really, the programs have had such an unbelievable effect on both of my children.

So Tamara has been using the CDs, too?

Tamara has used the relaxation program a couple times, and she says it helps her calm down a little. She wanted to hear the sleep CD, because she was curious. So I let her listen to it one afternoon. She got halfway through, took the headphones off, and fell asleep for about an hour.

Was she trying to fall asleep?

No, she just wanted to hear the CD. While she listened to it, it seemed like I could see her body go limp, because just before she listened, she was very hyper. She is fairly hyper in general, and I saw her whole body just go limp as though she was really relaxing. Then she turned over and went to sleep. She said she likes it and wants to use it more.

So has she started using the CDs at night, too?

I was going to suggest using the sleep program, but she suggested it first. She said she wanted to try something on her own. So she used the program and she fantasized not having stomach cramps and not being afraid of school and not having the frequent bathroom attacks. I saw her whole body relaxing and she drifted off in a daze. After that, she started using it off and on.

So she hasn't been listening on a regular basis?

No, not like Heather, at least not at first.

Not at first? Has she since started listening to the sleep program more regularly?

Yes, now she's using it nightly.

And what brought that about?

Her diarrhea stopped.

How quickly?

Within a week. The doctor was amazed when we told him what had happened. And as quickly as the diarrhea stopped, her attitude of being afraid to go to school stopped. She would tell me, "I'm not going to have diarrhea today and I'm not going to have stomach cramps. I'm not going to call you because I'm going to have a good day," and it worked.

She had some other gastrointestinal problems in the past, didn't she?

She had three bleeding ulcers.

Any problems with that now?

No. And if she gets uptight, she just retreats into her room and listens to a relaxation CD.

Have there been any other benefits?

She's no longer vomiting either. She used to have problems with vomiting; I don't think I told you about that.

No, you didn't.

She hasn't even complained of severe stomach cramps. I think she went back to listening to the CDs because there were so many stresses going on. The move, the new school, the diarrhea, stomach cramps, and headaches. She hasn't even been having headaches now.

So she listens to the sleep program every night now?

Yes. And now she'll even listen to the relaxation program in the morning.

What about her nightmares? Has she still been having them?

Oh, no. They've pretty much stopped now. And she wakes up feeling much better in the morning.

And her oppositional behavior? Did you notice any difference in how well she minds you?

Only a little bit, but it has certainly made a big difference in how she feels about school, which was a sudden change when she started using the programs. She's now looking forward to going to school in September, which was never the case because she hated school before.

So you think the program use improved her attitude about school?

Well, now she looks at herself, thinking, "Maybe I am pretty and I can get along with those other kids, and I have nothing to fear from them." I think it's helped her self-confidence and self-esteem. I think she has a ways to go, but she's made a good start. She did a tremendous job with herself, by using the CDs this summer.

What about her general activity level? You said she's a very active girl, to the point where you were wondering if she might have Attention Deficit Hyperactivity Disorder?

Yes.

Have you noticed any change in her level of activity or behavior during the day?

She is calmer. She can sit down and watch TV. That's been one of the biggest changes I've seen in Tamara, even though she's going through a hard stage at 13. Her biggest change now is she can sit down at the table and write for about an hour or two or watch TV. And she's even started reading . . . and she hated reading.

When did that start?

Guessing, I would say about a month and a half ago, right after she started using the CDs regularly. Now she uses them every night. They both have their own CD players and their own headphones. I also noticed that Tamara is learning to eat slower, which was another problem. She is learning that it's okay to sit there and relax. You don't have to be running or doing something every minute. It's okay just to be with yourself. I think that was an important lesson Tamara had to learn, and she did that by listening to the CDs and relaxing.

You said that her attention span is longer?

Absolutely.

Can you give me an example?

Well, now she'll sit and watch TV for an hour or two, if she really likes the programs. With reading she could do it for about a minute before, and now, I noticed last week she was reading downstairs and she read for a good 45 minutes without putting the book down. I don't know if she realizes this, but she's getting interested in reading different types of things, too.

Has her reading time increased more than her television time?

Yeah. She's reading more. She's spending more time in her room than in the den. There are certain things she likes to watch, but she'll give it up and go to her room and read and she's never done that before. To me, this is a miracle.

So you'd say you've noticed some very definite changes as a result of using the programs?

We've had very good luck with them. And besides using the programs with my children, I've used them myself; the relaxation program for my headaches, which are much better now, and the sleep program, too.

And how long does it take you to fall asleep?

I get to the stream. I've never finished the CD.

You've listened to it for a couple months and you have never heard the end?

I've never even heard the middle of it.

Do you think you'll ever sit up and listen to it all the way through?

I tried. A couple nights ago I had a bad night and I thought I would listen to the whole program. I was sitting with the night light on, and I got to where the stream is and I thought, *"I'll just lie down now because I knew I would be able to hear the whole CD,"* but I only got to the point where I was leaving the stream and I drifted off to sleep. I'm dying to know what's on the end of it.

Thank you very much for sharing your experiences with me. Perhaps we can continue this at a future time?

I'd be happy to.

❦ • ❧

Two Years Later

❦ • ❧

It's been two years since we last sat down to talk about your children, and since then, you have been through a very challenging time.

Definitely.

It wasn't long ago that your younger daughter was diagnosed as having a brain tumor and had to undergo surgery. Would you tell me a little about that?

Yes. My seven-year-old daughter, Heather, wasn't doing very well and was in the hospital for a work-up. They called me from the hospital and told me that she was quickly getting worse and they needed me to get down there right away. I ran out of the house and got there as fast as I could. I was really scared about what I was going to hear. When I got there I was told she had a very malignant brain tumor and that they were going to have to do surgery right away. I was devastated. I was hysterical at times, and I knew I needed something to relax me. I just couldn't go into her room falling apart like that because I needed to try to help her to relax.

So what did you do?

I went home quickly and got the relaxation program for me and the *Magic Carpet* program you had just given me for her. When I got back to the hospital I played the relaxation program, and it was enough to help me relax some. I then took it into her room and played it for both of us. Now, whether she heard it or not, I really don't know because she was pretty out of it, but I think she heard at least some of it because she started relaxing.

You felt you could see her relax?

Yes. And then immediately after her surgery, while she was in intensive care, I played *Magic Carpet* for her. The first few days after surgery, they couldn't give her anything for pain so she needed something to relax her.

Intensive care units are not very restful places.

Oh, it's very noisy. Plus they had a little boy next to her with all kinds of equipment and doctors in and out all day and all night. And they were waking Heather up every hour to take vital signs, and she would just be crying and she had no medication for pain. So in a situation like that, you really don't know what to do. You feel helpless. I thought it couldn't hurt to play *Magic Carpet* for her. I asked permission, and they said okay. It was such a relief, because I would see her relax and then fall asleep. We were using it six or seven times every day and also during the night.

Would it consistently relax her?

Yes, every time. It wouldn't put her to sleep, but it would relax her and the crying and the whimpering would stop and she might drift off for a moment, or at least rest for a little bit.

And at night, were you able to help her sleep?

When she was moved to Station 6B, she was having problems sleeping. She would wake up with a headache or she would just wake up from irritation of the incision, which itched. That was when I brought in a better CD player that allowed her to listen to *Magic Carpet* with headphones. I couldn't believe it because she became much more relaxed and she could go to sleep with it, almost every time she listened. When she was awake she was in quite a bit of pain and she was irritable and nervous.

What happened with that?

Finally, they were able to begin some pain medication. They started with Tylenol and that didn't do much. So they switched her to Tylenol with codeine, and that didn't work very well either. So that's when she started using the *Magic Carpet* whenever she was in pain. They were able to stop the Tylenol with codeine, and just give her regular Tylenol which, along with the program, was enough. Then in a short while they stopped the Tylenol. She hardly took any pain medication. Maybe some Tylenol once a day, where she had been taking Tylenol with codeine every four hours.

Did her physicians think this was out of the ordinary?

Well, everything was extraordinary with Heather right from the beginning. They said she was going to come out of surgery in a coma, and she didn't. They said she was definitely going to have a problem walking and she would need physical therapy and she didn't. And yes, they didn't understand how she got off all the pain medication so fast. They weren't saying that it was the CD that did it, but they were wondering to the point that they said they'd like to try it with other patients.

When you say, "they," who do you mean?

At Huntington Memorial Hospital, Dr. Hobart, her surgeon, said she thought it was probably the CD. She said it was unbelievable how many amazing things happened with her and that she would like to try the program with some other children. And then several of the nurses on the floor were very surprised by how well she responded. What I think was that it relaxed her and once she was relaxed the pain improved.

So now you're going to City of Hope for radiation? Do they know about Heather's program use?

From the first day we started going to City of Hope, I suggested that we use a CD in the radiation and simulation room. That's where they prepare the children with markings of the body and pictures, and they said okay. Heather had to go in the simulation room for extensive x-rays and marking of her body to get her ready for radiation therapy and we tried everything to calm her down.

They gave me permission to use the CD over the intercom; they were ready to try anything to calm her down. So we took advantage of it because she was one nervous child. She was in the body cast for two hours and we had to get her calmed down so they could take an x-ray. She had to be perfectly still. They had wires and things all over her.

*Did you feel the **Magic Carpet** was effective under those circumstances?*

Yes. In fact, it put her to sleep on the table, which surprised everyone. Nancy, Heather's nurse, had tried several CDs and said she would like to try yours with her other patients, too.

And has it continued to be effective through Heather's treatments?

Well, as a matter of fact, she did some pretty amazing things at City of Hope when they were giving her radiation treatments. They use medication to sedate children when they're getting radiation therapy. They told me I would have to stay at the hospital until it wore off. We used the medication once and it really didn't do much for her; it just seemed to make her dopey. We got into the practice of using *Magic Carpet* right before we'd go to the hospital so she wouldn't be so nervous.

She became very familiar with the program and was able take herself into her own imagination without actually listening to it. Nancy and the technicians were amazed at what she could do. She would slide into her body cast, which was the hardest part for her, and then she would become so relaxed that she wouldn't move. In fact she'd fall asleep. It would only take her a couple minutes and she'd be totally asleep.

The preparation was longer, but the actual radiation only took a few minutes and she would be perfectly still. If I didn't wake her up, I think she would've slept on that hard table, in the cast, for quite some time. Radiation therapy went on every day for eight weeks.

Did she actually sleep through most of her treatments?

Oh, yes. It got to the point where as soon as she hit the table she would be out. The hospital staff said they had never seen anything like it. They always have to medicate kids when they put them through that, but not Heather. And it made it nice for us because we didn't have to wait around for medication to wear off after her treatments. We could just go home.

Has Heather been waking up during the night at home at all?

She used to have problems waking up, but now she doesn't. If she does wake up, I just use the sleep program to put her right back to sleep. She hasn't awakened now for about a week. Just maybe, real quickly to go to the bathroom and she goes right back to sleep.

How long does it take her to fall asleep now?

She's out in about five minutes.

What does she say about her dreams now?

She has pleasant dreams now. Everything is fun. She's playing on the beach or in a pool; just pleasant things. And she says her dreams are all in color.

And during the day, has she been using the adult relaxation CD?

Well, during the day she uses it when she starts feeling worried. She takes the CD player with her up into her room and relaxes. I've noticed that she's not so uptight; she's not so scared about her health. She now seems much calmer. I think it has a lot to do with the program because I've really seen a difference. And with the headphones it makes it seem so real. It's like you're really on the beach. It's like, you can shut everything out; you don't hear anything but the voice and the background sounds of the stream, the birds, and the beach. She loves it so much she uses it for many things.

Like what else?

Well, the radiation made all her hair fall out, which is hard and kids make fun of you. It's hard to handle when you're only seven years old. When she was feeling bad about that she would go to her room and listen to the relaxation program, and it would seem to give her self-confidence. And then she didn't care what she looked like because she knew who she was and she didn't care about what other people thought.

You could see a clear difference after she used the programs?

Not only me, other people, too. She's a totally different child now and other people have also noticed the same thing. After radiation, she would use *Magic Carpet* and take a nap. When she was ready to play she could confront those other children who would tease her. It also seemed to help her cope with school where children would make fun of her because she couldn't learn as fast as them.

So she has been using the CDs for how long now?

Two years and two months.

Do you feel the programs have become more effective, less effective, or are about the same?

I think they're much more effective. It seems like a skill that she just keeps getting better at with practice. Now she knows that if she has a hard time, she can use the CDs, and if the CDs are not there, she can remember what's on them and she can do it herself.

She's learned to do it by herself?

Yes, she's gotten really good at it, too. Sometimes she doesn't feel like using a CD, so she visualizes herself on the beach with her toys. She just imagines she is on the beach and she goes right to sleep. So she is starting to be able to do it by herself. I can't believe it, but she's able to.

So you think it's even more effective now than when you first started using it with her a couple of years ago?

Oh, most definitely. Both of my children have changed dramatically, and all for the better. In fact, we all have changed through our use of the programs. All of us have benefitted.

I'm so happy to hear it. Thank you very much for all of your feedback.

You're welcome.

PAIN AND MEDICAL ILLNESS

As Heather and Tamara remind us, one of the most difficult challenges for parents to face is injury or illness in their children. Pain and disease were both significant factors in young Heather's experience, for one, and as her mother, Susan, explained, the devastation impacted her other daughter, Tamara, as well. And Heather, to this day, is alive and well. She overcame tremendous odds and earned the name "miracle child" at City of Hope.

THE MIND-BODY CONNECTION

Relaxation and visualization techniques, like those employed in all of my AudioMagic 3D audio programs, have been found to alleviate pain associated with various childhood illnesses and medical issues.

Mainstream science and medicine increasingly acknowledge the mind-body connection, as evidenced in the correlation doctors now typically find between anxiety and stress in many, if not most, medical illness. In the past, the term "psychosomatic" minimized and invalidated a person's experience of various physical symptoms, but more and more we recognize that, in a very real and pronounced way, both the cause and cure of most physical afflictions directly involve the mind.

THE STRESS RESPONSE VERSUS THE RELAXATION RESPONSE

We now, in fact, recognize stress and anxiety as one common aggravator of pain from any cause. Simply put, anxiety and stress trigger the body's "stress response," otherwise known as the "fight or flight" syndrome, a contracted physical state that typically heightens the senses, including the sense of pain. It only makes sense, then, that conscious, intentional relaxation can significantly restore one's ability to overcome painful sensations.

Think of a child about to receive an injection from her doctor. The parent or guardian present (or the doctor himself, or a member of his staff) will typically try to distract the child's attention from the injection site as the needle is inserted in order to minimize the experience of pain, for muscles tensed in anticipation increase the pain resulting from insertion of the needle. If you've tried this diversion yourself, you know it usually works quite well as the mind allows the muscles to relax with the focus diverted from the injection site. This common experience provides a prime example of the psychosomatic (mind-body) principle in action, showing how the mind and body are inextricably linked.

Virtually all parents have also experienced this link through the effectiveness of reading a child a bedtime story. As the tale absorbs the imagination, and as the imagination displaces the tensions of the day, deep relaxation follows and helps the child fall asleep. As it turns out, this same story-induced relaxation also helps strengthen the immune system and reduce sensations of pain. The act of daydreaming, incidentally, has a similar effect.

VISUALIZING FREEDOM FROM PAIN

This psychosomatic phenomenon has undergone considerable research in recent years (though not nearly as much as is called for), such as that described in a University of Arizona study, headed by the world-renowned Dr. Andrew Weil, on the use of guided imagery and relaxation techniques in the alleviation of Recurrent Abdominal Pain (RAP). A study of 94 cancer patients, published in 1995, revealed that those who were given visualization training as part of their healing reported experiencing less pain than those who weren't given the training. One year later, another study revealed the benefits of guided imagery in alleviating postoperative pain among children.

It is widely believed that children are, in fact, better than adults at employing visualization and relaxation techniques to alleviate pain and other physical problems, probably because children, more comfortably than adults, employ their imaginations and have yet to cement certain suppositions and preconceived notions in their minds about "reality." As good fortune would have it, a child's characteristically "wild" imagination and penchant for make-believe play can be one of the greatest assets in combating various physical ailments.

What Else Visualization May Help

Patients have experienced many therapeutic benefits using these techniques to deal with all sorts of medical conditions, including:

- headaches (including migraines)
- nausea and vomiting
- high blood pressure
- muscle pain (neck, shoulders, lower back)
- dental pain
- ear, nose, and throat pain
- asthma
- phantom limb pain
- HIV-related neuropathy
- heart-related chest pain
- digestive difficulties (including acid reflux and irritable bowel syndrome)
- cancer (and the symptoms associated with chemotherapy treatment)
- diabetes
- infections
- postoperative recovery from surgeries

Research now shows us that positive imagery has quantifiable effects on the physical body, namely in the release of immune-system-enhancing endorphins in the brain, as well as a marked rise in T-cells ("fighter cells") also involved in combating disease and infection. Deep relaxation also tends to make the mind more open to suggestion, this susceptibility forming the very foundation of more defined relaxation and visualization techniques such as hypnosis.

Pain and Sleep

Another obvious, though often overlooked, correlation between pain, the mind, and healing is that pain often impedes restful sleep, a significant aid in the body's healing process; with pain disturbing a patient's restful sleep, the healing process is naturally interrupted, too.

How to Help Your Child Relax and Visualize the Pain Away

Parents can facilitate this healing relaxation for their children in a number of ways:

- Encourage, for example, deep abdominal breathing
- Consider another technique for reducing discomfort and bodily tension called Progressive Muscle Relaxation, which essentially involves imagining each muscle in the body, one by one, relaxing
- Don't overlook gentle massage, proven to promote deep, healing relaxation

Parents can also facilitate pain relief through visualization as well by encouraging the child to imagine the pain or disease as a tangible object that can then be eradicated by a benevolent force (such as a rotten apple eaten away to nothing by an army of friendly bug helpers, or a black blob consumed by white light), or by encouraging the child to imagine herself in a soothing environment and pleasurable circumstances (such as floating on a raft on a calm, blue lake or engaging in a favorite sporting activity). Bubbles popping, stormy nights giving way to clear and sunny days, re-experiencing a funny moment encountered on TV, in a storybook, a movie, or real life, and stuffing one's pain or illness inside a magic box are all common and useful visualizations. Engage all the senses in the visualization—sight, sound, taste, touch, smell—to enhance the beneficial effects.

Meditation, hypnosis, and biofeedback are a few commonly practiced methods of relaxation and visualization, and doctors worldwide are increasingly incorporating these tools into their patients' pain management programs. But there are no hard and fast rules for practicing relaxation and visualization on one's own. There is no right or wrong way to do it, so long as you perceive the techniques as beneficial. Positive thinking is also a component of consciously harnessing the mind-body connection.

In simple and wonderful truth, relaxation and visualization can be used to great effect as both analgesic (for relief from pain) and anesthetic (for prevention of pain). In most cases, the mind-body connection is only partially effective for ameliorating the physical ailments and symptoms people experience, but it is nevertheless a significant part. Parents can indeed help their children accomplish a great deal in the healing process—including overcoming sleep troubles—by incorporating relaxation and visualization techniques in their children's program of recovery.

Chapter 13

Howard/Maya

Interviewed:	Howard
Child:	Maya, age 24, maturational age 12
Complaints:	*Anxiety*
	Insomnia
	Guilt
	Agitation

☙ • ☙

Please introduce *yourself.*

I'm Howard. I'm a psychiatric social worker.

Please tell me a little about the client you're here to discuss?

I have a 24-year-old Indian woman named Maya who is mentally retarded and has a very severe case of anxiety and difficulty sleeping.

And if you were to estimate her maturational age, would you guess it to be?

Intellectually, I'd say she is around age 12, or early teens in her thinking.

What sort of treatment has she been receiving for her anxiety so far?

She was put on Thorazine for extreme agitation.

How long has she been on Thorazine?

She's been on 150 milligrams of Thorazine at night for about a year.

And had she shown any psychotic symptoms?

At first, some staff thought that there was probably some psychosis involved, but I don't think so.

Why do you think she ended up on antipsychotic medication then?

She's extremely anxious and feels tremendously guilty about things and has real catastrophic thinking about the future.

I wonder why somebody chose Thorazine over an anti-anxiety agent, though.

I'd have to go back and check her chart at this point, but I think her high degree of agitation made her appear psychotic. She acts out in very agitated, childish ways. She used to throw things. She would break windows. I don't think her doctors even tried anti-anxiety agents with her. They must have suspected a psychotic process, but we haven't really observed any in over a year and a half. But the Thorazine pretty much immobilized her. In fact, she was overmedicated.

How long has she been here in the United States?

About five years, but she's been back and forth between India and here. When she was in India, she could not obtain the Thorazine. They would put her on an alternative medication by injection.

Do you know what she was on in India?

Well, when she went over there this last time, she took a two months' supply of Thorazine with her but she ran out. And they put her on another medication that just agitated her more. She just came back to the United States and she has lost some ground.

So she tolerated the Thorazine, even though she's apparently not psychotic?

She had been off the Thorazine for a while but she is very agitated and not sleeping well. We have the choice of putting her back on Thorazine or trying something different.

What is her sleep problem?

She ruminates. She stays up and ruminates about everything. Worries about the future, feels guilty about the past.

How long is she taking to get to sleep?

She says she takes hours to fall asleep. And then it's not restful sleep because she tosses and turns all night. Often she gets back up and walks around at night. She'll just be agitated, up wandering. Sometimes she says she even comes in the middle of the night to wake up her brother at 3:00 in the morning to talk about things that are upsetting her.

You said she is only getting how many hours each night?

Maybe six at the most. She does not sleep easily at all. It's toss-and-turn sleep—very anxious.

༄ • ༄

After speaking with Howard, I gave him the *Magic Carpet* and *Playhouse on the Beach* CDs to try with Maya. I chose children's programs even though she was 24-years-old because Howard judged her maturational age as only about 12. He stopped by soon thereafter to report on her progress.

THREE WEEKS LATER

So you tried using the **Magic Carpet** *program with Maya?*

Right. But first I listened to it myself so I would know what I was giving to her.

And you thought that it might be more appropriate to try a children's program rather than an adult program?

Yes, because Maya has borderline intellectual functioning. She has an IQ of between 67 and 80 on the various indices. So it seemed more appropriate to start her out with a children's program. I thought it was something she could relate to.

So you reviewed it first. What was your experience with it? How many times have you listened to it?

I listened to it once, and the one time I listened I had a very emotional experience. I started crying during it, which was totally unexpected, because I'm not the type of person who usually cries. It just triggered all sorts of childhood emotions and feelings, body feelings that I hadn't felt since childhood.

Why do you think you cried?

It was sort of a joyful feeling and a sad feeling at the same time. Sad because it represented feelings that I hadn't experienced for a long time. They had been buried.

So, you realized that you had kind of lost part of yourself?

Yes, sad because I realized I had lost part of myself, but happy at the same time because I was filled with a joyful feeling.

Has that experience affected you since then in any way?

I think it's still affecting me.

How long ago was that?

That was about three weeks ago.

How has it affected you?

All the animism in the CD kind of put me back in touch with nature, and I'm sort of reaching to more sensitively integrate myself with nature now, and I'm enjoying the pleasures of life more, maybe the subtler things that I had lost awareness of before.

Do you find yourself feeling more?

Yeah, as a matter of fact, I have. Even my wife and I are becoming more childlike together, which is a lot more fun. It's very subtle. This is after only one listening. It was a very profound experience.

So you went on to give this program to Maya.

After my experience with the *Magic Carpet* program, which really validated it for me, I was looking forward to trying it with her.

So what happened?

At first she had poor concentration and gave up trying, and I just encouraged her to keep listening in order to try to relax a little more and get into it to the extent that she could. And little by little, she started falling asleep before the CD was finished. And this has only been after a week and a half of listening.

What does she say about her sleep now? How many hours is she able to sleep?

She's sleeping very well, about eight hours continuously. And she's not getting up during the night and she's falling asleep before the CD is over. And this is very impressive because here is a 24-year-old woman who had to wake people up to talk about what she was ruminating about. She's not doing that anymore.

Is she any different during the day?

I can't really tell yet. She was in India for six months this time, and she is still working through returning this last time. She's readjusting to America, readjusting to living with her two brothers, who have had a hard time dealing with her symptoms, so this is just the beginning again of readjustment. We're going to have to follow her a little more.

That'll be interesting. Thank you for sharing your experiences with her and I'd like to check with you in the future.

Let's do that.

∽ • ∾

ONE WEEK LATER

∽ • ∾

It's one week later now, and you're still using **Magic Carpet** *with this patient?*

Yes.

OK. And you found **Magic Carpet** *to be effective in terms of her sleep problem?*

Yes, after a few days of program use she was able to go to sleep before the CD finished, which was quite quick. Now that another week has gone by, she's reporting that she's sleeping very well every night, listening to the CD, and drifting off very quickly.

So this new sleep pattern has been maintained. Any reports of improvement in her daytime behavior?

It's a little early to tell yet. I need to get objective feedback from her brothers. She feels she is still having a lot of communication problems, but her behavior, she reports, has been a lot more under control.

Well, thank you very much. I'd like to continue to follow up on this case.

My pleasure.

ONE MORE WEEK LATER

It's now been another week since we talked.

Right. Maya reported that she discontinued using *Magic Carpet* last week and she says she's had no problem sleeping anymore.

Despite the fact she is not using the CD now, she goes to sleep quickly?

She reports that she goes right to sleep and doesn't have any problems.

How is her therapy coming along? What's going on in general with her?

She's struggling with some issues. She's thinking about moving out on her own, away from her family, which is very significant, because they've been living together for a long period of time. But she wants to move out on her own now.

Has she brought up those kinds of issues before?

Actually, she hasn't. Her plan was to live with her brothers forever, and now, even though she's a little anxious about it, she's now planning on getting her own apartment. That's a real significant change for her.

Anything else to report?

No, that's about it. But I have to say she has made some rather remarkable and unexpected improvement and all without medications.

Thank you very much for discussing this case.

You're very welcome.

One more thing. You mentioned on the phone this morning that last night you used the adult sleep program yourself. Would you mind telling me more about that?

I had a particularly disturbing series of events happen last night and felt like it was going to be real hard to relax and fall asleep. And I put on the adult sleep CD, and even though I was still thinking about the problems, listening to the CD in the background, it still worked. I felt my muscles turn into butter, and just drifted off and caught myself in that half-in-and-half-out dream state and reached over and clicked off the machine and went right to sleep. And that was after a particularly difficult night.

Did you feel any differently when you woke up? Anything unusual?

Yes, I did. I felt more centered, and not upset about the events of the previous night. I felt better able to handle them.

Better than you expected?

Much better than I expected.

Really?

Much better. I anticipated waking up very intensely upset over what had occurred. And the events were the same, but the way I was handling it was quite different.

Thank you.

My pleasure. Really.

ADULT USE OF CHILDREN'S PROGRAMS

This interview reveals about the programs an interesting and unexpected application quite different from those we've explored to this point, namely, their effectiveness in use for adults as well as for children. Many of the adults interviewed in this book had reviewed the children's programs, either prior to or along with their children's first listening, primarily in order to monitor and understand what their children would be hearing. But in this most recent of cases, we find the practitioner actually having used the programs for his own benefit, with results certainly as compelling as some of the children we've studied.

STIRRING UP EMOTIONS

Howard, an experienced psychiatric social worker, had a profoundly moving and deeply personal experience listening to *Magic Carpet* himself prior to recommending it to Maya. In fact, you'll recall, he literally started to cry and reported feeling both sad and joyful at the same time, which, for him, I consider a very positive response to the program. I am confident that this visceral reaction of Howard's occurred because some aspect of the children's programs touched a core part of his being that was hidden by all the obstructive and inhibiting constructs of age and maturity.

In his own description of the experience, he even referred to childhood emotions that had been "buried." This burying of emotions recurs as a common theme in human experience. And the very unburying, experiencing, and—in the best of cases—resolving of these emotions form the basis of certain traditional adult psychiatric therapies.

LOSS OF SELF

The "losing" of oneself occurring at some early point in life is the very source of many mental and emotional disorders persisting throughout one's adult life. And it is often the "finding" and embracing of those lost parts of us that facilitates the greatest resolution of such problems. This pervasive phenomenon helps us begin to understand how and why a program directed towards children can have such potent benefits for adults as well—benefits as lasting as they are profound.

RECONNECTING: WITH THE CHILD WITHIN AND WITH MOTHER NATURE

Let me mention a couple of other points Howard made before I move on to Maya's experiences.

First, *Magic Carpet* helped Howard and his wife to be more "childlike" in their interactions together. Presumably he's referring here to a greater sense of lightheartedness, playfulness, and receptivity to the wondrousness of life and the world in which we live. Second, this development leads us to Howard's other pertinent observation: the powerful effects of reconnecting with nature through use of the programs.

Much of our adult stress comes not from the natural world but from civilization, a collection of human-devised constructs. Therefore, by evoking the simple beauty and bounty of our natural environment, we are better able to reconnect with our essential source, our "soul" or "spirit" if you will, devoid of those previously mentioned obstructive and inhibiting constructs of man-made society.

EMOTIONAL INTELLIGENCE

Let's move on, now, to Maya. You'll recall, although 24 years old, she had an estimated maturational age of half that. This is more common than one might think (if not as dramatic a divide). Many adults have what's termed an "emotional intelligence" moderately to excessively lower than that which would be considered "appropriate" for their chronological age. I believe it's safe to assume that most people reading this have at least some understanding of, and experience with, people walking around in bodies older than their "personalities," or maturational levels.

Even those of us whose emotional intelligence lines up in more appropriate and balanced accord with our chronological age can still relate to the feeling of that "inner child" always being with us, of carrying the child we once were around with us throughout the whole of our lives. To this child within, these programs speak. And because of this inner child, programs like these, although designed specifically for children, nonetheless often appeal to us "grown-ups," too.

BREAKING DOWN EGO BARRIERS

As adults, when stressed, we typically revert back to fundamental reactions and coping mechanisms developed early in life, in a sense temporarily "regressing" to our younger selves. It is this part of us that can be so helpful for wounded adults to reach in order to heal their deepest pain. And it is therefore to this part of us that efforts such as psychodynamic or insight-oriented psychotherapy are often directed.

I believe the simplicity of tone and the vividness of the imagery in these programs can help break through many of the barriers our armored and world-weary egos build up against our own healing, betterment, and positive change. As I wrote in the *Introduction*, children are superior to adults at receiving and integrating the benefits of relaxation programs like these, precisely because they have yet to build up obstacles, such as cynicism and doubt.

But that doesn't mean adults cannot reap the rewards of these programs (as it likewise does not mean that children can't be hindered by their own budding cynicism and doubt—especially when observing the adults around them).

Receiving and integrating as an adult the benefits of a children's relaxation program (or any such system designed to improve the lives of children) merely takes a willingness to let down one's guard and open up to the possibility of positive change. And this receptivity anyone of any age can permit at will. William Taylor Coleridge, late in the 18th century, in discussing the relationship between the reader and the written art, wrote of such a "willing suspension of disbelief."

These programs, designed specifically to benefit children, can help adults willingly suspend disbelief to overcome and reprogram negative patterning that has been dragging them down and holding them back for the better part of their lives, and in some cases even more effectively than programs geared toward adults.

In the final interview that follows, we meet another adult who used the programs herself, right along with her children, and who received healing benefits at least as profound as those her children received.

Chapter 14
Frances/Clarissa, Danielle, and Tanya

Interviewed:	**Frances, age 36**
Complaints:	*Mood swings*
	General anxiety
	Depression
	Anger/Rage
	Migraine headaches
	High blood pressure
	Insomnia
	Nightmares
Child:	**Clarissa, age 13**
Complaints:	*Worry/Nervousness*
	Resistance to reading
	Bedtime resistance
	Separation anxiety
	Low self-esteem
	Trouble falling asleep
Child:	**Danielle, age 15**
Complaints:	*Negativity*
	Trouble expressing feelings
	Poor academic performance
Child:	**Tanya, age 17**
Complaints:	*Low self-esteem*

How old are your children?

Tanya is 17, Danielle is 15, and my baby, Clarissa, just turned 13.

And your youngest is the one having difficulties?

> Clarissa is a constant worrier. She worries about all sorts of things that most 13-year-olds wouldn't be concerned about. She came home from school saying, "Mom, I'm so worried about my friend, Tasha. She's Buddhist and I'm afraid when she dies she's going to go to hell, and I really like her." And I said to her, "Don't worry, just pray for her."

Is she also having problems falling asleep?

> All the time, since she was around 6 years old. She goes to bed about 10:00 and she's often still awake at midnight. So it takes her at least one to two hours. In fact she's usually still awake when I go to bed, so she's always begging me to let her get in bed with me to sleep. And I end up saying, "Now look, you've got to go to sleep now. If you don't go to sleep . . . ." I have to threaten her with taking something away. She needs an incentive to go to sleep.

How has her behavior been during the day?

> She has always been the kind of kid where if any little thing happens to her, it just knocks her on her back. The smallest disappointment just causes her to well up with tears, and she feels destroyed. So she avoids trying new things.

And how is she doing in school?

> Well, she's always been a good student, but she doesn't like to read. She has a high reading level—actually, she reads at a high school level—she just doesn't want to read. She has no interest in reading. Like I keep getting notes from school saying she isn't completing her reading logs. Students are supposed to read and then comment on what they read.

How about the rest of your girls?

> Well, Danielle's always been a pretty negative person, always closed-off emotionally. I think a lot of it may have to do with how explosive I've been. I think she's sort of been conditioned to keep everything inside for fear of how I'm going to react. It's made her real sneaky.

Sneaky?

> Like she won't tell me anything. She doesn't clue me in to anything about her life or her problems or how she's doing. Even when she's feeling good about something, she doesn't bother to fill me in about it.

This seems like a good time to move on to talking about you some. You've been experiencing some difficulties of your own.

> That's right. You've read my file. I'm a wreck.

Explain a little about the specific symptoms you're experiencing, both on and off medications.

Sometimes I feel so sick inside that I won't even leave the house, won't take a shower, won't brush my teeth, and won't comb my hair. It can get really bad.

How about your sleep patterns? How much sleep do you normally get?

Well, out of 24 hours I probably sleep about 18 and this is because of the medication I've been taking. But when I'm awake, I'm anxious all of the time and have to deal with feeling angry a lot.

And when you aren't taking medication how long do you sleep?

When I don't take the medication, my anxiety is out of control and I can go days without sleeping. Sometimes I can't even keep a sentence together and then my anger will come up again. I overreact to everything. I'm just over the top, all of the time. When I do take the medication it helps me to sleep and to organize my thoughts, but I'm too tired to do anything, and I'm still anxious and angry a lot. I struggled with this dilemma when they tried to send me back to work. I just couldn't function, on or off the medication, and that was going on when I was just being re-trained. I wasn't even answering phones yet, and I needed to be ready to give a lot of information to people. So there was no way I could do my job, and that's when they finally put me on disability.

How long had you been struggling with intense anger?

About six years, maybe even longer.

Were there things in your life that brought that on?

Yeah. I was being abused both physically and mentally. I was a single mom and I was stressing. I couldn't handle what life was bringing to me. I was trying to raise three girls by myself. I was going through a divorce, and I was trying to find work but I didn't have a car. Everybody has it tough, I know that, but it was more than I could handle. And as my anger built up I got really scared for my kids. I felt the potential for me to become an abusive mom, like what I went through with my own mother, and I wasn't going to let that happen. I was determined to protect my children, even if I had to protect them from me. That's what I was thinking. And that was right before I was diagnosed as having bipolar disorder.

What happened then?

I ended up in a new relationship, but we broke up soon after because he just couldn't deal with me. You know, when I'm okay, I'm really okay, but when I'd get suicidal, he just couldn't handle it. I turned to the left, as they call it in my neighborhood, and there was no bringing me back.

So, that was the state you were in when I first started treating you, and you were taking a number of medications?

Yes, I had been taking Risperdal, Lamictal, Wellbutrin, and Celexa for three years, except during times I couldn't afford them, and even though I'm functioning very well, they aren't helping with everything.

Like what?

I'm still not getting the kind of rest I need. I still have nightmares. I still can't get restful sleep, even though I'm taking the medications. My body finally got kind of used to them so I'm not as sleepy as I had been in the past. Instead of sleeping 18 hours I'm now sleeping maybe 10.

And you have said it's not a very restful 10 hours either. Is that right?

No, not restful at all. I'll usually be up at least a couple times a night walking around the house all groggy, checking on the kids, checking the doors, going back to bed, getting up to see if I left a light on.

Are there any other problems you are struggling with?

Yeah, I'm also taking Inderal for high blood pressure. I weigh 300 pounds, so I'm obese and I have high blood pressure. I also get migraines a lot.

How often are you having migraines?

At least once a month, usually more. They usually happen around my menstrual period. When I was working, I used to get them so bad that I couldn't even see my computer screen. The light made my eyes ache to the point that I couldn't stand it. I would get nauseated and throw up. I had to take off from work pretty often when I had them. And I've continued to have them. It's depressing.

Has depression been something you have struggled with often?

Depression has been almost constant with me in the past. I have tried to kill myself five times. My first suicide attempt was when I was just a teenager.

❧ • ☙

After speaking with Frances some more, I gave her the *Magic Carpet* and *Country Friends* CDs to try with Clarissa, as well as a couple of my adult CDs, *Natural Relaxation* and *Natural Sleep*, to try herself. She returned four months thereafter to tell me how it all went.

❧ • ☙

*So, I gave you **Magic Carpet** and **Country Friends** for your youngest at the same time that you started using the adult programs.*

I came home that day with this bag that you gave me with the CD player and the CDs and also the Magic Massager you gave me.

Oh, the Magic Massager! We love the Massager! My girls have had such a great time with it. It's so cute how they massage each other, and are always bargaining for more. "I'll do this or that for you if you'll massage me for another 15 minutes." Usually they work it out, but sometimes I've heard them say, "Oh, you are asking for too much, I'll just massage myself." It's such a nice way for them to get closer to each other. I think it's brought them closer in a number of ways. When they start using it I can hardly get it away from them.

Anyway, so when I brought the CDs home I tried to make it as positive as possible and said, "I'm going to start listening to these special CDs to help me relax and sleep and you get to listen to your own special CDs." And she was like, "Really?" Anything that I do, Clarissa wants to do, so she was happy. She started by listening to *Magic Carpet* and she really liked it. She started sleeping better right away. Now, the other girls are a little older but they all sleep in the same room, so when Clarissa plays it on her boom box, they all hear it. Before long the older ones were saying, "We've heard *Magic Carpet* too much, it's for kids." But whenever I check on them, they're all asleep before it's over. I don't check on them nearly as often as I used to because they're asleep so fast—just knocked out.

How has Clarissa specifically responded to the program?

Her nighttimes are different. She actually likes going to bed now. She hasn't asked to sleep with me since she started the programs. She may get up in the morning and come in and cuddle with me, but that's all. And it's a lot more than just the sleep issue, too. She doesn't need me so much in general. She's much more self-sufficient now. She used to be kind of clingy. She was never an independent spirit; always needed to have someone with her everywhere she went and everything she did. I'm not going to say it's gone completely, but it's greatly improved. Before, I couldn't leave her at home by herself. Not that she wasn't trustworthy; she just got too anxious being alone. If I was going somewhere, she always asked if she could come along. Now she's happy staying home by herself. It's just not a problem any more.

Anything else?

The other day, I took Clarissa with me to college and she sat there doing her homework while she listened to *Country Friends* with her headphones on. She says it helps her to concentrate. I wouldn't have thought that would work.

So have you noticed any other changes with Clarissa since she started listening?

Confidence. She recently got up the nerve to try out for cheer squad and she made it. And not only did she make it, she has been making up routines and the last couple weeks they put her in charge.

Are you saying that before using the programs she wouldn't have had the confidence to do that?

She would have been just dreaming about doing something like that. She wouldn't have even considered trying. Now, she doesn't care what others think so much. Even with

Chapter 14 Frances / Clarissa, Danielle, and Tanya

the coach, she keeps getting more and more confident. Like Clarissa started showing up with new routines she had worked out and her attitude was kind of, *"Hey coach, let me show you something I've been working on."* Just very confident, as if it didn't matter if the coach liked it or not. And now the coach has been approaching her, asking if she'd be willing to work out new routines when they need them.

With her increased confidence, they've moved her out in the front line and everything. Before her moves were unsure, but now you should see her, she's fierce and vigorous and hitting all her moves exactly. And her facial expressions have even changed. She has this big smile, she sticks out her tongue, she winks, she just shines. And this is all really new. She just didn't have that kind of self-confidence and poise before. And honestly, this all started right after she started listening to the programs.

Has her program use seemed to have any effect academically?

She reads now. Within the past four months this has happened. She's very focused when she reads now. She's even getting her reading logs done without any prompting. Before, she never read for fun. Now she's always asking me to take her to the library for more books. Around Christmas vacation, she started reading *Nancy Drew* mystery novels. She's started to realize that she has missed out on a lot because she wasn't reading.

Have the programs had any effect on your other children?

Well, Danielle seems like she may be getting some benefits. She's never had a problem going to sleep, but she has also been listening to *Magic Carpet* because Clarissa plays it on speakers. Well, right after she started listening, she suddenly began to enjoy school. Suddenly, I didn't have to prompt her anymore. She organized her notebook and began keeping everything really neat. Whereas before, she was scoring 20s out of 50, now she's getting 38 on up. Before she was just, "Whatever . . . I'm going to be a photographer, I don't really care." But now it's like she wants to work, and that's new.

Also, she's becoming much more positive. It's a pretty remarkable change. She's not being sneaky anymore either. She's been more open. She's been telling me everything. She doesn't seem to worry about how I'm going to react. This may have something to do with the fact that I have calmed down. She doesn't mind sharing her feelings with me. It feels like the bond between us has strengthened.

And what about your 17-year-old? She's been in the bedroom listening to the programs, too?

She has no problem sleeping. So there's been no change there. But she's always been very unsure of herself and that *has* changed. An example is her Tahitian Island dancing. Before, she would only dance if it was some kind of performance that was set up. Even if we begged her to dance for us, she wouldn't do it. Now she'll dance in front of anyone, anytime. She's very relaxed about it now. And when she dances—what a difference! Now she's completely into it. You know, it's kind of a sensual dance, and before she was reserved. She's not just going through the motions now, she's feeling it. It makes it much more exciting to watch.

She's gotten a whole lot more confident in general. I've seen it in the way she interacts with her friends and also with me. You know how I was in the past. Well, she's always been very careful not to invoke my rage. But lately, we joke around, and she doesn't act afraid of me anymore. And we've gotten a lot closer. She's more willing to tell me how she feels. But that goes both ways. I'm able to talk to her about how I'm feeling. Before I used the programs it was a lot harder for me when I felt so anxious about everything. Now that I'm calmer, I can tell her how I feel, too.

In fact, I was just talking to her about my concerns about her going off to college. I told her that I worry about the decisions she's going to be making about pledging and drinking alcohol and all the other temptations. I tell her, "I worry that you won't remember what you're there for." And I can tell her this now because I'm calm, and I know I won't get upset and overwhelmed.

Before, all I could do was try to not do anything that would make me feel more anxious. And she reassured me. She said, "Mom, you have taught me well. And I'm not going to drink and I'm not going to have sex. And I know why I'm going there, and it's to get an education and become a social worker." Anyway, she has been sharing stuff that she normally wouldn't. She's a very private person, and she's been opening up, and that's new for her.

Has there been any change in the way your daughters act toward each other?

Yes. They don't argue as much. You know sisters bicker, but it's been really mild lately. The biggest change has been that they seem happy for one another, when something good happens to one of them. They've never been happy for each other like that. And they have gotten closer. Now it's possible that the oldest going away to college has something to do with this. They realize they're not going to be the Three Musketeers anymore, but still, it seemed to happen right after they started listening to the programs.

And everybody is more into a routine now. They all go to bed and get up without me having to boss them around. Everybody enjoys going to bed now.

Even you?

Yes, even me. When I first started listening to the programs I listened to one and then another, and I was relaxed but still awake, but pretty soon I couldn't even get through one of them. And right around then, I quit taking Risperdal and Wellbutrin and Lexapro, because I couldn't afford my co-pays. Sorry, I didn't let you know, but there really wasn't anything that could be done about it. I only continued the Lamictal, but I was able to sleep—no problem. I was amazed.

Oh, I wanted to tell you about something I did that has been really helpful. Right around the time you gave me the audio programs, I made my bedroom into a place where I really wanted to be. I rearranged the whole room and made it feel nice and romantic.

I got rid of a bunch of junk. I put flowers around my bed and set up some soft lights. And when I started using the programs, my feelings and the feeling of my room began to match. It made it all more believable. Before it was like, "Oh, I really don't feel like taking a bath." And it was the programs that made me feel different. I started looking forward to going to bed.

I take me a nice relaxing bath every night now with all my little bath salts. I brush my teeth and floss, and comb my hair and put on my nice warm fluffy pajamas. And every night I look forward to this ritual that I do for myself. And then, to top it all off, I get in my nice soft sheets under my two comforters and I put my headphones on, and I'm in heaven, because I know I'm going to go drift to sleep in paradise and I'm going to stay asleep—like I don't have a care in the world. It's like I have a date with myself every night, and with God.

When I wake up in the morning, I feel like I've been on a spiritual journey. I really look forward to it. Kind of like, *"I've been out in the rain all day, and it's cold, and I've been dealing with traffic and grouchy people, and I get home and I can't wait to take a nice warm bath and then sink into my cozy bed."* That's how I feel now. I never used to look forward to going to bed. Now I can't wait.

How long did it take before you felt you were sleeping normally?

My sleep was better right away, but in about two weeks I was falling asleep within 15 or 20 minutes, sleeping through the night and waking up in the morning feeling completely rested and refreshed.

So, have the programs had any effect on your anxiety? Have you felt a shift?

Major shift. Like back then, I was experiencing serious road rage. One of the worst cases of road rage you've ever seen. If someone tried to cut me off, or whatever, I'd follow them to their home. It got to the point where I couldn't be in the car alone. People had to drive for me. It was that serious. That's just not happening anymore. I have no more road rage. I'm not the same person. Now, my kids say, "Mommy, why didn't you honk at that guy? Why don't you use the horn anymore?" And that's not what they used to say. Before it was, "You're not going to follow that car are you?"

But that's what I was doing and that's dangerous. You don't know what's going to happen because people are crazy! Now if someone cuts me off, I feel like, *"He saw me, he didn't care, it's not personal. It's not like he knows me. Oh well, what am I going to do? Follow him and try to strike up a conversation? Like there's going to be some real communication between us? I don't think so."*

I was having road rage even when I was taking Risperdal, which is a pretty powerful tranquilizer. We're learning about psychopharmacology in my psychology class, and we're talking about medications I've taken. I don't even need most of them now. There's no need for them, because I'm just not doing that anymore and that's just one of the changes that I've gone through.

What's been happening with all the medications you were on?

For the past three months I have only been taking Lamictal. In fact I haven't even needed to take the Inderal. My blood pressure has been normal. I have been taking my blood pressure weekly, because I give blood, and it's been normal the whole time. And another thing, I'm not having migraines since I started your programs.

None at all?

Nope, not one. Not since I started your programs.

And what's been happening with your depression?

Gone.

It's gone?

That's right.

Could you tell me more about that, please?

I can say that my depression was gone by Christmas, so it took about two months. Christmas is usually a really hard time for me. And this was one of our poorest Christmases. Usually, it's so hard for me because I can't buy the things that my children really need, but this Christmas was a breeze. It was like, "Okay, no problem kids. We don't have a big tree, but we can use this little one. And let's go on the Internet and find ways that we can make our decorations. And let's make presents for everybody."

And instead of me worrying about what I didn't have for people for Christmas, I wrote poems and baked pies. We made ornaments from paper. We learned how to make 3D snowflakes and decorated the tree with them. On Christmas day I cooked a wonderful meal, and I hadn't done that for ages. I had a guest over. I hadn't done that in forever. It was one of the best Christmases we've ever had. And usually around Christmas I'm so stressed that I feel awful. It was awesome.

It sounds like there's a lot that's new.

In the last four months there have been so many wonderful changes, and it's all been from the inside out. I keep a journal, so I've kept pretty good track of the changes I'm talking about. And I know when they happened, which was right after we all started listening to the programs.

You know, I can talk about all these changes that we've gone through, but I don't think you can really understand how dramatic it has been. I wish you could have seen what it was like around our house four months ago and you could then see what it's like now. I think that's the only way you could really understand what I'm trying to explain to you.

It's just amazing. Utterly amazing. And the idea that it all goes back to being able to relax—just being able to calm down. It's that easy. There's something to be said for being able to relax.

There's also something to be said for getting a good night's sleep.

That's for sure. I think it's the most valuable resource our bodies have for rejuvenation. A little mini-vacation of sorts. I've never been on a vacation my whole life. I've never gotten away from it all. Never taken my kids on a vacation. And I think it does something to you when you never get away, when you're always under the gun, pressure on you all the time. And, in fact, your body gets programmed to always be on alert, and you kind of get frozen in that state and feel helpless.

I started college right around the time that you gave me the programs, right? And one of the classes I'm taking is Psych 101. People have been sharing really openly in there and I've told them quite a bit about me. I was so excited last week to give a report as to how far I have come. Starting in October, when I first saw you, and now it's February and so many things have changed.

But anyway, what I was going to say was, in psychology class we studied how circus elephants are trained. When they're young, they attach them with heavy chains to a large stake in the ground. They struggle and pull at it but they can't break free, so they just give up trying. And from then on, even when they grow up to be these huge, strong animals, even a tiny thin rope will keep them there. As soon as they feel the slightest resistance, they just give up, even though they are now strong enough to pull the whole circus tent down. They no longer believe in their own strength.

It's learned helplessness and I can see how it has kept me stuck where I am. But it doesn't have to be that way. I'm poor, I'm a black woman, I live in the ghetto . . . . And without a break from all the emotions that weigh us down, it's easy to believe in limitations that aren't really there. When you go on vacation and get away from your usual way of thinking you have a chance to relax and see yourself differently. When you never go on vacation, when you never relax, you tend to keep thinking in the same old ways. You tend to just focus on survival and remain stuck.

And this is a way the programs have helped you?

Exactly. The sleep I get now is so different than before. The sleep I got before just wasn't restful. I used to have the craziest dreams—nightmares all the time. I'd wake up and the dreams seemed so real that I'd just be crying and it was hard to pull myself out of it. And I don't have nightmares now.

When I enter your 3D world of sound, it's so real that I actually feel like I'm there on that tropical island. And when I'm on the hillside overlooking the ocean, on the trail, or by the stream, or down on the beach I'm not that single, poor, black woman in the ghetto; I'm a child of God with as much potential as anyone else to create the life I want. It's up to me if I reach my goals or what I let stop me. No matter what's going on during my day, I know what awaits me. Each night I have a mini-vacation to look forward to. Each night I feel like I'm the richest person on earth. I do.

I never really enjoyed sleep before. It was just something I did because my body just had to. Now it's something I do because I love doing it. And there's a lot to be said for being able to step back and take stock. Yes, I live in the ghetto. And yes, I'm poor, and yes, there's no gas in my car, and there's no money in my bank account. But you know what? That's just how it is right now. It's not how it's going to be forever. And I'm not that elephant tied to the stake. If that elephant knew how powerful he was, he could just break loose and run out of that tent and be free. And that's how I feel right now; like nothing can stop me.

And I feel that way because I'm able to take stock of my life every night. It excited me when I learned about the autonomic nervous system, and that it could be reset. It's almost like praying for forgiveness, and having your slate wiped clean and being able to start all over, fresh. So it's almost like when I go to bed it wipes my slate, my day, clean. All the trash and all of the gunk, all that stuff, I don't absorb it anymore, it's all wiped clean. Before, I slept but I wasn't rested. I was still carrying around a bunch of crap. Before, when the medicine used to put me to sleep, I slept, but I wasn't rested, the crap was still there. I wish I had better words to describe this.

You're doing fine.

It's just . . . I don't wake up with all the stress that I woke up with before, the pressure of the world just weighing me down. I don't have that anymore. It all goes into the recycle bin, and when I wake up I'm ready for the day.

I used to go for as long as three days without taking a shower. Now when I get up I always take a shower. I want to do my hair, and I put my makeup on and I like to look pretty. I don't just put an outfit on, I want it to coordinate. I don't want it to just match; I want it to be fashionable. And my art teacher gave me a compliment, she said, "You're really a sharp dresser," and I hadn't heard that in years.

You're expressing your beauty.

I *am* feeling beautiful. I'm feeling like I'm an expression of the Most High. And I'm not fixing myself up to impress anyone. I'm doing it because I want to feel beautiful, because I'm tuning into my real nature, and it's beautiful.

You know, I'm originally from the country, and whenever I'm in a natural setting I feel close to God. So every night when I'm walking through nature or I'm on that beach, I'm with God. And the 3D sound makes it so real that I actually feel like I'm there. I don't get very far in the programs at night before I fall asleep, so sometimes I listen during the day, so I can be awake and enjoy being there in nature.

And you find that helps you, too?

It sure does. You know, I've had a hard time trying to explain what happened to me when I used your programs. I guess they're kind of like hypnosis, not exactly, but kind of, and you know what happens if you tell someone you are doing hypnosis? The image that comes to mind is of someone swinging a watch and saying, "Your eyelids are getting heavy," and they imagine someone acting like a fool and clucking like a chicken every time a certain word is said. You know that's what people think because of the entertainment industry. So if you say you are doing hypnosis, people just tune you out. I've kind of given up trying to explain what I've been doing to people. And when I tell people I'm not the same person, they don't know what I was like before anyway.

So you find that these positive changes have been showing up in all different areas of your life?

And especially at school. I tried going back to school a couple times in the past, but I got so anxious that I just couldn't do it. The first time I couldn't even get through orientation and the second time I only attended one biology class and I never went back. I was so anxious about the idea of taking tests, which has always been such a problem for me in the past, that I just couldn't see how I was going to do it. Well, I just finished my first quarter and I made the President's List.

What does the President's List mean?

I had a 4.0 grade average—straight A's. I've never done anything like that before. The last time I had good grades was in junior high school when I got mainly B's. Sometimes I'd get an A. But I haven't been in school since dinosaurs walked the earth, so getting straight A's was really something. It's a small Christian college with really nice teachers and I'm sure that kind of support helped. Besides being less anxious, I think the fact that I can sleep now is a big factor. I'm able to organize my day, and I'm alert. I can focus. I'm definitely more relaxed, too. Now I go into tests with a whole new attitude. I say to myself, "I know this material, and I can do this." Before, no matter how hard I studied or how well I knew the material, I'd just panic.

So would you say there has been a major shift in your confidence level?

Has there ever—a huge shift! I used to always worry about what other people thought about me. Now, I don't really care so much. I feel like I've been freed up from worrying about that. Another big shift has been my motivation. I remember in the past, when I was reevaluated for my disability, the examiner asked about my daily activities and almost all of my answers were, "I'm not motivated to do that." I felt that way about everything.

Now, I'm a different person. I just went to a community newspaper and asked them if I could write an article. Would you believe that I was invited to write a regular column? Here's the newspaper with my first one. I don't want to toot my own horn, but it's good. I already have my next six planned. I'm completely excited and motivated. You can't imagine how different this is for me.

I'm not saying that your programs are a miracle drug, but you have to wonder with all the things that have happened to me since I started using them. It's pretty amazing. My blood pressure returned to normal, my migraines are gone, I can sleep, my anxiety and depression are gone. I'm just so thankful—it's been an answer to my prayers.

Just learning how to relax is so important. I can't help but wonder how different my life might have been if I'd been able to use the programs years ago. Maybe I never would have been on disability. But "if" is the biggest word in the dictionary.

Indeed.

My next stop on this journey is making my body healthier. I weigh 300 pounds. I can say that now, but before I used to cry about it. I don't want to weigh so much. I want to be active, and I want to feel better. And that's my next challenge. The fact that I've gotten this far makes me know I can do it.

Even though now I don't care so much about what other people think of me, I want to lose weight. You know before, I kind of liked having the weight on me because I wasn't so attractive to men. There was a time when if a man approached me it was like, *"Okay, I'm cute? Well, why not?"* I really wanted to be around someone who thought I was cute and then I'd be stuck with some jerk.

I've made some poor decisions when it comes to men. It got to the point that I didn't want to feel cute, so I wouldn't have to deal with them. At least that was my excuse for gaining weight. So it seems like there's a man issue mixed in there somewhere. It's probably important that I deal with that. So I need to lose this weight for me. I want to feel healthy. I don't want to use any issues I have with men as an excuse any longer.

Good for you.

You know, I stopped buying all that crappy food I used to buy, and I'm now getting healthy snacks. I'm making a lot of changes. I'm avoiding fried foods now and I'm eating a lot more vegetables. And I'm also trying to get to where I enjoy exercising. I know that's an important part of this and I'm determined to do it now.

Is there anything else you'd like to share in this interview?

You know, I just wish I could take others on a tour of the dreams I have at night. It's hard to describe. I enter a world that's so wonderful. The programs take me into a world of nature that comes to life in a magical way. And from there I go on my own personal adventures. I have written about this in my journal, trying to describe what it's been like, but it's hard to do because it's so different from normal experience in this world.

When I put on a CD it's like my body just flips a switch. Like I said, at first I could listen to two CDs. But now, in 10 minutes, I'm not in this world any longer. These programs are awesome. I'm not sure you realize the implications of what you have created here. I'm sure you had an idea of what you expected them to do when you created them, but I doubt you could've imagined the effect they would end up having on people.

Look at me. When you consider all the medications I was taking and all the problems I was having, and now how different my life is, it's like a miracle. Most doctors would have looked at my diagnosis and my thick chart and just refilled my prescriptions and told me to go home and keep taking them. What else could they do? When I quit taking them in the past, I just fell apart.

But you gave me your programs and you encouraged me to see what I could do to help myself. And when I couldn't afford my medications I ended up taking a leap of faith, and the depression and anxiety didn't come back—unbelievable. I know that with bipolar disorder the only thing predictable is it's unpredictable, but so far so good.

I'm not sure you can really understand what all of this means to me. You gave me tools that I can use any time I need them, and they really work. You have empowered me. It's a skill I'll always have. I no longer feel like I have to depend on all those medications to just keep me calm enough to get through the day. Now I only take one medication, and I can't ever remember feeling this good. I'm not just functioning; I'm beginning to live the life I want to live. I start my days with enthusiasm, I'm productive and calm, and I'm enjoying what I'm doing most of the time. And when night comes, I look forward to going to sleep and getting the kind of rest that I've always needed.

When you look at my chart, you see someone with bipolar disorder, post-traumatic stress disorder, and generalized anxiety disorder, and you think, *"What a messed up girl."* But I don't match my chart anymore. And that's an accomplishment that I can hand back to you. You know, the way you have put these programs together, with the 3D sound and all, is pure genius. At least I haven't seen anybody else doing anything like this.

It's a pretty novel approach, no doubt, and I really do love working with the 3D sound, which is so perfect for my purposes. The soundtrack just sort of carries you along and your mind starts to fill in the pictures and pretty soon it turns into a kind of waking dream—sort of like virtual reality. And because it feels so real, it may have a lot greater impact on your subconscious mind, which probably reacts as though these little adventures in relaxation are *real—part of your life story. And because the subconscious doesn't deal with time in a linear fashion, perhaps it allows you to kind of re-write your personal history. In the same way that you return to times past or visit the future in your dreams, your subconscious mind may place these experiences of relaxation in the present, past, or future, so in a way it may be an opportunity to re-write the story of your life.*

Sure feels like it's helped me re-write my *entire* story. It's so wonderful to be able to say I'm a changed person and that I'm free from my past and finally creating the life I want for myself. And it's so reassuring to know that the programs will be available for me and my children the rest of our lives. I just know that I'll be able to handle whatever comes my way. Hallelujah!

Thank you so much for sharing your experiences.

Thank you for making it possible.

It's been my pleasure.

~ • ~

LOW SELF-ESTEEM

In this interview, both Frances and her daughters experienced problems of low self-esteem. It probably won't surprise you that this is a common issue that many people, young and old, face. What may surprise you, however, is how much sleep plays a role in these mental/emotional states.

Sleep and Self-Esteem

A 2004 study of over 2,000 Illinois students found that as children get increasingly fewer hours of sleep per night—as is typical with children advancing through their middle school years—they become increasingly prone to feelings of low self-esteem and depression. While acknowledging that emotional issues such as these are common in adolescents, researchers still concluded that decreased sleep was at least partially responsible and, conversely, that increased sleep could help mitigate feelings of depression and increase self-esteem.

The Role and Benefits of Self-Esteem

Self-esteem has been found a critical part of a person's success in life, whatever paths they may pursue, whatever their goals may be. Self-esteem helps people form healthy relationships and it helps them feel a sense of purpose and motivation to contribute to their world.

Threats to Self-Esteem

I've already discussed the issue of self esteem from a number of angles including the profound effect bedwetting and obesity can have on it, from shame and guilt. Furthermore, as you saw in the commentary on academic performance, reduced and disrupted sleep can hamper the development of a child's cognitive abilities. And when a child falls behind his classmates, self-esteem suffers, too.

Seven Pillars of High Self-Esteem

Nathaniel Branden, Ph.D., author of *The Psychology of Self-Esteem* and *The Six Pillars of Self-Esteem*, outlines six specific practices, the commitment to which can help increase a person's self-esteem:

- conscious living
- self-acceptance
- self-responsibility
- self-assertiveness
- purposeful living
- integrity

To Dr. Branden's list, I would add a seventh pillar: ***adequate restful sleep***.

In addition to improved quality of sleep and increased sleep duration, other factors that can help raise one's self-esteem include regular exercise and a balanced diet. As luck would have it, these factors also help increase sleep duration and improve quality of sleep.

The bottom line on self-esteem and sleep is that taking care of oneself is a key element of self-esteem and, in turn, adequate amounts of restful, healing sleep are key to taking care of oneself.

Part III
Other Considerations

Chapter 15

Strategies and Solutions for Childhood Insomnia:
Sleep Hygiene and Beyond

So far, I've concentrated on DreamChild *Adventures and on interviews* with some of the people who used the programs to significant benefit. In this section, I'll present some additional views on sleep dysfunction and traditional strategies that are taught in one form or another by most experts in the field of childhood sleep disorders for resolving or preventing these problems. You can, of course, use the audio programs along with these suggestions in order to create the most effective treatment possible to meet your individual needs.

The information that follows will simply introduce and summarize a number of strategies for you. You will then be in a much better position to determine what other resources may be of interest as you further refine your child's overall sleep program. You'll learn how to establish new patterns, habits, and routines that may help both your child and you to sleep better at night.

Sleep Hygiene

If there were a single concept that most closely encompassed all of these healthy sleep patterns, habits, and routines, it would be "sleep hygiene." Common, in fact, among all of the strategies and solutions outlined in this chapter—and more, in this entire book—is this pervasive concept of sleep hygiene, and an active awareness of it.

Sleep hygiene refers to the set of habits and guidelines that promote consistently restful and sufficient sleep at night and complete alertness during the day. It's what you can do, and in some cases *should not do*, to help your child sleep easily and well.

Like dental hygiene, sleep hygiene isn't just for children; it's for everyone, regardless of age. And like dental hygiene, instilling good sleep hygiene habits early on in life will promote the retention and sustaining of those good habits throughout one's lifetime.

Sleep hygiene can even help people avoid a bevy of the sleep-related disorders discussed throughout these pages. The clearest sign that someone has poor sleep hygiene (or could at least use some improvements in the area) is if they experience trouble sleeping at night and/or sluggishness during the day.

Childhood Sleep Problems that Can Be Sourced Back to Poor Sleep Hygiene

This would be a good spot to bring back to mind that list of childhood sleep problems I outlined in the introduction to this book:

- bedtime resistance
- anxiety about sleep
- sleep onset delay
- nighttime wakings
- inadequate sleep duration
- difficulty waking in the morning
- morning moodiness
- daytime sleepiness

Every one of these issues can be traced, at least in part, to a lapse or gap in some aspect of proper sleep hygiene—and by the same token, every one of these problems can be alleviated, again at least in part, by making the appropriate adjustments in sleep hygiene.

Benefits of Improving a Child's Sleep Hygiene

Even anxious children can experience transformative improvements in their sleep through adjustments in their bedtime habits and routines—so much so that it can leave them better prepared on mental, emotional, and physical levels to handle their anxieties in a more positive and healthy manner.

Guidelines to Good Sleep Hygiene

As I go through the various guidelines and practices incumbent in good sleep hygiene, many items may be familiar to you from other parts of the book. That makes the following list a quick and handy reference for good sleep hygiene for children. Note that while many of these items are applicable to adults as much as children, the focus in this list is specifically on good sleep hygiene *for children*.

Bedtime Schedule

The first rule of good sleep hygiene is to create a bedtime routine that works for your child and you, and then *stick to it*. Inconsistency in a child's bedtime routine is most often at fault for any sleeping troubles that she experiences. Conversely, instituting regularity in bedtime practices has the most profound effect on reducing, or eliminating altogether, sleeping difficulties.

The Body Clock and Circadian Rhythms

Why is consistency so important? Because sleep and waking cycles need to act in harmony with all other body cycles, such as body temperature, metabolism, dietary schedule, and hormonal activity—what are collectively known as the "circadian rhythms." Our bodies are designed to naturally seek out what's known as a state of "homeostasis"—that is, the condition wherein all body systems find balance. In order to achieve that homeostasis, all these circadian rhythms must sync smoothly with one another.

Think of a bedtime schedule like setting your child's "biological clock"; set it right and your child's bodily rhythms begin to naturally run like clockwork.

How to Establish a Bedtime Schedule for Your Child that Works

To best establish a comfortable and effective sleeping/waking framework for your child, it helps to attend to her other daily circadian rhythms with as much vigilance as you do her sleeping/waking rhythms. Find consistency in the flow of your child's entire day, including schedules of eating, playing, napping, bathing, exposure to light and dark, and so on. Start with the events that already typically occur at the same time each day, and work from there. Perceiving your child's sleeping schedule as part and parcel of this larger set of circadian rhythms empowers you to create synergy in these rhythms and promote that optimum state of homeostasis in every waking and sleeping moment.

What follows next are some practical suggestions on how to establish a bedtime schedule that works. First of all, as implied above, to be complete, a bedtime schedule must include both a regular bedtime *and* a regular waking time. And integral in determining these times, of course, is making sure they are practical and realistic for both your child's and your other life schedules.

What's more—and what many parents fail to realize or, if they do realize it, fail to enforce—is that this bedtime schedule should be consistent seven days a week. If you must adjust it for weekends, then don't adjust it by more than an hour in either direction, or else you'll defeat the whole purpose of trying to instill a natural circadian rhythm in your child. Her physiology simply will not know when it is time to sleep or be awake. And this goes double for teenagers.

Common Pitfall: Your Own Schedule's Irregularity

Adults, of course, find this framework a challenge because their own schedules usually differ from weekdays to weekends—and in many cases from weeknight to weeknight. This irregularity in their own schedules makes it particularly difficult for parents to enforce a regular bedtime schedule for their child each and every night of the week, but it makes it no less necessary. Children need to be coached into a successful adulthood (again, this might go double for teens.)

Optimal Sleep Duration for Children

At the same time, in order to be effective, the sleeping and waking times you set must not merely be consistent and practical, they must also enable your child to get just the right amount of sleep needed—not too little and not too much—which is critical. The ideal amount of sleep at any given age varies widely between individuals, and adequacy of sleep should be determined by a careful evaluation of symptoms, but some general sleep guidelines are as follows:

Ages 3-5: 11-13 hours per day
Ages 5-12: 9-11 hours per day
Ages 12-18: 9-10 hours per day

Sleeping soundly at night and living an active, alert waking life can become second-nature, a healthy habit that may be carried throughout one's lifetime.

BEDTIME ROUTINE

The second rule of good sleep hygiene, and just as important as the first, is setting up a regular bedtime routine for your child, about a half-hour long, leading up to bedtime itself, which involves comforting and familiar activities that are also relaxing.

WHY A BEDTIME ROUTINE IS SO IMPORTANT

One significant reason children function best with a certain amount of structure is that uncertainty, not surprisingly, has been shown to foster anxiety in children ... and anxiety is the greatest enemy of sleep. But children only experience this sense of structure, once it's established, if you consistently enforce it. When you make an exception, even a rare one, you encourage resistance to the very rules you want followed; then both you and your child will feel frustrated.

It definitely takes effort to set, enforce, and adhere to a consistent bedtime routine, but it takes considerably more effort to deal with a child who doesn't have such structure and consistency in her life. So while your child may not particularly welcome the idea of a clear and consistent bedtime routine or schedule, especially at first, you can take heart that the benefits for all concerned will quickly become apparent and, in time, she may even grow to enjoy it and look forward to it.

WHAT NOT TO DO 30 MINUTES BEFORE BEDTIME

Thirty minutes before bed is the time for her to start winding down, not up. To be avoided during this critical time period are:

- heavy emotional conversations
- TV
- video games
- active, rough-and-tumble play or cardiovascular/aerobic exercise
- caffeine (chocolate, caffeinated teas, and some sodas)
- lots of liquids (water, juice, milk)*
- big meals and sugary snacks*

[* *A note on these last two items*: It turns out certain light snacks can actually help a child, once she falls asleep, to stay asleep. Foods with predominantly carbohydrates and proteins (such as milk and cookies), and foods with tryptophan (milk, turkey) both fall into this category. *Just remember to keep bedtime snacks light.*]

Good bedtime routine activities include:

- taking a warm bath
- reading a story together
- quiet, relaxing family time

- listening to tranquil music, nature sounds, or a relaxation CD
- stretching

As children grow older you can be more flexible with bedtime routines, which may grow to include a walk outside, a chat on the back porch about the day's events or future plans, or perhaps playing a board game or card game or doing a puzzle together. Older children may want to retire to their room to read, listen to music, or work on a favorite hobby before retiring for the night, and possibly listening to a sleep program.

Whatever activities you and your child decide upon, the cornerstone of your child's bedtime routine is that she knows what time she is to slip into her pajamas and brush her teeth, what time to be in bed, and how much time she can spend on in-bed activities such as reading or listening to a sleep program.

THE FOUNDATION OF GOOD SLEEP HYGIENE

These two "rules" then—a regular bedtime schedule and a regular bedtime routine—comprise the foundation of good sleep hygiene. From there it's only a matter of refining various habits, behaviors, circumstances, and beliefs. For your convenience, I've divided those refinements into two categories: *Environmental Sleep Hygiene* and *Daytime Sleep Hygiene*.

ENVIRONMENTAL SLEEP HYGIENE

Certain qualities of the setting in which you put your child down to sleep can play a significant role in the quality of her sleep:

- **set a bedroom temperature that's comfortable and will remain consistent throughout the night**, erring on the cooler side as it's more supportive of healthful sleep than an excessively warm room (that being anything over 75 degrees); and keeping that temperature consistent throughout the night can help avert nighttime wakings
- **make the room sufficiently dark**; a small nightlight is okay, if needed, but too much brightness interferes with restful sleep
- **ensure sufficient ventilation/air circulation**, such as by cracking the door open or using a ceiling fan set on low; refrain, however, from leaving a window wide open all night for both safety and health reasons (*additional air quality solutions follow at the end of this list*)
- **provide your child a quiet sleeping environment**, for reasons that should be obvious
- **shut off the television** and, what's more, take the television out of your child's bedroom; recall from *Bedtime Routines* above that all television-viewing should cease at least 30 minutes before bedtime anyway
- **keep the bed for sleeping**, in other words refrain from getting your child in the habit of associating her bed with anything other than sleeping, such as playing, reading, eating, or watching TV; for this reason, the value of children's custom theme beds and playhouse beds that have become somewhat popular of late is questionable

- **dress your child in comfortable pajamas/nightclothes**, as the more comfortable she is the easier time she'll have falling asleep and staying asleep
- for the same reason, **provide your child with a comfortable mattress and pillows, bedsheets, and blankets**
- **keep alert for dust, dust mites, and other allergens commonly found in beds and bedrooms**; helpful air quality solutions include:
  - keeping pets out of children's bedrooms
  - replacing old carpets and pillows/bedding/mattresses
  - cleaning out ducts and furnace filters
  - employing an air conditioner or HEPA air filter

DAYTIME SLEEP HYGIENE

Many of the factors that influence your child's sleep the most don't even occur at night. On the contrary, a variety of habits and behaviors that have a major impact on her sleep occur in broad daylight.

The following are suggested daytime behaviors supportive of good sleep hygiene:

- **expose your child to sunlight first thing in the morning**, as soon as possible after waking, as it helps to set her circadian rhythms for the rest of the day (and long-term for the rest of her life); additionally, ensure your child gets sufficient exposure to natural sunlight on a daily basis
- **avoid naps** (with the exception of very young children), as it can both lead a child to be less sleepy at bedtime and disrupt her natural circadian rhythms, or sleeping/waking patterns
- **discuss your child's medicines with her pediatrician**, as some children's medications (including prescription drugs, over-the-counter medicines, and all-natural/herbal remedies) could have side effects that interfere with your child's restful sleep; if your child is using such a medication, your doctor can usually help you find adequate alternatives devoid of these side effects
- **don't use your child's bedroom for punishments or time-outs**, as a child must feel comfortable, safe, and happy to be in her bedroom in order to fall asleep easily and sleep soundly—all of which are prevented when she starts associating her bedroom with punishment
- **monitor the content of your child's television viewing, Internet surfing, and video game playing**, as exposure to excessively violent, disturbing, or confusing images could be responsible for many sleep disturbances, such as nightmares
- **confront bullying or other prevalent emotional issues in your child's daily life**, as any number of daily stressors—from being subjected to bullying on a daily basis, to experiencing trouble in school, to facing emotional troubles at home like a divorce, a death in the family, a move, or sibling rivalry—could directly impact your child's sleep; exploring the suggestions given in *Chapter 17: Strategies and Solutions for the Problem of Anxiety* would also fall into this category of good sleep hygiene

Consider these the *Four Cornerstones of Good Sleep Hygiene*:

- Bedtime Schedule
- Bedtime Routine
- Environmental Conditions of the Bedroom
- Daytime Behaviors and Habits

Improvements in your child's sleep patterns likely won't happen overnight, but once you begin implementing good sleep hygiene practices in your child's life, you're bound to notice positive results in their due course.

If you do implement these suggestions and your child isn't eventually getting a complete and restful night of sleep on a nightly basis, then it's time to reevaluate your practices and make the appropriate adjustments where it seems appropriate until your child is getting that complete and restful night of sleep every night.

BEYOND SLEEP HYGIENE

As you undergo this process of reevaluating and refining, you may start by examining the *Four Cornerstones of Sleep Hygiene* as they relate to your child's life. But do keep in mind that these aren't the only factors that could affect your child's sleep for better or for worse. The remainder of this chapter is devoted to those additional factors beyond sleep hygiene that could help you help your child to get the regular good night's sleep she needs.

SLEEP ASSOCIATIONS

One of the foremost authorities on children and sleeping is Richard Ferber, M.D., and in his seminal work on the subject, *Solving Your Child's Sleep Problems,* he outlines a philosophy on helping children develop healthy sleeping habits that is still widely taught and practiced today.

According to Ferber, creating and stridently adhering to rituals and routines regarding bedtimes, pleasant practices that make a child look forward to bedtimes—and more, the right bedtime routines and rituals for their long-term well-being—is essential not only to helping a child develop good sleeping habits but in preventing a slurry of developmental problems and further sleeping difficulties in the future.

Ferber asserts that consistency is critical to ingraining positive sleep patterns and associations, and avoiding the adoptions of negative ones. This concept of "associations" is at the core of Ferber's philosophy on the importance of establishing consistent bedtime routines. "We all learn to fall asleep under a certain set of conditions," he notes. What for adults entails the right pillow, a particular side of the bed, a certain position, and reading, watching TV, or other bedtime ritual, begins in infancy with the particularity of conditions and circumstances under which a child learns to fall asleep and sleep soundly.

Pivotal among these life-essential bedtime associations, says Ferber, is the habit of sleeping alone—of temporary separation from the parents. Says Ferber, "Sleeping alone is an important part of his learning to be able to separate from you without anxiety and to see himself as an independent individual."

All childhood sleep experts address the importance of sleep associations. Note the cardinal rule:

All children should fall asleep under the same circumstances they will experience when they awaken during the night.

NIGHTTIME WAKINGS

Notice that I said *when* they awaken, not *if* they awaken. We all experience about five brief wakings during the night. We change body position, check our environment, straighten our blanket, or reposition our pillow. If all is well we return to sleep quickly, usually without remembering we were awake. But if you awaken to find things not as they were when you fell asleep, such as a missing pillow or a light on, you'll suddenly find yourself wide awake assessing the situation.

In order to fall back to sleep after nighttime wakings, children quickly develop the habit of needing the same circumstances around them as when they first fell asleep. If you allow a child to fall asleep on the couch in the den with the TV on, for example, and then you carry him to bed, he will awaken to a changed environment and may be unable to fall back to sleep on his own. He may begin to cry instead or come to your bedroom complaining that he can't sleep and want you to do something about it. And, of course, this isn't a time when you particularly want to be up with him because you also need your sleep.

ROCKING YOUNG CHILDREN TO SLEEP

A disrupted sleep association, for example, often becomes a problem for very young children who are regularly rocked to sleep and then laid to bed after they are asleep. They awaken to a new circumstance and react to the parent's absence and the absence of rocking. Although a young child will enjoy the relaxing comfort of rocking, or of a little back rub, take care not to establish a habit of his falling asleep *while you are doing it*. Be sure to stop and leave the room before he actually falls asleep. And don't lie down in bed with your child until he goes to sleep, because you will not be there when he awakens.

LEAVING THE LIGHT ON

If you leave the child's bedroom light on while he falls asleep and then turn the light off after he falls asleep, he awakens to a disrupted association that demands assessment and, consequently, alertness because someone (or some*thing*) has clearly altered—been in control of—the environment while he was asleep; the assessment may thus short circuit to anxiety over loss of control and further disruption of sleep.

RELAXATION AIDS AND SLEEP ASSOCIATIONS

In order for your child to sleep well at night, he must learn to fall asleep alone under the same conditions he will experience upon waking during the night. Disruption of sleep association, however, does not appear to apply to the use of audio programs as relaxation aids.

But audio recordings in the natural world have a beginning and end; a child quickly learns that the audio program will end (unless you've set the machine to repeat—an *inadvisable* action). Relaxation and receptivity to sleep are the goals of the program, not prevention of the natural occurrences of brief wakings. The relaxed child, secure in his environment, returns to sleep even when not listening to a program because things are as they should be. Thus, even restless children tend to experience deeper sleep after using the programs, with a reduction in the number of anxious nighttime wakings that lead to disruption of sleep.

Further, if your child has developed the habit of needing you present in order to fall asleep, you may find the sleep programs particularly helpful. The programs become a transitional experience that keeps him company, entertains him, and then, naturally, puts him to sleep. With time, he learns to fall asleep on his own without endless episodes of crying or begging for "one more story."

TEACHING YOUR CHILD TO FALL ASLEEP ALONE

If your child continues to insist that you be present when he falls asleep, you may wish to institute a behavioral program designed to eliminate this habit. As mentioned above, you must establish conditions for falling asleep that will be present when he awakens during the night. You will need to make a concerted effort to establish reproducible sleep associations, and it must be done consistently or it is likely to fail.

Begin by asking yourself how long you can listen to your child cry before feeling that you have to do something. It is best to start slowly and can be as short as a minute, but you will achieve your goal more quickly if you begin with five minutes. Each night at bedtime, and after nighttime wakings, your child must fall asleep alone, without your presence in the room. Gradually, you will need to let your child cry for longer periods of time, before returning for a few minutes to check on him. When you return you can pat him on the back, reassuring him that everything is all right, that you care about him, but *always leave the room while your child is still awake.*

You will need to continue this until he finally falls asleep while you are out of the room. If the child has not gotten back to sleep, but the crying has stopped or has eased to mild whimpering, *don't go back in.* On the first night, you might want to make fifteen minutes the longest time that you wait before returning, if your child is still crying. On subsequent nights, progressively increase the time that you wait before returning. If your child awakens crying during the night, begin the same procedure again, waiting for five minutes and working up to fifteen. The same procedure can also be used during naptime.

Use a gradual approach such as this. Your child needs to learn that you are nearby and taking care of him; he can only learn this through experience. He will eventually conclude that it isn't worth fifteen or twenty minutes of crying just to have you return briefly, and in the process he will learn to fall asleep alone and in bed.

By the end of the first week, your child should be sleeping better, and by the end of the second week, he will likely have fallen into normal sleep patterns. For older children who have been sleeping poorly for many years, the changes may take a little longer, but this procedure should nevertheless work. If the child is old enough, you can explain that you will do your pleasant bedtime routine together and then you will leave the room with the door open.

IF YOUR CHILD LEAVES THE BED DURING THE NIGHT

If your child gets out of bed during the night, take him back into the bedroom, put him into bed, and tell him that he must stay in bed or you will close the door for a while. If he gets out of bed again, put him back to bed and close the door for about a minute. Don't lock the door, but if he tries to open it, hold it closed (locking the door can be very scary and counterproductive to this new learning process). You want him to learn that the door being open is under his control, but that you cannot be manipulated. Keep in mind that you are trying to help him learn to calm down and fall asleep on his own. If you lose your temper, threaten him, or spank him, the situation will only deteriorate. You want an atmosphere of support and caring, not one of fear and punishment.

If your child continues to get out of bed, increase the door closure time to three, and then, five minutes, which should be the maximum time on the first night. If he stays in bed, open the door after the time is up and give him a word of encouragement. And if your child gets out of bed later, after a nighttime waking, follow the same pattern you used at bedtime, beginning with one minute.

Don't be surprised if the first few nights aren't easy, but be assured things should get much better after one or two weeks. Practice consistency, since your child needs to learn exactly what to expect. Don't make the mistake of thinking that it won't hurt if you ease up for just one night. Such a lapse could easily delay your success for an additional week or longer. Research has shown that "intermittent rewards" occurring only one out of ten times can sustain undesirable behavior. So you won't be doing your child any favors by making such an exception. In fact, quite the opposite; you will simply extend a surely frustrating process for both of you.

Throughout this process both parents should alternate, although you don't need to adhere strictly to an every-other-night schedule; this alternation simply shows the child his parents are of one mind in this bedtime issue. Your child should expect both of you to respond the same way to any of his actions. During this process, if at all possible, avoid the use of a sitter, but if you must use a sitter, let your sitter put your child to bed in the easiest way possible. Thus, the exception falls on the sitter and consistency remains the bastion of the parents—the normal nightly family routine.

CO-SLEEPING

In the previous section we covered a traditional sleeping arrangement wherein the child sleeps alone. Our discussion regarding bedtime routine in that section assumes the desired outcome leads to the child's learning to successfully fall asleep and remain asleep in his own private space. In this section on co-sleeping, however, we'll take a look at a rather different sleeping arrangement, one in which the child sleeps in the same bed as his parents, and we'll also examine some of the adjustments parents must make if this strategy is to work for all concerned.

I take no stand on the subject in these pages, but rather attempt to present you with an evenhanded view of both sides of the debate as the tide continues to ebb and flow, with many childhood sleep experts saying that most American parents today engage in co-sleeping with their babies at least sometime in their children's lives, although most parents won't admit it.

Cultural Opinions on Co-sleeping Over Time

Consider cultural shifts of opinion. Before the 20th century started taking form, even our own culture accepted co-sleeping as the norm. But, swiftly, opinion began to turn the other way, disfavoring it. As recently as 1999, in fact, a U.S. Consumer Product Safety Commission (CPSC) Report recommended all children younger than two years old never be permitted to sleep in bed with their parents. The report cited, among other horrifying statistics, that over three-fourths of infant deaths occurring under three months old are caused by a sleeping adult inadvertently rolling on top of the infant and suffocating it. Interestingly enough, however, that same CPSC report implies approval of co-sleeping for children over two years old.

Experts still vociferously debate the wisdom of having a child with sleep difficulties sleep in the parents' bed with them. *Harm or benefit?* It depends on which expert you ask.

The Two Holdouts: U.S. and Europe

As it happens, the United States and Western Europe, for the most part, are currently the only places in the world with a great aversion to co-sleeping. One study found that out of 186 non-industrial cultures, not a single one encouraged children under age 1 to sleep alone. In fact, in Central America, Asia, and Africa the common perception holds that in countries shunning co-sleeping, parents actually neglect their children.

Separation Anxiety: Necessity or Not?

"She must learn," Ferber says, "to tolerate separation from you when you are out of the room or when she is left with a sitter, at day-care nursery school, or kindergarten. And she must learn to accept separation from you each night when she falls asleep."

For most babies and many children, the separation anxiety of being left alone to sleep at night is so strong as to lead to the baby or child crying, sometimes ceaselessly until one of two things happens: the baby cries himself to sleep or the parents come in to comfort him.

The notion of this separation anxiety and whether it is a necessary stage in a child's healthy development or an unnecessary trauma detrimental to that development is at the crux of much of the debate between advocates and opponents of co-sleeping.

Latest Research on Crying

Contemporary research on crying has started to indicate that, despite popular assumptions:
- it could be dangerous for a baby

- it could be extremely traumatizing for the baby with possible long-term consequences
- it does not benefit the strength of their developing lungs
- it does not always tire all babies out until they ultimately fall asleep
- it should not be ignored under the common misperception that parents might "spoil" their children if they are too attentive

WHAT FERBER'S OPPONENTS SAY

Ferber's detractors label his paradigm as the *"Let them cry it out"* model, though Ferber would be the first to correct them. Indeed, Ferber does believe that confronting this separation anxiety and not kowtowing to it is instrumental to a child's healthy development, but that is not to say he advocates leaving a baby alone to cry himself to sleep.

FERBER COUNTERS

On the contrary, Ferber concurs that doing so, while it may be effective, is "unnecessarily difficult."

Rather, he promotes a gradual system of leaving the crying child alone for progressively longer intervals of time, starting with extremely short intervals, of course, before stepping back into the room briefly to reassure the child she hasn't been abandoned. He says, "Your child has to learn some new rules, but he won't understand them at first. He should know that you are still nearby and taking care of him And he can only learn this through experience."

As Ferber makes pointedly clear, the focus, and sole purpose, of the parents' returning to the room in the increasingly spread out intervals is to comfort the child, show her they haven't abandoned her, and that they still care for her. The purpose is not to help the child fall asleep; that she still has to do on her own. For this to work, *the parents must always leave while the child is still awake.*

He asserts, "If your child is 'too afraid' to [sleep alone], and you deal with his fear by letting him into your bed, you are not really solving the problem." You will help your child far more, says Ferber, by helping him get to the root of his fear and working through it.

THE FAMILY BED: EXPERTS DR. JAY GORDON AND MARIA GOODAVAGE WEIGH IN

Pediatrician Jay Gordon, M.D. and sleep-researcher Maria Goodavage are among those who disagree fervently with Ferber, arguing that his advice runs counter to raising a healthy and well-adjusted child. Instead, they advocate the "Family Bed" paradigm, suggesting that parents tuck a child into the parents' own bed every night, only referring to it as the family bed rather than defining it as the parents' own separate personal property. Gordon and Goodavage argue that such a practice helps the child develop a much-needed sense of safety, security, and comfort at nighttimes.

FERBER'S ARGUMENT AGAINST THE FAMILY BED

In Ferber's book, he voices a strong argument against the family bed which asserts that the practice is a psychopathological response to parental guilt, that, in fact, parents who have their child sleep in bed with them become more withdrawn emotionally from their children, and that they may practice co-sleeping to avoid dealing with an unhappy marriage. He even warns that a co-sleeping child may compete with the same-sex parent for the affection of the opposite-sex parent.

Further, he explains that, in general, all people sleep better when they're alone in bed, citing studies showing that one person's movements and arousals throughout the night stimulate more frequent nighttime wakings and changes of sleep states in another person sharing the same bed.

He argues that children who sleep in the family bed grow up more needy than their peers who sleep in their own beds, which suggests that the practice of co-sleeping, rather than relaxing and reassuring a child, can actually cause him to feel anxious and confused instead.

Co-sleeping advocates like Gordon and Goodavage call such beliefs outdated and unsupported, citing more recent evidence which shows that children who sleep in a family bed, in truth, grow up to be more well-adjusted adults than their peers who sleep alone.

WHAT ABOUT SECURITY OBJECTS... BLANKETS, TEDDY BEARS?

Ferber does allow that a security object—a "special toy or favorite blanket" may be used to help comfort him during the separation from his parents, giving him a sense of some measure of control over his world when he is unable to effectively exert his control on the parents.

This allowance of Ferber's, however, opens up a whole new can of worms on the other side of the debate which points out a dangerous contradiction in teaching children to value and depend on things more than people for comfort from life's stresses.

CO-SLEEPING AND SUDDEN INFANT DEATH SYNDROME (SIDS)

In *Good Nights*, Gordon and Goodavage, outline several points that studies have revealed about the benefits of co-sleeping, including potential protection from Sudden Infant Death Syndrome (SIDS).

Others, however, have suggested that this consequence of co-sleeping—protection from SIDS—occurs because the baby spends more time in light sleep than in deep sleep, as she is constantly stirred by her parents' frequent movements throughout the night, and is therefore more able to rouse herself awake when her breathing pauses or her body temperature drops.

HOW DEEP IS THEIR SLEEP (IS YOUR SLEEP)?

Does a child sleep deeper or lighter when in his parents' (or "family") bed or is there no correlation at all? Will each child sleep as lightly or as deeply as she sleeps, regardless of whose bed she sleeps in? Alas, not enough research has been done to answer these questions conclusively.

PARENT-CHILD SLEEP SYNCHRONIZATION

A study conducted at the University of Notre Dame Mother-Baby Behavioral Sleep Laboratory did, however, make the startling discovery that a baby sleeping between its two parents at night entered the same sleeping and dreaming stages at almost the same times as her parents throughout the night. Researchers concluded that this "synchronization" could be instrumental in helping the baby form healthy sleeping habits.

This synchronization may take place in other areas of the parent-child dynamic as well. For example, whether during sleeping or waking, when a parent and a child make skin-to-skin contact, the parent's heart-rate and body temperature seems to adjust to appropriately stabilize the baby's heart-rate and body temperature.

OTHER BENEFITS OF CO-SLEEPING

Other discoveries Gordon and Goodavage report that support the practice of co-sleeping cover a wide range:

- from the most predictable—that babies sleep better in their parents' bed
- to the most unusual—that babies who sleep in a family bed don't practice the dangerous "head-banging" behavior seen in many of their solitary-sleeping peers
- to the utterly astonishing—that young children who sleep beside their parents grow up to be more independent individuals. As this argument goes, rather than forcing independence on a child by discouraging a sense of dependence, independence is fostered by satisfying the child's natural need for dependence.

Family and sleep experts, like University of California psychiatry professor Thomas Anders, M.D., assert that the practice of co-sleeping also promotes greater closeness amongst family members.

Study of this co-sleeping phenomenon in premature and fragile babies in particular has revealed that such a practice helps those children "sleep more deeply, cry less, breathe better, grow faster" and be sent home from the birthing hospital sooner than they otherwise would have been.

Gordon and Goodavage point out that science now has evidence that babies are in fact supposed to sleep close to their parents. And despite continuing skepticism regarding repercussions on the restfulness of the parents' sleep, a survey of parents who have already engaged in the practice of co-sleeping found 98% of them proclaiming they would do it again should another infant come into their lives.

CO-SLEEPING AND BREAST-FEEDING

Other studies have shown that mothers who breast-feed sleep better when their baby is in the bed with them at night. As more and more mothers practice breast-feeding their babies rather than bottle-feeding, the incidence of co-sleeping has risen at about the same pace, with current statistics showing that approximately 80% of babies who are breast-fed at least periodically sleep in the family bed. This practice makes even more sense in that breast-fed babies typically require more frequent feedings than their bottle-fed peers.

A Shocking Turnaround: Ferber Rethinks

Now here comes something that nobody expected—even Dr. Ferber himself ultimately came around to accept the potential value in co-sleeping. In an interview for a 1999 *New Yorker* magazine article titled, *"Sleeping with the Baby,"* by co-sleeper John Seabrook, Ferber actually softened his position on the subject, recanting his assertion that co-sleeping hinders a child's development of independence and individuality, indicating it was a "blanket statement."

He further clarified his current philosophy. Parents should find whatever works best for them and their child, and it's not the same for everyone. He still believes in many cases co-sleeping is the wrong answer, but sometimes it works perfectly for parent and child, and is therefore the right course of action for that family.

Ultimately, a Choice

So there you have it—a general picture of both sides of the ongoing co-sleeping debate. With all this in mind, if you are in a situation in which you are realistically considering co-sleeping with your infant, you'll want to do it properly, healthily for you and your child both. That is why the next part of this section is directed specifically at you.

Making the Family Bed Safe

For starters, one caveat most co-sleeping advocates are careful to make is that any parents considering implementing the family bed dynamic in their household first ensure that their bed is made *safe for a baby to sleep in*. In *Good Nights*, Gordon and Goodavage lay out a very clear set of safety guidelines for creating "The Safest Sleep."

Among the suggestions for creating a safe family bed are:

- using only a firm mattress or futon (nothing too soft)
- using as big a bed as you can afford (a king-size if possible)
- keeping the bed away from walls (as babies can become trapped between the mattress and wall, and then suffocate)
- making sure any headboards or footboards are secure and snug against the bed, with no gaps in which the baby could potentially get trapped (or just don't use a headboard or footboard at all)
- making certain any gaps in a slatted headboard or footboard don't exceed 2⅜" (to keep the baby's head from slipping through)
- using only light blankets, layered if necessary, for adequate warmth (but avoiding at all costs thick, downy comforters and duvets)
- keeping long hair tied back securely
- always positioning the baby on her back
- not letting your baby sleep or take naps alone in your bed or the family bed (though if you must, being sure to install guardrails and possibly bolsters, too—an alternative to this being to wear a sling for your baby to nap in)

An alternative style of family bed is a three-sided crib that attaches to the bed, keeping the baby in her own space but well within close reach at all times. Another option, called a "snuggle nest," prevents parental rollover.

The most extreme method of creating a family bed, yet also considered the safest, is to place the mattress on the floor and make sure all pillows and blankets are nowhere near the baby's head. If the mattress is not placed on the floor, just keep in mind that the lower the bed to the floor, the safer for the child.

When Not to Co-sleep

Beyond the safety of the bed itself, proponents of co-sleeping also advise that if one of the parents in the family bed has their sleep detrimentally affected by the practice, it should be discontinued immediately, as the negative impact on that parent could most assuredly impact the child as well. Gordon and Goodavage also warn that if a parent sleeping in the family bed has been drinking alcohol, using drugs, or taking prescription medications, the baby should not sleep there.

Note also that obese parents ought not share their bed with their children under any circumstances because of an increased risk of suffocation.

Co-sleeping and Nighttime Wakings

Remember, of course, that nighttime wakings are as common for babies as they are for you, and any literature to the contrary is usually based on outdated data, mostly coming from the 1950s when babies were formula-fed and left to sleep alone.

Co-sleeping and Sex

Regarding another common (but little-discussed) concern, parents considering implementing a family bed in their household might worry that co-sleeping could impact their sex life. And while this is a completely valid and justified concern, the solution to it is not to forego having a family bed at all, but rather to come up with new, more creative ways to find intimate alone time. Removing sex from the bedroom could actually turn out to add some spice and playfulness to a couple's sex life.

Where to Place the Baby in the Family Bed

There is some debate among co-sleeping proponents about where to place the baby in the family bed, some arguing that the baby should be placed next to the mother only, as the mother is typically more conscious of the baby's presence, even while asleep, others arguing that the baby be placed between the two parents so that there is no concern about the baby rolling off the bed or mattress. Both sides of this debate agree, however, that if siblings share the family bed, they should not be placed side by side but rather have at least one parent lying between them.

Transitioning a Child from the Family Bed

Finally, a few words on how best to help a child as she grows up to make a healthy transition from sleeping in the family bed to sleeping alone in her own bed. Sometimes this is easy, such as when the child herself requests the change be made. And many co-sleeping proponents suggest that parents simply not worry about it until the child herself brings it up. (This, by the way, often happens spontaneously around age 6 or when a new baby enters the household.)

Other times, however, more deft and graceful handling of the situation is in order, lest you promote undesirable behaviors like clinginess and severe separation anxiety. Gordon and Goodavage offer several suggestions on making that transition as smooth as possible:

- wean the baby from breast-feeding first before trying to wean her from co-sleeping
- start the conversation with your child well before the time when the transition is actually to take place, giving her something to look forward to
- build or redecorate your child's "new" bedroom and, if it hasn't already been done, furnish it with the bed in advance of making the transition in order to start getting your child excited about having her very own space
- start off by placing your child's new bed (or a separate futon or floor mattress) pressed alongside the family bed for a while
- offer to move her into her sibling's bedroom
- break the night up in half, either starting with your child in the family bed, then moving her to her own bed once she's asleep. But this should only be done if no sleep issues arise—remember the sleep associations rule—or starting your child in her own bed and giving her permission to crawl into bed with you when she wakes during the night
- provide a subdued nightlight in the child's bedroom
- prohibit potentially frightening TV shows or movies prior to bedtime
- practice for nighttime with daytime naps

One other possible method of helping your child make such a transition—and one of some controversy—involves rocking or nursing a child to sleep and then laying her down in her own bed, the arguable problem with this being that the child may come to depend on this ritual for getting to sleep. In addition, and as mentioned previously, if that child has trouble sleeping, then waking up in a different setting from where she fell asleep could upset her and make it harder for her to get back to sleep.

A Two-Week Plan for Weaning Your Child off the Family Bed

A final alternative Gordon and Goodavage offer to all of these suggestions is a modified version of the let-them-cry-it-out-alone method described at the beginning of this section. Note that it should only be attempted by desperate parents with children in perfect health over the age of 12 months. It goes like this:

- Nights 1-3, let the child sleep in the family bed, or alternatively, in a crib placed in the same room as the family bed. At any time throughout the night when the child wakes, give her some TLC and a feeding, then lay her back down while she's still awake to fall back asleep on her own, being careful not to let her fall asleep in your arms
- Nights 4-6 are the same as the first 3 nights except without the feeding
- Nights 7-10 are the same as nights 4-6 except now you're not even to pick up the child at all when she awakens during the night. Just talk to her, touch her gently, rub her back, but do not pick her up
- For up to one week more feel free to rock, cuddle, and feed your child to sleep if she insists, but do not feed her or pick her up during the night once she is down
- After this final week put the child down to sleep while she's still awake

Children can usually be weaned out of a family bed situation once they reach 2 or 3 years of age, around the time that children actively seek out independence from their parents naturally. Babies who are consistently deep sleepers, however, could make a smooth transition as young as just a few months old.

MEDICATION FOR SLEEP PROBLEMS

When a child continues to suffer from sleep problems and a family thinks they have tried every avenue, they may end up asking their pediatrician or family physician to evaluate their child for sleep medication. So, are there times when this is an appropriate course to consider? If you have no interest in exploring the use of sleep medications with children, you may wish to skip this section. But if you would like to know more about the use of medication, let's consider some important facts.

REASONS FOR AND AGAINST USING MEDICATIONS

We're now going to examine the two sides of the ledger: reasons that support medication use for pediatric insomnia and reasons that argue against it. As a caveat, however, medication should only be considered if a child demonstrates *significant difficultly in initiating and maintaining sleep.*

There are a number of *sedatives* or *hypnotics* that are currently prescribed by pediatricians and child psychiatrists. In determining their appropriateness for your child, your doctor would take a number of personal variables into account, things like your child's age, and the presence of psychiatric or developmental problems (ADHD, autism, mental retardation, blindness, pain).

And then there is the question of related stress for everyone in the household. Is Dad about to lose his job because his son's sleep problem is keeping him awake? Is the family likely to face eviction a short while later if this continues? You may laugh, but in clinical practice these kinds of dilemmas constantly arise. So there may be times when a child's sleep difficulties can present an emergency that predicates a quick solution, like that which medication offers.

Sleep Medications for Kids when There's No Emergency?

But should medications be considered in the absence of an emergency simply because nothing else is helping? This is where it gets a bit trickier, especially because the research necessary to evaluate the effectiveness and safety of sleep medications for childhood insomnia hasn't been done. In fact, there is less research on this than on any other area of pediatric medication use. Additionally, it's not helpful that the efficacy, tolerability, and safety of these drugs in children are largely unknown. So doctors are forced to make a number of assumptions and extrapolate from adult use of the same medications, adjusting dosages based on age, size, and so forth.

Rebound Insomnia

A significant drawback of many prescription sleep medications is that they set the stage for "rebound insomnia." Thus, if you use the medication regularly, when you discontinue use, sleep for one or two nights will probably not be as good as it would have been if medication had not been used. Rebound insomnia reinforces the belief that medications are needed on an ongoing basis, when, in fact, that may not be true.

Studies on Sleep Medications in Children

The few studies on sleep medication in children have led to mixed results, though on the positive side, most studies have not reported significant adverse reactions. Ultimately, therefore, doctors must base their decisions on their own clinical experience with the medications.

Deciding Whether or Not to Medicate

Other considerations regarding childhood sleep problems will also enter the picture:
- type and severity of the problem
- duration of the problem
- frequency of the problem
- occurrence of previous failed attempts at conventional behavioral therapy
- other specific therapeutic strategies

Managing a Child on Sleep Medication

When a physician makes the decision to prescribe a sleep medication to a child, a number of factors need weighing in determining how best to manage the case. A careful history should be taken to try to verify the cause of the sleep problem and contributing factors leading to it, along with an evaluation of how the sleep disturbance is affecting the health and daily functioning of the child. And, as mentioned above, the impact on the family, including parental exhaustion, must also be considered.

You might find the following topics of interest, although some of the terms are fairly technical. This list has been reprinted, with permission, from *A Clinical Guide to Pediatric Sleep: Diagnosis and Management of Sleep Problems*, a textbook for primary care physicians.

Once the decision to include pharmacologic management has been made, additional specific issues to consider include the following:

- **Potential benefits of pharmacologic intervention** must substantially outweigh the risks. Although no drug currently available is "perfect," agents should be selected to maximize the benefit/risk ratio
- **Pharmacotherapy combined with behavior therapy** should be used, as this strategy is far more likely to yield long-term success
- **Adequate sleep hygiene**, including sufficient sleep, a regular sleep schedule, and appropriate bedtime routines, should be part of every management plan
- **Selection of a specific pharmacologic agent** should be made according to the type of sleep problem. For example, primary difficulties with initiating sleep require use of a medication that has rapid onset of action and a very short half-life, whereas sleep maintenance problems may require a somewhat longer acting agent. [The term "half-life" is a measurement of how long a medication remains in the body.]
- **Selection of medications should also consider specific patient variables**, such as age, presence of comorbid medical and psychiatric conditions, and use of concomitant medications that may interact with sedative/hypnotics
- **Treatment goals** should be clearly outlined and measurable (sleep onset consistently less than 30 minutes, improvement in mood and attentiveness)
- **Duration of therapy** should be the shortest possible time interval to achieve results. The duration of therapy should be discussed and clarified with the family before initiating medication
- **Dosing should be initiated at the lowest level** likely to be effective and titrated up as necessary
- **Timing of medication** should minimize "morning hangover" or persistent grogginess. In general, this means choosing an agent with the shortest possible half life
- **Side effects** should be reviewed with the family as well as the child or adolescent as appropriate
- **Monitoring** of efficacy and side effects should take place frequently and systematically
- **Particularly in adolescents**, both the possibility of interaction with other substances (alcohol, marijuana) and the potential for abuse of medication should be considered
- **Abrupt discontinuation of pharmacotherapy** should be avoided, as this is likely to result in rebound symptoms and changes in sleep architecture. In some cases, as with antihypertensive alpha-agonist clonidine, abrupt discontinuation may be dangerous (rebound hypertension)

So as you can see, a physician who decides to treat your child with a sleep medication takes on quite a burden of responsibility. And keep in mind that some childhood sleep experts, like Dr. Richard Ferber, are outspokenly cautionary regarding the use of sleep medications in kids:

In my practice, I see far too many young children who have been given powerful medications in an attempt to relieve sleep disorders that could have been corrected by other means. In many cases, whatever the child's problem, the medication only makes matters worse. Also, the child's daytime behavior and ability to concentrate and learn may well be compromised.

Specific Medication Used in Pediatric Insomnia

There are currently no sleep medications that have been approved by the U.S. Food and Drug Administration (FDA) for use in children, and manufacturers do not provide suggested doses for use in children. All this is to say that, while in some cases medications can be useful, parents should first understand that, in part because there are no clear guidelines for dosages for children, there are certain risks involved. Anyone considering giving their child medications for these problems should do so only as a last resort, and only under the proper supervision of an appropriate physician specialist.

Having said that, I'll describe the following medications you'd most likely encounter should you start looking into this option for your child.

Antihistamines

This group of medications are sold over-the-counter and include Sominex, Nytol and Unisom, which contain diphenhydramine (Benadryl) or doxylamine. There has been little research on the sedative effects of antihistamines, even in adults, but a recent study indicated that, although sleep is often improved initially, after several days the effect wears off for most people. In addition, daytime sedation is a common side effect which can impair concentration and coordination. Other common side effects include dry mouth and constipation. Certain children, however, may experience the opposite effect of the desired reaction, possibly resulting in greater alertness, restless behavior, and worsened sleep.

Benzodiazepines

This group includes a large variety of agents commonly prescribed to adults for the treatment of anxiety and insomnia. Examples include Valium (diazepam), Klonopin (clonazepam), Ativan (lorazepam), Xanax (alprazolam), Halcion (triazolam), and Restoril (temazepam). The primary difference between various benzodiazepines is the length of time that they remain in the body (and exert their effect). Primary side effects include daytime sedation (if a longer acting agent is utilized), cognitive impairment, and rebound insomnia. Major drawbacks include suppression of "slow-wave sleep" (the deep, more restorative sleep) and their abuse potential.

Chloral Hydrate

Many years ago this was a popular sleep agent, but it is rarely used now except in a single dose for medical or dental procedures. Studies have shown that it tends to lose its sleep-inducing effect after several nights and its safety in long term use is questionable.

Clonidine

This medication is used primarily to treat daytime hyperactivity in children with Attention Deficit Hyperactivity Disorder (ADHD) and to treat hypertension (high blood pressure) in adults, although some physicians still use it to induce sleep in children. Other potential side effects include dry mouth, low blood pressure, irritability, and irregular heart beat.

Melatonin and Melatonin-Like Agents

Melatonin is a hormone that is naturally secreted in the body during nighttime hours and is instrumental in maintaining the normal 24-hour sleep/wake cycle. As people age, there is a tendency to secrete less of this hormone, which makes older people more susceptible to sleep phase (sleep cycle or circadian rhythm) problems, which are also caused by jet lag. Melatonin may be helpful in these circumstances and perhaps in adolescents with delayed sleep phase (late to bed, late to rise), but use in children has been poorly studied. This over-the-counter agent is not regulated by the FDA. And just because melatonin is a "natural hormone," that's no assurance of its safety for children. Potential side effects include low blood pressure, headache, light-headedness, and possibly seizures.

A rather new addition to this category is Rozerem (ramelteon), which affects the same receptor sites in the brain as melatonin but five times more powerfully. This mechanism of action allows it to be advertised on television as "not habit forming." Side effects, although rare, include daytime sedation, dizziness, nausea, headache, fatigue and insomnia.

Desyrel (trazodone)

This is one of the more commonly used medications to treat insomnia in adults. Originally developed as an antidepressant, and used decades ago for that purpose, it is popular with many physicians because of its low abuse potential. Its primary side effect is daytime sedation, which has a high incidence of occurrence.

Second-Generation Sleep Medications (Ambien, Sonata, Lunesta)

Several medications have been developed specifically for the treatment of sleep disorders with the goal of providing agents that might be more effective, and have fewer side effects and abuse potential, than the older benzodiazepines. These medications have minimal effects on "sleep architecture," meaning they do not suppress deeper, more restorative sleep. On the negative side, some people engage in activities such as eating, driving, or making phone calls while on these medications, and later have no memory of the events (amnesia). Other potential side effects include daytime drowsiness, headache, dizziness, tolerance (requiring higher doses), confusion, and sleep walking.

Ambien (zolpidem) was the original member of this group and continues to be widely used. Sonata (zaleplon) is unique because of its extremely short duration of action, which means that it has little tendency to cause morning sedation. This makes it ideal for people who have trouble falling asleep, but unhelpful for those who tend to awaken during the second half of the night. Lunesta (eszopiclone) is the newest member of this group. Advantages include the virtual absence of rebound insomnia (though it is minimally present with Ambien and Sonata), long action, and infrequent daytime sedation.

Valerian Root

This is another over-the-counter agent and is considered a dietary supplement as opposed to an actual medication. Preparations made from this plant may reduce the amount of time it takes to fall asleep and improve sleep quality, but it's not clear what the active ingredient is and the potencies may vary from preparation to preparation. Research on its use in children is limited, but one study did show it to be safe and effective in children ages 6 to 12 using an average dose of 600 mg.

Medications, or even food supplements, for sleep in children should always be used under the supervision of a physician. Occasionally, giving a child short-term (one to two week) drug treatment may serve to break a cycle of poor sleep and allow a more normal pattern to emerge after the medication is stopped. But medications should never be used as a substitute for the appropriate alternative interventions that have already been discussed. It is much better, and in the long run will be much more successful, to take the time to help your child learn how to sleep without drugs. In addition, developing effective strategies and new habits will allow you and your child to develop more confidence in dealing with problems that may emerge in the future without feeling that you need to immediately "head for the medicine cabinet."

If your child has been prescribed medication for the treatment of a medical condition such as epilepsy, asthma, or ADHD, and it seems that the prescribed medication itself may be causing sleep problems, discuss your concern with your doctor. There are several approaches that may be helpful, such as altering the dose or timing of the drugs, and the use of alternative medications.

CHAPTER 16

MEDICAL CAUSES OF SLEEP PROBLEMS

The following are some of the chronic medical conditions that frequently cause sleep disturbances:

- diabetes
- asthma
- headaches
- skin irritations
- any condition that causes pain

Colic, incidentally, is the most common cause of sleep problems in the youngest of children, but since it occurs exclusively in the first few months of life, it is out of the age range for which I am offering advice.

When chronic conditions are present, parents usually know of them; if effective treatment occurs at this stage, sleep problems can be minimized.

CHRONIC MIDDLE EAR DISEASES AND SLEEP

Chronic middle-ear disease often goes unrecognized, yet is easy to treat. It is caused by the buildup of fluid in the middle-ear cavity behind the ear drum, when the fluid does not drain satisfactorily. This fluid can become infected, and the infection can, in turn, cause extreme pain; but even when not infected, middle-ear fluid can cause sleep disturbances. Fluid buildup can cause temporary hearing loss and, if present for an extended period, the hearing loss can become permanent. Any evidence of sudden hearing impairment or unexplained ear pain is good reason for a doctor's visit to determine if there is a middle-ear drainage problem.

HEARTBURN AND SLEEP

One final source of nighttime pain that can cause insomnia is gastroesophageal reflux, commonly called heartburn. The valve that holds food in the stomach and prevents it from coming back into the esophagus may not function well, which can result in pain. But pain caused by reflux is more likely to be present when a child is active than during sleep. So if a child is not also complaining of stomach/chest pain during the day, nighttime pain is unlikely. However, when this condition is present it can be easily treated, resulting in improved sleep.

ADHD (ADD) and Sleep

Attention Deficit Hyperactivity Disorder (ADHD), sometimes referred to as Attention Deficit Disorder (ADD), is a neurological condition characterized by inattention and impulsivity, which may or may not be associated with hyperactivity.

In recent years, researchers have noticed that the symptoms of chronic sleep disturbances overlap indicators used in diagnosing ADHD, namely:

- daytime sleepiness
- short attention span
- irritability and low frustration threshold
- trouble modulating emotions and impulses

These observations led to a wider investigation into the link between ADHD and sleep, and in those investigations many correlations were indeed found.

Children with ADHD have trouble "winding down" enough to get to sleep. Their minds are still racing, even though their bodies may be tired. Truly, it's a thin line between sleep-related symptoms and the symptoms of ADHD.

Which Came First: The ADHD or the Sleep Disturbances?

Because these two issues—sleep and ADHD—are so intermeshed, it often becomes quite difficult to discern whether ADHD is the cause or effect of a sleep problem. And while it may seem obvious that treating ADHD could lead to better sleep patterns, it is also equally true (albeit, perhaps, less obvious) that treating sleep difficulties and sleep disorders can also help reduce the symptoms of ADHD and improve one's ability to function well despite the diagnosis.

If Your Child Has Symptoms or a Diagnosis of ADHD

If your child has been diagnosed with ADHD or you have observed your child displaying symptoms of the condition, be sure also to have your child checked out for any diagnosable sleep disorders, as effectively correcting one of these problems may be necessary to correct the other.

The Genetic Component of ADHD

ADHD has a very strong genetic component and, in fact, is usually an inherited disorder. And yet this etiology does not satisfactorily explain what appears to be a dramatic increase in children who seem to suffer from this disorder. The number of school-age children who now meet the criteria is rather extraordinary and is estimated at between five and ten percent. Recently published research reported an increased incidence of ADHD when a child's mother smoked and/or used alcohol during pregnancy and with early exposure to lead.

THE DIETARY COMPONENT OF ADHD

Lastly, it is worth noting that some people also believe diet is a factor in ADHD. The first solid evidence to support this view was provided by research done at the University of Southampton in England in which 300 children from the general population were studied. The results were reported in the medical journal *The Lancet* in 2007, and the researchers concluded that artificial colors in the diet resulted in increased hyperactivity in children. The issue of diet and children's behavior remains hotly debated and will require additional research to clarify the relationship.

OBSTRUCTIVE SLEEP APNEA

In the past, snoring in children was usually dismissed as nothing more than an annoyance to those who had to endure listening to it, but now we know snoring can actually indicate sleep apnea, a significant breathing problem which occurs, of course, during sleep. This is a condition that requires medical attention.

WHAT IS OBSTRUCTIVE SLEEP APNEA?

Obstructive sleep apnea (OSA) is characterized by repeated and prolonged obstruction of air through the throat during sleep. The most common cause is enlargement of the tonsils and adenoids in the sides and back of the throat. There is also a strong correlation with obesity, although OSA can occur without either of these factors present. The intermittent obstruction can be partial or complete and may occur for varying lengths of time.

SIGNS AND SYMPTOMS OF CHILDHOOD SLEEP APNEA

When it is happening, the child will be snoring, struggling to breathe, and at times gasping for air. "Apnea" actually means the absence of breathing, and in adults with this disorder their breathing often stops completely. Children are more likely to have only a partial obstruction, yet just the struggle to breathe can cause partial wakings and lack of deep, restorative sleep.

Airway obstruction leads to multiple brief arousals from sleep, resulting in daytime sleepiness. Abnormal breathing during sleep disturbs restful sleep, and could explain why the affected person doesn't feel rested in the mornings upon waking or during the day and can affect a child's daytime behavior and ability to learn.

In children, sleepiness often manifests itself differently than how it appears in adults. Instead of yawning and appearing sleepy, children may develop any number of behavior problems such as difficulty concentrating, forgetfulness, difficulty learning, irritability, and hyperactivity.

WHEN IS SLEEP APNEA MOST LIKELY TO OCCUR?

Episodes of sleep apnea happen most commonly during REM (rapid eye movement) sleep, when dreaming is taking place. And because most REM sleep occurs during the second half of the night, parents may be unaware of their child's apnea episodes, unless they observe them closely in the early morning hours. Episodes most likely occur, too, when children sleep on their backs.

DIAGNOSING CHILDHOOD SLEEP APNEA

Sleep apnea is now routinely diagnosed in adults, although many doctors still fail to recognize it in children despite its common occurrence. Sleep apnea is present in approximately two percent of children of preschool age, but there is scant data on its prevalence among other age groups. (Snoring occurs nightly in approximately 10 percent of all children and occasionally in about 20 percent.)

If you suspect OSA, ask your pediatrician for a referral to a pediatric sleep specialist, or at least a pulmonary specialist who is familiar with childhood sleep apnea. An evaluation should include a visit to a pediatric ear, nose, and throat (ENT) specialist and probably an all-night evaluation in a sleep center, preferably a pediatric sleep center, in order to make the final diagnosis. Some childhood sleep experts recommend that all extremely obese children receive an all-night sleep study because of the high incidence of OSA in this group.

DOES EFFECTIVE TREATMENT EXIST FOR SLEEP APNEA?

Fortunately, treatment for obstructive sleep apnea usually succeeds. If enlarged tonsils or adenoids are responsible, surgical removal is usually very helpful. If OSA is being caused by facial or oral abnormalities, surgery, again, is often the solution. If obesity is the primary cause for the obstruction, an effective diet and exercise program is the clear solution, although it can be a difficult one to implement, as I observed in Chapter 10. This may require well-coordinated medical management with a nutritionist and counselor, and perhaps a support group.

If such interventions cannot be implemented or, for any number of possible reasons, they fail, then use of a continuous positive airway pressure (CPAP) device may be indicated. This treatment is provided by a machine that blows air through a tube connected to a mask the child wears while sleeping. Some children find a mask that covers the nose uncomfortable, but this therapy can be extremely effective. As children grow and their airway enlarges, some will outgrow their OSA. For others, if they can eventually lose the necessary weight or undergo the necessary surgery, the device may no longer be needed.

BRAIN DAMAGE AND SLEEP

A child who suffers from neurological impairments may present somewhat of a special challenge because of potential preexisting damage to the mechanism that controls the act of falling asleep or staying asleep. Such a disorder is usually quite obvious and occurs in children with mental retardation, seizures, blindness, or deafness. Although sleep medication may be appropriate for neurologically-impaired children, non-medication interventions have also proven effective and should be among the first strategies employed with them.

Chapter 17

Strategies and Solutions for the Problem of Anxiety

Sleep-related anxiety symptoms, **bedtime resistance,** trouble sleeping through the night, and frequent and recurring nightmares all indicate the possibility of anxiety. Fortunately, some of the same methods that are most powerful in reducing anxiety are equally potent in eliminating sleep-related difficulties, and vice-versa.

The Sleep-Anxiety Link

Back in the Anxiety section in the introduction to this book, I quoted *Freeing Your Child From Anxiety* author Tamar E. Chansky, Ph.D., describing the at-once "diametrically opposed" and "inextricably-linked" relationship between sleep and anxiety. In that passage in her book, Chansky goes on to say, "Sleep is about letting go, and anxiety is about holding on. Working out a peaceful resolution between the two is an essential life-management skill." That is the ground we will now tread.

Fear versus Anxiety Revisited

To begin, I refer back to another statement I made in the Anxiety introduction regarding the distinction between anxiety and fear. I explained that fear is grounded in reality—some threat or danger triggers the fear. Anxiety, however, is formed in the imagination—based on an unfounded fear of some perceived threat or danger that doesn't really exist. But that's only part of the full picture. The other part involves the purpose of anxiety.

A Purpose for Anxiety

Regardless of how bad it feels and all the pains we go through to avoid it, not all anxiety is bad. And despite how purposeless it feels, anxiety does indeed have a purpose. This is because not all perceptions of threat or danger are unfounded.

The purpose of anxiety is to protect us. If a child using scissors to cut a shape out of construction paper feels anxiety about sticking himself with the sharp point, the child is going to be extra careful to avoid that injury. Anxiety in small and reasonable amounts helps prevent the dangers it predicts.

The problems come in when the appropriate action is taken in response to anxiety's signals or the perceived threat is no longer present—and the anxiety persists.

THE STRESS RESPONSE: HOW ANXIETY WORKS

So far in our discussion, we have gone over *what anxiety is* and *what anxiety does.* But in order to help our children deal with their anxiety, we must understand a bit more about *how anxiety works.*

As sharp a distinction between fear and anxiety as I've drawn, they have an equally distinct similarity as well. Anxiety, like fear, triggers the *"fight or flight"* response (also called the *stress response*).

I also mentioned earlier that anxiety produces very real and significant physical symptoms. Among the most pronounced of those symptoms are the ones directly associated with the *fight or flight* response:

- sweating palms
- dry mouth
- shallow breathing
- "butterflies in the stomach"
- rapid heartbeat

These and all of the other symptoms anxiety produces share a certain commonality—discomfort. Sometimes that discomfort can be so intense it crosses the threshold into pain. Children, in particular, often experience anxiety in just this way.

HOW CHILDREN EXPERIENCE ANXIETY

Children may not be aware that they are feeling anxious, but they will know if they have a headache, a tummy ache, muscle tightness, sleeplessness, or any combination of the above. An anxious child may experience dizziness, shortness of breath or nausea. In fact, because more often than not an anxious child's response to his anxiety is *flight*, or withdrawing inward, clinging to the known and avoiding the unfamiliar, anxious children often perpetuate their physical symptoms when they realize that such things can be used as legitimate excuses to get out of subjecting themselves to the very situations that produce the anxiety within them in the first place.

The imagined dangers that anxiety portends range from embarrassment and humiliation to physical harm and even death. And now we see that the heightened and exaggerated sense of danger that anxiety produces causes enough physical reactions in the body to make it seem as though the perceived danger had actually occurred. And well after the perception of danger is gone, the reaction may remain. Anxiety can, in fact, keep a child locked in that danger zone perpetually.

When a real danger is present, and fear kicks in, the physical symptoms that are triggered have a purpose. They prime the individual to take action—*fight or flight*—that will resolve the crisis, dispel the fear, and thereby relieve those symptoms. But in the case of anxiety, when there is no real threat upon which to act—to either defend against or evade—the child is left with these unresolved *fight or flight* impulses and all of their associated symptoms stuck inside him.

With no appropriate action he can take to dissipate his body's stress response, the child is left with no way to escape from these feelings, and a state of persistent, ongoing stress sets in. As we all know, the range of symptoms and diseases associated with stress are extensive.

THE TRUE ROOT OF A CHILD'S FEARS

Helping your child break this cycle and put an end to their torment requires, as you might expect, getting to the root of his fears. And here's where things get really interesting. Because it turns out that the triggers for a child's anxiety—school, socializing, separation from parents—are actually not at all what the child is truly afraid of. Rather it's the physical sensations of fear, the symptoms that anxiety produces—the *stress response*—that the child fears.

It is the anxiety itself that the child fears. *Nothing to fear but fear itself,* indeed.

Therefore, the more a child avoids these anxiety-producing situations, the more anxiety those situations, and thoughts of them, produce. But the less a child avoids the situations that provoke anxiety—in other words, the more he engages in the very situations that trigger the anxiety within him—the less anxiety those situations (and thoughts of them) will produce, because the child learns over time that there is little to actually fear—and more, that he is bigger than his fears. In the book *Keys to Parenting Your Anxious Child* (part of the Barron's *Parenting Keys* series), Katharina Manassis, M.D., F.R.C.P. calls this process *desensitization*.

This is not to say that helping your child to overcome his anxieties is as simple as forcing him into the situations that trigger it. There is more to it than that.

WHY REASSURANCE DOESN'T WORK

Regardless of a child's specific anxiety or its trigger, almost all anxieties children may experience convey a deep-rooted need to escape from their circumstances and feel reassured and protected. But attempts to reassure the child that the object of his anxiety is nothing to fear generally backfire, precisely because they focus attention on the object of the anxiety (the "trigger") rather than the anxiety itself.

It is next-to-impossible to convince a child that the danger doesn't exist when he perceives it so clearly to exist. Furthermore, coaxing a child to see that his fear is unfounded only serves to make him feel as though you don't understand what he's going through or that your see him as weak and incapable.

COMMON PITFALL: DOWNPLAYING IT

Since anxiety is something everyone experiences in some measure, parents often mistakenly downplay their child's worries, comparing them to the parents' own experiences of anxiety (now or from when they were a child), but a significant difference exists between the low-level anxiety that everyone experiences now and again, and chronic, pathological anxiety that interferes with one's life.

When an anxious child becomes aware that the people around him, especially those closest to him—parents, teachers, counselors—don't understand or relate to his experiences, he will not only end up feeling isolated but, ultimately, may feel hopeless regarding any possible recovery or experience of "normalcy." This, obviously, will undermine any efforts to help him.

How to Help a Child with Anxiety

Parents of an anxious child can take comfort, however, that they are in the best position of anyone to help their child. It has been proven that a parent's involvement in helping a child deal with anxiety is more effective than when that child is solely treated professionally (through a therapist or psychiatrist). As Dr. Manassis says in her book, "most therapists will spend one or two hours per week with your child. A teacher will spend perhaps 30 hours per week. That leaves 136 hours for you, the parents!"

So if a parent isn't to reassure the child, what then? The answer is to validate the realness of the child's feelings, whatever the perceived object or trigger. A child's feelings of anxiety are very real, even if the object of their fear is not. Before you can help a child cope with anxiety, he needs you to first acknowledge and validate the reality of his fears—not as being *justifiable* but as being *real*. Fear is an emotion; emotions aren't rational, but they are valid and real. And your child needs to hear you affirm that.

So instead of trying to convince a child that there is nothing to fear, acknowledge your child's fears (*"That must be very frightening"* or *"That sounds like it feels awful"*) and then see if, together, you might come up with ways to face down those fears. Don't ever underestimate the therapeutic value for your child of your mere acceptance of his problem and recognition of his feelings without judgment.

Besides showing the child that he has an ally in you, this also helps him take the first crucial step in freeing himself from anxiety, which is to recognize and accept that he has an anxiety problem. Once he owns the problem as his, he can then begin the work of confronting it.

Talking with Your Child About Anxiety

The best thing you can do as a parent to help a child with anxiety is to get him to talk about it. Since your child will undoubtedly be less able to rationally broach the subject of his anxiety while he's in its throes, it's better if you start taking the time to discuss his anxiety with him when he's not experiencing it. Even so, there's still the inherent challenge that since anxious children are keenly aware of the abnormality of their experience and fear criticism and embarrassment should word of it get out, they tend to avoid discussing their anxiety.

But without the child's own self-description of his anxiety, it's all guesswork on your part. Hearing about the child's own experiences, thoughts, and feelings in his own words reveals a great deal about the nature and causes of the anxiety. Plus, the very act of talking about his anxiety helps a child to diminish it.

The First, Biggest, and Most Powerful Step in Dealing with Anxiety

Fortunately, accepting one's anxiety is not only the first step in dealing with it but also the biggest and most powerful step. For just as with any bully, turning and facing an adversary instead of running away changes its behavior. Facing an anxiety problem means accepting its existence and committing oneself to conquering it; this cognition automatically and by its very nature diminishes the intensity, duration, and frequency of the problem.

Confronting one's anxieties may seem like a painful process, but it's actually quite the opposite. The water in the pool may look cold, but once you jump in, it's not bad at all. Likewise, the anxiety about the problem causes emotional pain. Facing the anxiety dissipates that pain—in large part—in and of itself; the water in the pool is not so bad after all. Confronting one's anxiety results in an immediate sense of accomplishment and improved self-confidence—an excellent launching pad for real healing and transformation.

A Support System

As we've seen, first and foremost in that healing, an anxious child must be taught that he is not alone—that he has the understanding and support of loved ones around him. Dealing with a child's anxiety together as a family issue and not just the child's problem is a powerful way to positively transform every one of the family's members individually and the entire family as a whole. What comes next is to teach the anxious child that he is never trapped—that he always has choices, always has ways out of the fear, that there will always be steps he can take to feel more safe and calm.

Separating the Child from His Anxiety

Among the most beneficial of those steps is learning to separate himself from his anxiety—that he is not his anxiety and his anxiety is not him. As the DuPonts explain in their books, it is quite difficult to observe an emotion and experience it at the same time, because observation creates an immediate separation between the observer and that which is being observed. So help your child to observe his anxiety. Discuss the varying intensities of different anxieties as they occur; discuss the circumstances which increase the anxiety and those which decrease it. In this way, together you objectify the anxiety and thereby help the child disassociate from it or, put another way, help him disentangle that knot of negative emotions from his self-identity.

The more a child can experience the distinction between himself and his anxiety, the more prepared he can become to face it effectively, proactively, when it does occur. He'll develop increasing control over his mental, emotional, and behavioral responses not only to the anxiety at hand but also to any future anxiety when it does occur

Empowering Children

He will begin to understand that anxiety is not a black-and-white condition that he can turn "on" or "off" like a light switch, but that it exists on a continuum, sometimes small, sometimes great. He will begin to understand that there are certain times, places, people, and situations that tend to trigger his anxiety, thereby empowering him to prepare and behave accordingly. He will learn that, while fear chases you when you run from it, when you turn and face it, it dissipates—all by itself. None of this necessarily rids the child of his anxiety, but it at least helps him claim that vital seat of control over his responses and behaviors. This alone goes a long way towards restoring (or establishing) a child's confidence and self-esteem.

Only the person experiencing the anxiety—only the child himself—can recognize and tackle the problem. This is a difficult lesson for both parent and child to absorb. You can help, certainly, and your child will no doubt be glad to accept all the help you have to offer. You can help the child recognize the problem and accept his responsibility, and you can give him permission to go for it. But you cannot face down the anxiety for your child—no matter how much you may wish you could, and no matter how much your child would like you to. It is the child's issue to deal with, and ultimately only the child holds the key to the relief the child desires. And your child must understand this as clearly as you do, for true lasting relief.

Children need to understand that their anxiety feeds on their fear. If they refuse to give in to their anxiety and the uncomfortable feelings it presents, then the anxiety has nothing to feed on and either retreats or it withers away and dies. Notice, again, that it is not the object of the fear that the child must learn to overcome but the feelings of fear themselves that the anxiety produces. In this way, a child (or adult, for that matter) can confront any object of fear by addressing the fear itself and not the object.

MISSION ACCOMPLISHED?

Perhaps an even harder lesson that children also need to understand is that, while anxiety may go away for good, that isn't usually the case. While the child can beat back the anxiety, the victory is likely temporary. The anxiety will probably ebb and flow throughout his lifetime. So while it is *possible* on the one hand to be permanently rid of a given anxiety, it is more likely that anxiety will periodically return. The victory lies not in having vanquished the foe, but in having the confidence that you can face it down if it shows up again. And this knowledge helps foster that confidence.

We don't solve anxiety problems by making big, bold changes, but rather by small, reasonable, and realistic ones, consistently over time. "Curing" anxiety is an ongoing process that requires gradual steps towards the greater goal of complete freedom from anxiety which, alas, we may never totally achieve. In a sense, then, this is a journey with a nebulous terminus: we see we've rounded what we thought the last bend, the station is just ahead; we chug along until, all of a sudden, we realize we've overshot the station—*oops, no problem just back up a little, now forward a little. Ah, there we are.* Importantly, we realize we are the engineer. We are in control of this journey which we now see has more than one terminal. We can go on boldly from here. Thus the journey of life continues far off into the future, and we're in control. *All aboard that's comin' aboard!*

So even though anxious feelings likely will reappear, the more a child practices not giving in and not feeding fear with fear, the less uncomfortable the discomfort and painful the pain, the shorter its duration, the less paralyzing effect the anxiety produces. The better a child gets at practicing not feeding anxiety with his fear, the less able anxiety is to take hold of that child and cause him to do its bidding.

As Dr. Manassis says, by acknowledging the reality of the child's fears and empowering him to manage them proactively, "the result is a child who feels understood but also ready to face a challenge."

RELAXATION

Instrumental to those ends, and bringing us back full circle to the *DreamChild Adventures* programs, is learning to relax.

The range of tools and techniques popularly used to help children overcome anxiety is vast and varied, including goal setting and goal completion, incentives and dis-incentives, role-playing, parties and other social events, extracurricular activities, fitness and exercise, diet and nutrition, and anti-anxiety medication (under a physician's proper supervision, of course). But no single tool or technique is more ubiquitous in anxiety texts, both those written for children and for adults, than relaxation.

THE RELAXATION RESPONSE

The "relaxation response" is the opposite of, and the solution to, the "stress response." As Dr. Manassis defines it, the relaxation response is "the body's automatic physical response when sensing no danger. It is designed to reduce a person's level of stress when in safe situations."

A moment ago, I mentioned that action can be taken in response to genuine, legitimate fears in order to avert the danger and decrease the symptoms associated with the stress response, but that with anxiety because there is no actual danger to avert no such action can be taken. Action *can* be taken, however, to dissipate the perceived threat of imminent danger, which would also help assuage the symptoms of the stress response. That action, of course, is relaxation, and it is something that can be induced and even self-induced.

That is because relaxation is a function of the parasympathetic, or voluntary, nervous system, whereas the stress response—*fight or flight*—is a function of the sympathetic, or involuntary, nervous system. That means the stress response is something that "happens to us," that is "beyond our control," while relaxation is something that we can make happen, that is within (some measure of) our control.

BENEFITS OF RELAXATION FOR CHILDREN

When so much of handling anxiety involves talk and self-talk, a child might appreciate some lessons in honest-to-goodness action he can take to combat his anxiety. That is, besides just confronting the feared situations head-on, of course—a task made much easier by approaching it from a relaxed state of mind and body.

Relaxation promotes improvements on a mental, emotional, and physical level; a powerful combination when you consider that anxiety is a problem with mental, emotional, and physical components.

Relaxation also helps a child to distract himself mentally from his anxieties, which by itself alleviates much of the emotional discomfort associated with them. Another way, more intentional perhaps, of "distracting" the mind is giving it something positive and proactive to focus on. Similar to the DuPonts' assertion about it not being humanly possible to observe your pain and feel it at the same time, Dr. Manassis points out that when the mind is focused on one thing, it can't worry about another; it's just not humanly possible.

That is one reason why sleeplessness and anxiety go hand-in-hand. Because all during the day an anxious child has plenty of stimulus around him to distract him from his fears. But at night, when it's just him and his thoughts alone in the dark, all those suppressed fears from throughout the day can now resurface. Relaxation can provide that distraction.

Beyond that, however, since the true source of an anxious child's fears, as we now know, are the physical symptoms of stress and anxiety, not the actual life circumstance that seems to provoke it, the physical benefits of relaxation techniques can have a profound impact on a child's experience of fear and, thus, his anxiety.

COMMON RELAXATION TECHNIQUES

Common techniques for achieving relaxation that are outlined in many books about anxiety, and for that matter, most books about relaxation as well, include:

- *deep abdominal breathing*—consciously breathing down into the belly (activating the parasympathetic nervous system) rather than the chest (activating the sympathetic nervous system)
- *progressive muscle relaxation*—focusing on relaxing each individual muscle or muscle group in the body, one at a time (sometimes tensing the muscle first before relaxing it, in order to better isolate it and distinguish the way it feels relaxed from the way it feels tensed)
- *visualization*—conjuring up pleasant and relaxing images in the mind (sometimes amplified by then imagining the sounds, smells, and tactile sensations of the pleasant visualization as well)

Since parents can only make themselves so available to help guide their child through these processes, and since it may take a while, depending on his age, for the child to develop these skills himself, a relaxation CD is a solution many parents may turn to for empowering their child to get guided support for relaxation on their own, on demand. All of the above-named techniques, by design, are woven into the *DreamChild Adventures* programs.

A CAVEAT: THE CHILD'S VOLITION

The one caveat about all of these relaxation techniques, however, is that the child has to want to do it. As you may already know too well, you cannot force a child to relax. You can only guide, facilitate, and encourage.

THE SLEEP-RELAXATION LINK

Sleep—and more specifically, a deep, restful, and uninterrupted sleep—is a fundamental aspect of relaxation, a key component in achieving and maintaining a relaxed state of body and mind. Without a regular good night's sleep it is inordinately more difficult to relax oneself and therefore inordinately harder to manage one's anxiety. Securing those deep, restful, and uninterrupted nights of sleep consistently, then, can become your child's first line of defense against anxiety.

DIETARY RELAXATION AIDS

Diet and exercise may also play a significant role in helping your child relax and combat anxiety. As Dr. Chansky explains, "Anxiety tends to creep in when our defenses are down, when we're sick, stressed, or sleepy."

In terms of diet, the key factor is avoiding caffeine, which for children means avoiding chocolate, black tea, and many types of soda. Caffeine is a stimulant that activates the sympathetic nervous system (fight or flight, the stress response), and because of that may facilitate a state of anxiety and hamper efforts at relaxation. Other than avoiding caffeine, simply maintaining a generally balanced diet has three powerful benefits. It helps the body become:

- better able to defend itself from illness
- more easily able to manage stress and anxiety
- more receptive to those efforts

EXERCISE FOR RELAXATION

In terms of exercise, the benefit to anxiety-sufferers is that physical exercise causes the body to release endorphins into the bloodstream. These neurochemicals are, as Dr. Manassis explains, "the body's natural painkillers." In addition, she reminds us, cardiovascular exercise over time reduces blood pressure and heart rate, which also make it easier for a person to relax and stay relaxed. What's more, exercise helps tire children out, making it easier for them to get to sleep and sleep well at night.

ANXIETY DISORDERS

As we've seen, when anxiety rises above what is considered "normal" or appropriate for one's age group to the extent that it pervades day-to-day living, setting up seemingly insurmountable limitations, then that anxiety surpasses the mere problem stage and rises to the level of a full-fledged Anxiety Disorder. No exploration of anxiety would be complete without a discussion of these disorders and the current knowledge on their relationships with sleep and relaxation.

Anxiety disorders are the most common of all mental disorders in children, afflicting about one in every eight children, with a current total estimated at about 19 million in America. Anxiety disorders fall into six different types:

- **Generalized Anxiety Disorder**—one common symptom is feeling extremely tense and having trouble relaxing; adequate restful sleep is essential for helping children with this disorder, and intentional physical relaxation is particularly beneficial
- **Social Anxiety Disorder**—teaching a child with this disorder relaxation techniques for calming himself before entering social situations can be extremely helpful
- **Obsessive-Compulsive Disorder (OCD)**—keeping a child's stress level low is paramount with this disorder; a common symptom of stress, as you know, is inadequate restful sleep

- **Specific Phobic Disorder**—again, deep relaxation is extremely beneficial in helping kids combat the symptoms of fear caused by this disorder (the most common, incidentally, of all anxiety disorders in children); visualization also proves highly beneficial in combating phobias
- **Panic Disorder**
- **Post-Traumatic Stress Disorder (PTSD)**

In Dr. Cynthia G. Last's book, *Help For Worried Kids*, she describes the first four of these as common "anxiety disorders of childhood," with panic disorders and PTSD less commonly seen in children. She does, however, add one other common childhood anxiety disorder to the list: **Separation Anxiety Disorder**. Most interestingly, as it affects our conversation on sleep, common symptoms of this disorder include trouble sleeping alone and trouble sleeping away from home.

These disorders all share in common a sense of worry. Further, many people with anxiety disorders suffer symptoms from several of the above-named diagnoses. Regardless of diagnoses, however, there are essentially two types of anxiety associated with every anxiety disorder:

- anxiety felt leading up to the situation
- anxiety felt during the situation

The former, the anxiety felt leading up to the situation, is almost always the more drawn out and paralyzing form of the two.

DIGGING FOR THE ROOT CAUSE OF A CHILD'S ANXIETY

With all our talk about the stress response, it is important as you try to sort out the root causes of any child's anxiety to keep in mind that anxiety disorders are not necessarily always directly related to a particular stressor. Sometimes the disorder *is* the stressor, caused by a combination of biological factors (genetics) and psychological factors (upbringing/environment)—more on these in a moment. A specific stress could simply trigger an existing anxiety disorder, while not being its actual cause. In fact, studies have found that children and others with anxiety disorders share in common an increased sensitivity and subsequent reactivity to stress.

MEDICAL ASSISTANCE FOR ANXIETY DISORDERS

Whatever your suspicions about a particular child's condition, a thorough examination by a trained professional is the only way to know for sure if he is suffering from an anxiety disorder, as there are many other conditions that present the same symptoms as anxiety. As far as that goes, a child can simply be "anxious" (prone to anxiety) without necessarily having a particular anxiety disorder—and it is, in fact, the more common situation. Regardless, diligent and proactive attention is essential.

And, in either case as well, broaching the subject with a trained medical professional can help direct you to the proper treatment options and self-help literature most appropriate and beneficial to your child. Such an awareness of the specific nature of your child's anxiety will also enable you to proactively discuss your child's condition with the teachers, mental health professionals, and other significant adults in your child's life.

Fortunately, as Dr. Chansky points out, "Anxiety disorders are the most treatable psychiatric condition."

Hereditary Anxiety: The Role of Genetics in Childhood Anxiety

Before closing with the silver lining in the dark cloud of anxiety, a word on genetics and heredity. Insofar as the *Nature-Nurture* paradigm is concerned, anxiety is a product of both.

Some people are genetically-predisposed to anxiety. Jerome Kagan, Ph.D. described a trait he called *behavioral inhibition* that can be observed in children beginning as early as 21 months of age. As Dr. Manassis explains in her book, *behavioral inhibition* occurs when "the usual tendency for young children to explore their surroundings appears inhibited."

If one of the parents has anxiety, it's more likely that their children will have anxiety than if neither parent did. Some people innately react to even the smallest things with intense responses while others are genetically programmed to be relatively unaffected by adversity, able instead to "go with the flow," or to "roll with it"—whatever happens *happens*. Do not let this revelation discourage you.

Despite a child's genetic predisposition for anxiety, the way he is raised is of paramount importance in determining how that child will respond to the world in the face of it.

Only with great difficulty can one rid oneself of anxious feelings, especially when it is part of one's genetic predisposition. But every person—including a young child—has the potential to take charge of his responses to anxiety by changing his thoughts and choosing his behaviors.

The Silver Lining on Anxiety's Dark Cloud

The silver lining in the dark cloud of anxiety is that it is considered, and rightly so, to be a disorder of "quality people." This is because an anxious person is simply more prone to consider other people's feelings. People with anxiety also think more than non-anxious people do about the consequences of their actions, and even though that thinking is riddled with uncomfortable emotions, anxious people usually wind up acting in ways that protect other people's feelings.

A bully, for example, doesn't have problems of anxiety, and therefore does not care about hurting other children, while a child with anxiety is very unlikely to brazenly and intentionally hurt another person. Also, while incessant worry about getting into trouble may cause a child pain and discomfort, it keeps that child from getting into trouble.

Better People

As such, an anxious person's anxiety actually makes him a better person, a better friend, son or daughter, sibling, and schoolmate. People with anxiety are typically some of the nicest people around. Properly channeled, anxiety can promote appropriate behavior as much as it can promote inappropriate behavior when improperly channeled. Bestowing on a child this understanding of the positive side, the brighter side, of anxiety and the goodness that comes from it, can help an anxious child tremendously in overcoming the guilt, shame, and self-deprecation that typically comes bundled together with his anxiety.

As mentioned earlier, a child with anxiety is prone to believe that there is something wrong with him. But these previously mentioned positive qualities that anxiety can foster may reveal to that same child that there is also something especially "right" with him, too, and in a way, something "better" about him than his non-anxious peers. This can help a child to feel better about himself—a major step on the road to recovery from chronic anxiety.

Showing consistent appreciation for these qualities that make your anxious child more respectful, courteous, thoughtful, introspective, caring, compassionate, obedient, honest, and more, helps your child to see himself with new, more forgiving and self-loving eyes.

A Self-Feeding Cycle: For Worse or For Better

As you've seen repeatedly, anxiety and sleep disruption are tied together inextricably, each one contributing to the other. Fortunately just as anxiety feeds on itself, so does relaxation. A state of relaxation literally alters the brain's responses to various stimuli. Dr. Chansky refers to the work of Jeffrey Schwartz, M.D. and Sharon Begley, who, in their book *The Mind and the Brain*, discuss how the brain is constantly reprogramming itself to supply the greatest amount of neurons to the pathways and regions of the brain we most frequently use.

So if (hypothetically speaking, of course) you've lived in a state of anxiety and sleeplessness most of your life, your brain becomes programmed to support what it perceives as a chronically heightened state of stress and threat of danger. In other words, it becomes ever-easier and faster for the brain to make the connections and associations that trigger the stress response and maintain it. But if you start practicing relaxation, over time and through frequent repetition your brain will start to reprogram itself to support a more relaxed state of being, making the relaxation response ever-easier to achieve and maintain.

You literally can reverse the brain's tendency to react anxiously to various situations simply by practicing relaxation. Truly, the relaxation response is the antidote to the stress response. Relaxation helps diminish anxiety and it helps reduce impediments to healthful sleep. We, therefore, have come full circle to the *DreamChild Adventures* audio programs, powerful tools for undoing the strands of that self-tightening knot of anxiety.

Chapter 18

Summary: Nature-Deficit Disorder

*I went to the woods because I wished to live deliberately,
to front only the essential facts of life,
and see if I could not learn what it had to teach,
and not, when I came to die, discover that I had not lived.*

Henry David Thoreau, *Walden*, 1846

We've explored many subjects together in the span of this book, from fear of the dark, to television and resistance to reading, to divorce, death and dying, to self-esteem, along with many medical issues, all of it with the united objective of helping your child to have a good night's sleep.

A Web of Interrelationships

As we've roamed through these subjects, we've discovered that many of them—like fear of the dark, and death and dying—are inextricably interwoven in a dual cause-and-effect relationship.

Let me offer a simple (perhaps even simplistic) illustration:

- Issues around sleep can interrelate with issues of fear of the dark.
- Issues around sleep can interrelate with issues of death and dying.
- Issues around fear of the dark can interrelate with issues of death and dying.

For children, and even some adults, all three may interconnect—each one . . . sleep, fear of the dark, death and dying . . . with either or both of the others. So it goes with all of the influences—internal and external—in a child's life (and for that matter, yours and mine as well).

I by no means wish to imply any sort of unsubstantiated causation between any of these issues and any other. I do however wish to shed light on the viewpoint that no problem, no issue, no behavior or circumstance stands alone. Rather, each meshes with all of the other influences underlying all of the given problems, issues, behaviors, circumstances, and whatnot—namely, ***the person***. The individual person resides in the core of it all and, as it applies here and now, within the child.

Nature-Deficit Disorder (NDD)

To illustrate further, consider another condition in a child's life that may have a pronounced effect on his sleep and, *vice versa*, one on which his sleep may have a profound effect. Moreover, this condition affects and is affected by every other condition we've discussed in these pages—fear of the dark, television, resistance to reading, divorce, death and dying, self-esteem—and all the rest. This condition is the experience of nature—the forest, meadows, streams, lakes and oceans—the great outdoors. And if anything illustrates a seamless web of interconnected relationships, nature does.

Over eons of human evolution, lifetime after lifetime transpired in deep rapport with nature. Our everyday world drenched us in sensory richness and enlivened our every moment, which we human beings are—in a very real sense—physically "hardwired" to experience, by which I mean explore, relate to, learn from, and care for. Research conducted using my *AudioMagic* Nature Sound programs lends support to this theory (for more on this study, see Appendix H).

A fascinating book, published in 2008, makes a bold assertion about the effect of nature on our children . . . or rather, the effect of the lack of nature, these days: nature's absence, or, to put it another way—a *nature-deficit disorder*. Richard Louv, chair of the Children & Nature Network, and recipient of the 2008 Audubon Medal, has published seven books and has written for some of our nation's—and the world's—most prestigious periodicals such as *The New York Times, Christian Science Monitor,* and others. The seventh of Louv's books, *Last Child in the Woods,* at the time of this writing, is a best seller.

I find mention of the book's success relevant to this discussion of its contents because it reflects a prevailing interest in Louv's message, perhaps because it speaks so profoundly to our own experience. Louv asserts that civilization today in America deprives a whole generation of children of a relationship with nature that is vital if they're to grow into healthy and well-adjusted adults. And he warns that if we don't start taking conscious actions as a community of parents, educators, leaders, and guardians, we may, by standing aside, tacitly initiate countless generations of children growing up dysfunctionally, with no idea of the basis of their problems, much less of the knowledge necessary to remedy them. So, too, may our children grow up dysfunctional if we don't help them get their proper sleep and learn the intrinsic value of it.

Louv draws many strikingly similar correlations between the many issues a parent may face and this *nature-deficit disorder* he describes—its relationships with fears, anxieties, emotional intelligence, self-esteem, academic performance, childhood obesity, and, yes, with sleep.

For me, then, because of my own bent toward the healing efficacy of nature's beauty, I find an easy companionship between Louv's assertion and my interest in the sights, smells, movements, touch, and especially in the sounds of nature. It consequently seems only natural to me to weave 3D sound through the warp and woof of nature to create a comforter which helps children overcome sleep deficit dysfunction by experiencing the calming effects of nature. I hope this comforter promotes restful and restorative sleep and in turn helps children grow into healthy adults, who along the way will avoid the terrible void of nature-deficit.

Let's expand a bit, therefore, some of the parallels between the web of influences surrounding nature and sleep—or more specifically, between nature-deficit disorder and problems sleeping.

Television, NDD, and Sleep

Just a few generations ago, children grew up in a much different world. There was no television, for one. And most children grew up helping around the house and yard or, in many cases, the farm. They spent their regimented time in productive engagements, often directly involving nature—collecting wood, feeding livestock, weeding, and other chores. Their play time then was unregimented—that is, "unstructured, imaginative, exploratory"—and much more likely to involve the natural surroundings with which they already had such intimate rapport (playing ball, swimming in the river, riding bicycles). The kind of rapport that could help a child sleep better at night, fully wound-down from active, exuberant play, unafraid of the dark or things that go bump in the night, and eager to face the new day and the adventures it brings.

In my interview with Kenneth, his stepdaughter Pamela was having problems with anger which manifested in her relationship with her siblings (sibling rivalry) and no doubt had some of its roots in her parents' divorce (children of divorce). She wasn't reading (resistance to reading) and was doing poorly in school (academic performance). And she had trouble sleeping. Pamela suffered from nightmares, and wanted "to watch television all night," as Kenneth put it.

In *Last Child in the Woods,* Louv laments that kids flock to the TV partly because, despite our best efforts and intentions, we've actually conditioned them to avoid the outside, and how else are they going to get the healthy escape and fantasy they need?

Permit me to summarize several of the points Louv makes:

- We close down parks and develop over what was once public land, leaving children nowhere to go when we tell them to go outside and play. So kids fill the sidewalks and streets and loiter around convenience stores and in parking lots.
- By enforcing ever stricter regulations—building, community, environmental—children are hearing, in no uncertain terms, that their free-play is not welcome here, there, or anywhere. No words need be exchanged for them to get this message. It's being told to them loud and clear through unacceptably repressive conditions. So again, they retreat inside and turn on the television. Or they lie around and play video games. Or both.
- Likewise, children flee the structure many of their caretakers keep trying to impose on them. Not only does it run counter to the very nature of childhood and the purpose of play to regulate how a child plays (or doesn't play)—safety, etiquette, and good sense naturally aside—but it implants in children a terrible fear that can hold them back for the rest of their lives. The structures and strictures often placed on childhood play, and outdoor play especially, often come from a place of fear, usually, Louv says, of danger and litigation. This teaches children that it's not safe to be themselves, that it's not safe to go outside, nor to be on their own, separated

from their parents, or to learn to trust their judgment when facing the unknown. We inadvertently accelerate this process in response to shrinking reserves of buildable space, as developers press city councils for more building lots per acre. Then, as houses are built closer to one another, buyers demand more private space, and builders happily respond with larger houses, until we have subdivisions of 4000 square-foot houses crowded onto 5000 square-foot lots. Where else do children—and adults, for that matter—have to go but inside?

Thus, we set the stage for nature-deficit disorder.

Looking through the eyes of the child, do you find it any wonder that so many children retreat to the television? The TV provides them a sense of safety and solace, relaxation and imaginative, if artificial, stimulation, and autonomy that a relationship with nature would have done a better job at. Or as Louv himself might say, it is a poor substitute for the relationship with nature which every child requires to grow up healthy, happy, and prosperous.

Television, as babysitter and companion, in fact isn't a phenomenon relegated to just the home. We now commonly see a small TV installed in the back seats of automobiles to keep children entertained—read: *quiet and complacent*—not only on long car trips, but those as short as to the mall and back. Meanwhile a whole world zooms by, unnoticed, just outside the window.

TV does more than just lull us to sleep at times, and stave sleep off at others. It also keeps us sheltered from the real world, outside of the illusory one on the screen. A world that becomes increasingly threatening and intimidating the longer the separation lasts. We even now assume necessary the ubiquitous home alarm system to insure ourselves against unauthorized entry into our reclusive pavement palaces.

Louv cites University of North Carolina professor Robin Moore in pointing out that the sensory stimulation prevalent in our ambient natural environment is the predominant sensory stimulation each of us personally experience. Therefore, allowing children the freedom to explore the natural world, each in his own way, is instrumental in helping them to develop a clear sense of self and a healthy relationship to the world at large.

As with a lack of adequate sleep, although in different ways, a deficiency in a child's exposure to nature puts at risk his development of self-esteem, self-reliance, imagination and creativity, motivation, and ability to relate with others.

Which brings us to the subject of school.

ACADEMIC PERFORMANCE, NDD, AND SLEEP

A report entitled *"Closing the Achievement Gap,"* from the State Education and Environmental Roundtable, a study of environment-based models of education, concluded that a study of 150 schools nationwide for a period of 10 years showed that schools that taught environmental awareness produced students more adept in math, language arts, science, and social studies. Decision-making, critical-thinking, and problem-solving skills were enhanced. And behavior and attendance rates excelled.

A similar study in 2005, this time of 255 at-risk sixth graders, revealed that the students whose educational program involved outdoor activities and environmental studies displayed:

- a 27% increase in measured mastery of science concepts
- enhanced cooperation and conflict resolution skills

and also displayed gains in:

- self-esteem
- problem-solving
- motivation to learn
- classroom behavior

Exposure to nature and restful sleep seem to have similar effects on a child's academic performance, as do they on a child's weight (just as a child's weight affects her interactions with nature and her sleep).

CHILDHOOD OBESITY, NDD, AND SLEEP

It isn't hard to see the correlation between a child's exposure to the outdoors and childhood obesity. Besides the obvious health benefits of fresh air and sunshine, most of a child's activity held outdoors is active, aerobic activity. It's no secret that exercise is a key component in healthy weight management. And if most of a child's vigorous cardiovascular, muscle-building, coordination-developing exercise occurs out of doors, then it stands to reason that more and better out-of-doors environments for doing so is a key component in combating childhood obesity.

It also has the added benefit of giving a child what he needs to tucker himself out so that he can settle down for a deep and reinvigorating sleep without argument, without interruption. Here sleep and nature work together in a self-feeding, self-perpetuating cycle to help a child, among other ways, to achieve and maintain a healthy weight. And of course, what arrives fast on its heels might likely include improved mood and ability to relate with others, greater academic performance, and increased self-esteem.

Of course, with 80% of Americans living in cities, children face a difficult challenge in simply finding the space to have this need met. But the cost of not having it met is far more than cosmetic. Childhood obesity often leads to larger health problems. When we view childhood obesity as a life-or-death problem and not just a lifestyle problem, we see how vital it is that we do something about it. Earlier in this book we saw how improving a child's sleep habits is one action we can take to help protect them from these dangers. Spending time in nature is another one.

Fortunately, while many children may resist forced, intentional exercise, if given the space to run about and roam free, many will do a more than adequate job of exerting the energy bubbling inside them.

Case in point, Lia's daughter Ana was a restless child, doing anything to avoid going to sleep and when she slept, sleeping restlessly, tossing and turning and entangling herself in the bedsheets. Ana was also overweight.

Clearly, if Ana was lacking in physical exercise it wasn't from the lack of energy to do so. She had more than enough energy, more than she knew what to do with. It made her unruly and disruptive in school, to the point of forcing her parents' hand, with acts of stealing and violence, to place her into an even more structured and potentially stifling environment. The audio CDs might very well have provided Ana with a much needed reprieve from the outer world and given her a chance to feel more at peace in her own inner environment.

With that peace she became more able to function appropriately in the world she shared with other people. Eventually she even became motivated to start a diet, with no prodding from the outside.

Following on the progress Lia describes her daughter making, Lia is in an excellent position to give a newly inspired, self-motivated, and self-aware child like Ana more outlets for free, expressive, explorative play in her outer world, in nature, without so many boundaries, or rules, or structures. Along with the *DreamChild Adventures* programs introducing deep and restful sleep, increased exposure to nature could help a child like Ana develop greater harmony between her inner and outer worlds so that exercising and slimming down to a healthier weight might come more naturally.

This leads me to make a brief comment on self-esteem.

SELF-ESTEEM, NDD, AND SLEEP

In the case of Bobby, the son of the woman Alan was dating, the boy's poor sleep was associated with heavy television viewing, poor reading habits, academic difficulty, and poor self-esteem. Alan witnessed a turning point in Bobby's life, after using the audio CDs, when Bobby overcame his fears of nature, of all things, and the big, bad world outside, and started dirt bike riding and trying out for soccer. Alongside those benefits of restful sleep and exposure to nature, not least of which is self-esteem, came improvement in Bobby's reading skills and interest, a decrease in his television viewing, a more appropriate demeanor when relating to others, both authority figures and peers, and a greater passion for experiencing what the world and life have to offer.

Recent studies have shown that children's camps and programs based in adventure therapy and direct outdoor education have pronounced therapeutic value for troubled youths, by imparting leadership skills, academic prowess, confidence and self-esteem, strength of character, and ability to relate to others.

MEDICAL ISSUES

Louv's discussion of nature's beneficial effects on children with ADHD is strikingly similar to our earlier discussion of the effects of sleep on ADHD. He reports that some researchers recommend parents provide their children more access to "green space" because it may improve their "attentional functioning"—their attention span.

Louv then goes on to discuss, as we have already, the over-prescribing of stimulants like Ritalin (methylphenidate) and Dexedrine (dextroamphetamine) to solve the problem, rather than the restoration of a more healthful sleeping and waking environment, one more conducive to the child's development of attentional functioning and all the other skills needed to live a fulfilling life.

Divorce, NDD, and Sleep

"Divorce affects a child's whole world view," I wrote in the commentary on "Children of Divorce." In that discussion, we learned how children of divorce may struggle not only with sleep troubles but with reading abilities, academic performance, and interpersonal relationships with peers and authority figures. "It forces reexamination of the concepts of safety, stability, trust, and love," I wrote. These are some of the same qualities that a nature-deficit disorder seems to affect.

Throughout all of these examples—these issues—one message remains clear: nature is not a luxury. It's not leisure time. It's a necessity. It's vital for proper developmental growth and critical for maintaining a healthy life.

The same applies to sleep. It is not a luxury, and should never be treated as such. To say, *"I have no time for sleep"* or *"I have no time for nature"* is to fool only yourself. And worse, Louv suggests, doing yourself a disservice, and maybe even harm.

Louv attributes to a parent's "acutely tuned responsibility" the attitude that children taking time for relaxation and leisure is self-indulgent. That seems thoroughly counterintuitive, yes, but nevertheless it is a commonly held myth among today's "grown-ups" that work must always come before play. That our obligations are paramount, and only after those obligations are met can we permit ourselves the luxury of some down-time—some fun and relaxation. Of course, our children are going to model—to perpetuate—this myth in their own lives. After all, who else is there for the children as a model? As Louv describes it, a family hike may be more of a priority than many parents realize. Certainly such an activity is more of an instrumental factor in a child's overall health and wellness than it is a frivolous and self-indulgent luxury.

The Unseen Perils of Modern City Life

In his January 2, 2009, feature for *The Boston Globe,* "How the City Hurts your Brain," journalist Jonah Lehrer proposes that it is now, more than ever, imperative to bring nature back into our lives. He describes recent scientific research revealing that exposure to today's urban environments impairs some of our basic mental processes, and writes, "After spending a few minutes on a crowded city street, the brain is less able to hold things in memory, and suffers from reduced self-control."

Long-term migrational trends have, for the first time in human history, resulted in more people living in cities than anywhere else, and the nature-deficit impairment Lehrer describes may not be a mere coincidence. As I proposed earlier, we could be starving an entire generation of a much needed form of essential human nourishment. One could almost wonder if Lehrer were talking about nature here, or sleep.

As Lehrer writes, the overstimulation of urban environments forces one of the human brain's weakest spots to work itself into overdrive. This is the part of our brain that filters out irrelevant stimuli in order to help us pay attention to what matters. Excessive stimulation, like that which we find in modern cities, impairs the part of our brain involved in *paying attention*.

What's more, Lehrer goes on to explain, such "cognitive overload" also impairs our self-control, which is itself controlled by the same part of our brain responsible for paying attention; the same part of our brain, in other words, that's just been depleted by filtering out all the irrelevant stimuli in order to pay attention to what's most relevant in the moment. And when we think of self-control, we must also be reminded that this includes control over our emotions.

Put simply, our ability—or inability—to pay attention, and our self-control—or lack thereof—coexist in a self-feeding cycle either impaired or aided by certain qualities of our external environment.

URBAN VERSUS NATURAL ENVIRONMENTS PUT TO THE TEST

University of Michigan psychologist Marc Berman validated this impairment in an experiment wherein students were split into two groups—one sent to an arboretum, the other to busy city streets—and then put through a battery of psychological tests. Test results showed that those subjects exposed to the city streets suffered impairments not found in those subjects exposed to the more natural environment, including impairments in the areas of mood, memory, and attention.

We can now say with relative certainty that in contrast to urban environments, natural environments do not demand so much brain power—and specifically the powers of "controlled perception" to resist temptations—leaving both our ability to pay attention and to control our impulses intact, and more—rejuvenated and refreshed.

This is not to say that city-dwelling is inherently bad and rural life is inherently good. It is not to suggest that people abandon their city apartments and move to farmhouses in the middle of nowhere. On the contrary, it's much easier to bring nature to you.

THERAPEUTIC PROPERTIES OF NATURE

For example, we also know now that nature has therapeutic properties. Scientific research on the effects of nature on sick hospital patients has already made this evident. According to an article by Stephen Mitrione, M.D., M.L.A., on *Therapeutic Responses to Natural Environments*, studies have found that the design of a health care facility can influence many elements of patient care, including the rate of infection, the rate of errors made by health care providers, and the costs involved in treating a particular condition.

One of the most famous of these studies, conducted by Dr. Roger S. Ulrich, Ph.D., of the Center for Health Systems and Design at Texas A&M University's Colleges of Architecture and Medicine, revealed in Ulrich's 1999 paper entitled *Effects of Gardens On Health Outcomes: Theory and Research*, that patients in hospital rooms with garden views used less pain medication, recovered from surgery faster, and were discharged sooner than patients in rooms with no view. Nature exposure also proved to reduce these patients' levels of stress and anxiety—and those of their family and the hospital staff.

Lehrer cites a similar University of Illinois Landscape and Human Health Laboratory study in which director Frances Kuo found that women residing in public housing complexes could focus better when their apartment had a view of a courtyard filled with lawn, trees, and flowers.

This is not a new concept either. As Mitrione observes, therapeutic gardens in health care settings are as ancient as the Middle Ages. One theory behind this age-old phenomenon (the "biophilia hypothesis") says that our bodies respond to natural settings because our genes have been encoded by evolution to do so. In other words, areas with lots of vegetation and a steady, healthy water supply were the most advantageous for our species' survival.

Whatever the reason, thankfully, hospitals today are recognizing this nature-wellness connection and are starting to invest heavily in therapeutic landscaping and architecture.

A Heartening Realization

Meanwhile, we individual caretakers can take heart that all research on this subject suggests that even a limited sense of nature (like that from looking through a window) can have a powerful impact on one's psyche and—thanks to what we already know of the mind/body connection—one's biology. As Lehrer notes, "Even these fleeting glimpses of nature improve brain performance, it seems, because they provide a mental break from the urban roll."

Back to the Core Question: How to Help a Child Sleep?

So we revisit now the core question that brought me to research and write this book and brought you to read it: *How do we help the children in our lives sleep better at night?*

As we witness the soothing nighttime sounds of nature supplanted by the jarring shrieks and growls and roars of the city or the eerie moans and groans of the suburbs, we're left to wonder, how a child—or anyone for that matter—is expected to sleep under these conditions? And who in her right mind wants to awaken in the morning, only to leave the safety and security of home to venture out into all that?

The DreamChild Adventures 3D Audio Series

Thankfully—and predictably—it turns out many of the remedies for nature-deficit disorder are the same as those for sleep difficulties. And, once again, this brings us back to the *DreamChild Adventures* 3D Audio Series. In all of the cases discussed in this book, the *3D Living Sound* audio programs served to help those children sleep better at night, and seemed instrumental in the myriad improvements reported in a host of other issues they were facing. These programs have been carefully crafted to provide sleep and relaxation-enhancing benefits through a synergy of structural, cognitive, and suggestive elements. One of those elements—one which is prevalent throughout each of the CDs in the series—is the presence of nature.

COUNTRY FRIENDS

- *a car trip to the countryside*
- *a walk down an imaginary pathway through an enchanted forest*
- *a meadow with a farmhouse*
- *an interlude by the river for a meditation to the sounds of water, wind and birds*
- *reflected images on the surface of a pond*
- *a pathway to the ocean beach*

MAGIC CARPET

- *a playground*
- *a zoo*
- *farm animals*
- *a pathway through an enchanted forest*
- *Mother Nature's words of care and comfort*
- *a sandy ocean beach*
- *gently rolling waves*

PLAYHOUSE ON THE BEACH

- *a beach*
- *seabirds*
- *fish*
- *seashells*
- *an interlude of floating on the gently rolling waves*

Admittedly, an audio experience of nature, no matter how immersive, does not perfectly substitute for nature, but we can at least start with the simple observation that these and other nature-filled audio CDs make proactive use of what we are now discovering is a critical aspect of healthy childhood development.

The *DreamChild Adventures* 3D Audio Series in particular, recorded as it is in *3D Living Sound*, augments and enhances these benefits of audio exposure to nature measurably. As I briefly mentioned in the commentary on Resistance to Reading, University of Arizona professor of psychology, neurology, and psychiatry Gary E. Schwartz, Ph.D., studied the difference in effects on the brain from 2D audio and *3D Living Sound* by analyzing the EEG topographic brain–mapping data produced when subjects listened to recordings of the same sounds in *3D Living Sound*, stereo sound, and mono (or monaural audio).

As for the various subjects' direct experiences, not only was the *3D Living Sound* environment perceived as "more real" than the other two, but the difference reported between how the subject experienced the *3D Living Sound* was as vast a difference from the stereo sound experience as listening to stereo sound was from mono. Granted, we're not providing certain senses (like smell and touch) but that didn't seem to detract from the subjective experience of full immersion in a "real" nature experience which, it turns out, allows listeners to imagine the other senses, most particularly sight (as visualization).

Further, examination of the brain maps produced during these experiments revealed that the visualization area of the brain "lit up" considerably more when the subjects listened to the *3D Living Sound* recordings than when they listened to either of the others. These results show, again, that *3D Living Sound*™ has an even more pronounced effect on the brain (and dare I say the brain–body connection?) than do standard 2D sound recordings.

Commenting on his findings, Schwartz says:

> These data further support the hypothesis that the 3D tapes were more attention-getting, novel, and interesting compared to the stereo tapes. The fact that they show up on the left side and posterior (rear) regions (occipital) is consistent with the idea that both verbal imagery and visual imagery were activated by the 3D tapes. [NOTE: *at the time of Schwartz' studies, the* 3D Living Sound *audio recordings were produced on tape rather than CD; the relevant effects, however, remain identical.*]

It appears that the "virtual audio environments" of the *DreamChild Adventures* 3D Audio Series offer an added dimension of reality that effectively enhances the nature experience and, therefore, its many medical benefits.

Conclusion

What I hope to have conveyed in this book is that the *DreamChild Adventures* 3D audio programs are a proven effective tool for helping children achieve a deep state of relaxation and sleep, and with this change, they show marked improvement in many other areas of their lives, affecting their health and well-being on every level—mental, emotional, physical, and, perhaps, even spiritual.

I also hope this book has begun to make clear that everything a child experiences affects the whole of his being. And what's more—and this may come as a surprise to you—caretakers of children can interpret this revelation as liberating and empowering.

How?

By realizing that everything and anything you do to help your child in one area of his life will almost assuredly benefit him in all the other areas.

Every positive, proactive step you take makes a difference. It all helps, and more, it seems, than any of us will ever know. A plant brings life into a lifeless corner. A window brings sunlight into an otherwise dark room. A vegetable garden replaces a patch of dirt. A walk together, caretaker(s) and child, hand-in-hand, through the park brings together nature and people. And if there's no park, a walk around the block. Sit together on a porch, snuggled in a comfy chair, reading a book together aloud.

Or listen to the sweet *3D Living Sound* of nature and the soothing voice of a caring and trusted guide. This liberating revelation, this empowering awareness, allows you at any given moment to work with your child on those challenges and issues you feel most focused on at that time. There is no right or wrong way. There is only your way. Yours and your child's.

Remember: everything you and your child face is interconnected, interwoven—like a tapestry.

Follow the threads and you trace the fabric of a child's life. I encourage you now to allow your awareness of this fabric to drape over you like a warm, soft comforter that tucks you in for a good night's sleep. Because when you can see your children as they are, you have everything you need to help them sleep well, too.

A Personal Invitation

I hope that you have found inspiration in the stories of the many wonderful people who reported their results from using *DreamChild Adventures*, and I would like to invite you to participate in a similar manner. You will have the opportunity to write a Customer Review on the 3daudiomagic.com website and, if you wish, share your own story and insights with others. You will also have an opportunity to use a bulletin board through which you can communicate with other program users, to ask and/or answer questions.

I hope my book doesn't really end here so much as it begins something even more dynamic. I envision people actively taking part in helping one another, creating a support network of sorts, to welcome those new to this unique therapeutic offering and to advance each other's practice of these techniques. I also look forward to contributing to this growing community of individuals, as we learn, share, and celebrate each other's achievements on the road to lasting peace of mind for ourselves and our loved ones.

APPENDICES

Appendix A

A Brief Disclaimer

I *wish I could tell you* that all children who use the *DreamChild Adventures* programs will have results that are as dramatic as those reported in this book, but I can't. The cases cited were quite extraordinary in terms of both the scope and degree of improvements, and I can't claim they are a representative sample nor can I guarantee your child will experience similar results. Nonetheless, even with this unscientific sampling, the promising benefits are clear. Further, of all the patients who tried the *DreamChild* programs, not one has reported any significant adverse reactions.

In my clinical practice as a psychiatrist, I have enjoyed the opportunity to observe the effectiveness of the audio programs over many years. After comparing the results to traditional interventions, such as medications, to treat anxiety and sleep disorders, I find this novel approach offers tremendous advantages: safety, effectiveness, range of benefits, lack of side effects, and personal empowerment. Please understand, I'm not, by any stretch of the imagination, a purist when it comes to practicing alternative medicine. In fact, in my day-to-day practice, I rely on medications for the treatment of many disorders, but the 3D audio programs are one of my primary therapeutic interventions and have provided my patients success I could not have dreamed of without them. And keep in mind that medications and audio therapy are not mutually exclusive. In many cases, in order to achieve the best results with a particular patient, I utilize both.

Appendix B

Audio Equipment

These programs have been *professionally recorded* using state-of-the-art digital technology which offers exceptional sound quality. But in order to reproduce high-quality sound and achieve maximum effectiveness, the programs should be listened to with headphones of sufficient quality. Please keep in mind that the headphones provided with the average CD player or mp3 or mp4 player provide very poor sound quality. A modest investment in quality, lightweight, open-air headphones will add appreciably to the therapeutic experience.

If you would like to truly maximize the listening experience, I strongly encourage you to purchase the Sennheiser PX 100 headphone, which is what I used during studio mixing of the programs. This headphone is no longer being produced, but at the time of this writing could still be found online through various vendors (I cannot highly recommend purchasing its replacement, the PX 100-II). By listening with the Sennheiser PX 100, your child will experience remarkable sound quality with a very comfortable fit, and although no headphones are "childproof," this one is of very sturdy construction and likely to last a long time. Although ear cushions eventually deteriorate on any open-air headphone, they are easy to replace at low cost. A less expensive and excellent alternative is the Koss PortaPro headphone. While not quite as comfortable, the sound quality is nearly indistinguishable from that of the PX 100.

Appendix C

Hearing Risk

Now *I want to cover an issue* germane to any discussion of audio-based therapy, and likely to be a concern on any parent or caretaker's mind, and that is the attendant potential hearing risks.

Noise-Induced Hearing Loss in Children

Our children's hearing is quite sensitive (as is our own). Noise at extreme levels lasting for long periods of time can permanently damage the ears and cause irreversible hearing loss. Medically this is known as "Noise-Induced Hearing Loss" (NIHL). And in the case of a child, not only does it affect his hearing, but it can also affect his language development, social development, and learning abilities.

What Causes Hearing Loss?

While it is true that hearing damage can potentially be caused by short-term exposure to extremely loud sounds (an explosion), it is far more often the result of long-term exposure to moderately loud sounds for long durations at a time and/or over recurring periods of time. This slower, more common, and insidious method of harming one's hearing occurs through the gradual wearing out of the inner ear hair cells and the progressive weakening over time of their capacity for recovery.

But even in the case of the rarer, former cause of NIHL, it is still a measure of both loudness *and* persistence of the sound in question that determines the risk for permanent damage; NIHL is a cumulative problem. But how big a problem is it?

Statistics on Children's Hearing

The American Academy of Audiology revealed that around 5.2 million children in the U.S. between 6 and 19 years of age (that's 12.5%, or one in eight) have permanent ear damage and NIHL. And the National Institute on Deafness and Other Communication Disorders reports that since 1971 the number of Americans from age 3 and up who have some form or other of hearing loss or damage has doubled, and then some. The American Speech-Language-Hearing Association conducted a study in 2006 that showed over half the participating high school students reported having at least one symptom of hearing loss. "We'll be seeing many more instances of people having to use hearing assistance devices and at a younger age. Much like obesity, we may get to a point where there is a norm of poor hearing." (*In Pursuit of Silence*, George Prochnik, 2010.)

Statistics from the European Union are just as dire. According to a recent study, 5%—10% of people in the EU who listen to personal entertainment players are at risk of developing symptoms of noise-induced hearing loss after five years.

SAFE-LISTENING STANDARDS FOR CHILDREN

Unfortunately, although these statistics are quite conclusive, there are no agreed-upon standards for safe listening levels: OSHA has determined the maximum decibel level for safe listening is 90 decibels; the National Institute for Occupational Safety and Health and the Centers for Disease Control and Prevention say 85 db; certain scientific studies set the bar still lower, at a more conservative 79 db; and the Environmental Protection Agency recommends keeping exposure for any 24 hour period below 70 db.

To provide a reference point for understanding these numbers, here are a few comparisons:

- 120—150 db: loud music, firearms, fireworks, jet engines, ambulance sirens, jackhammers
- 80—96 db: MP3 and MP4 players through earbuds at maximum volume, night clubs, hair dryers, lawnmowers, snowmobiles, chainsaws, pneumatic drills, helicopters, the subway, busy restaurants
- 70—80 db: normal urban street traffic, alarm clocks, vacuum cleaners
- 60 db: normal conversational tones
- 40 db: raindrops
- 35 db: voices whispering

Two sets of safe-listening standards recognized by one or more qualified organizations follow at the close of this section. Before I present those standards to you, however, I must address their limitations.

VARIABLES: THE CRUX OF THE FORMULA

The problem, in a nutshell, is there are too many variables that can influence any individual's personal "safety zone"; therefore any singular definitive benchmark is doomed to have too-wide a margin of error. For example, one less frequently considered but highly influential variable is the variation in the "toughness" or "tenderness" of the listener's ears.

COMMON PITFALL: DESENSITIZATION

The danger for many young people in particular is that, as they continue to listen to their portable entertainment devices at loud settings, they become desensitized and raise the volume still further in order to restore what they perceive to be the level of loudness to which they are accustomed. This creates a vicious and never-ending cycle of increasing the risk and accelerating the advance of NIHL.

How Safe Are Portable Music Players?

Many people are very worried about today's breed of portable music players (or PMPs) which, like its predecessors, are eminently portable and has an extremely long battery life, but with the alleged potential for much greater and, therefore, more dangerous sound output. Some say this could pose a serious threat to the hearing of a whole generation; others say this is total panic and exaggeration.

So, to get a more scientific vantage point on the subject, we turn to a paper presented by Cory D. Portnuff, Au.D., Ph.D. and Brian J. Fligor, Sc.D. at the **2006 NIHL in Children Conference** entitled, *"Sound Output Levels of the iPod and Other MP3 Players: Is There Potential Risk to Hearing?"* Their presentation was based on findings from a study the two conducted to evaluate output levels of several popular PMPs to determine their risks to hearing.

In the study, Portnuff and Fligor examined five MP3 players from three different manufacturers, using with each player in turn each of five different models of earphones (including stock earphones). They then measured the full range of output levels, from lowest to highest, of each pairing (25 in all: 5 MP3 players x 5 models of earphones) while playing, in turn, each of five different genres of music as well as a set of pure tones.

What they found, across all MP3 player-headphone combinations, was the measured potential to produce sound levels high enough to cause hearing loss—"if used at high enough volumes for extended durations." That means the onus still rests on the listener (or in our case, the parent or guardian) to monitor volume levels and listening durations. Technology will undoubtedly continue to both help and hinder that process.

The Hand that Giveth... How Technology Helps and Hinders

Technology has already hindered that process by producing devices with greater music storage capacities and longer battery lives, increasing the potential duration of uninterrupted exposure to excessive sound levels available to us. On the other hand, technology has already innovated several ways to help parents to protect their children's hearing (*many of which follow later in this section*).

Before we leave the Portnuff/Fligor debate behind altogether, let me point out one additional, and unexpected, finding of the study: that the output levels across all player-headphone combinations consistently remained relatively comparable across the full spectrum of sound levels, with the greatest similarities at the highest volume settings. This tells us that, barring feature-enhanced devices and those specially-made for kids, there is little to no difference in sound output from one MP3 player to another, nor from one set of headphones to another.

Myths and Facts about Personal Music Players

In a May, 2009 article titled, *"Safe-Listening Myths for Personal Music Players,"* Brian Fligor and Deanna Meinke debunk some of the pervasive myths which have arisen out of the NIHL debate. Among those debunked:

- **that listening to music through earphones are a predominant cause of NIHL in children**—in truth, statistics suggest that the main culprit is more likely fireworks or firearms
- **that insert earphones (or earbuds) are more harmful than the kind that sit on top of your ears**—in truth, evidence exists that whether they sit on your ear or in your ear or even have so-called "noise-canceling" capabilities, the output level of a pair of earphones or earbuds has no bearing on a user's preferred listening level, which remains a relative constant regardless of device, influenced in any given moment more by background noise than much else
- **that the volume is set too loud if residual sounds can be heard coming from the earphones by other people in the environment**—in truth, even sound levels that are measured directly at the eardrum cannot be used as an accurate or definitive indicator of risk
- **that MP3 and MP4 players are more dangerous than portable CD players or cassette players**—in truth, the maximum sound output levels produced by MP3 and MP4 players are set to be equal to or less than that of portable CD and cassette players

How to Set the Volume on a Listening Device

Still, as a general rule of thumb, the volume on these listening devices should be set low enough that one can hear surrounding sounds and carry on a conversation at normal vocal levels. Alternatively, if you can stand it, keep the volume at around 65 db, the level of normal conversation, and you probably won't ever have to worry about your listening devices causing you noise-induced hearing loss. Also, if listening outdoors is planned, the volume should be set in a quiet setting indoors first, and left at that level when going outdoors, resisting the urge to raise volume levels in response to background noise in the environment.

Boston Children's Hospital researchers recommend keeping the volume levels on all listening devices to be used by children below 60% of their maximum setting. Other recommendations suggest setting the volume no higher than 20% below the highest setting.

A Couple of Caveats

Having said that, you'll get no argument from me that lockable volume controls are no panacea for parents to childhood NIHL. As we know, duration of listening is also a primary factor in NIHL, always, regardless of any decibel maximum. But that doesn't diminish the lockable volume control technology's viability in reducing risk—one small, but valuable component in a larger, preventative solution to NIHL.

I also will not deny that 85 decibels is not necessarily and, in all likelihood, most definitely not low enough to eliminate altogether the possibility of permanent hearing loss—especially in children. This number, 85 db, was derived in a study of adults (an OSHA study on workplace environments). Unfortunately, there is no definitive scientific word yet on whether children are more sensitive to noise and more sensitive to noise damage than adults, or if they are less so. As such, and in the face of vociferous debate, no one can say with certainty that any benchmark set for adult hearing would or would not apply for children's hearing as well.

However, as a doctor beholden first and foremost to the precept "Do no harm," I do not get to pick a side on this issue, as it is inherently incumbent upon me, regardless of who is right, to take every possible precaution to produce these therapeutic programs in such a way as to ensure that the hearing risks they pose remain at an absolute minimum.

More on Setting the Volume on a Listening Device

Also I offer the following advice for best setting optimal volume levels for safe, effective, and enjoyable listening to the *DreamChild Adventures Programs*: set the volume to what seems like the most realistic sound level for the actual real-life sounds being heard. In other words—if you hear a bird chirping, set it at the volume at which you'd expect to hear an actual bird chirping.

In setting the volume level as close to that of real life experience as possible, even if the recording plays the sound of a jet airplane soaring overhead or a motorcycle whizzing by, just as it is in the real world, that excessively loud sound won't last long enough to pose any real danger. Since the majority of our content is nature sounds, there is nary a sound loud enough or lasting enough to be concerned with. And more to the point, listening to nature sounds and soft vocal tones at a high volume isn't necessary to enjoy and benefit from the programs.

A Partial List of Recommended "Kid-safe" Audio Listening Products

For further support, I direct you to the innovation of several audio-listening products designed specifically with child-safety in mind (listed alphabetically):

- **cBlue Headband Headphones for Kids**—designed to fit growing kids, with a lockable volume control for setting maximum levels
- **Hamilton's "The Guardian"**—wired headphones which have a visible display on the exterior of the headphones that monitors listening levels and shows parents whether volume levels are dangerously high at any given moment
- **iHearSafe Safe Volume Earbuds and Headphones**—compliant with the 85 decibel maximum level set by the National Institute for Occupational Safety and Health and Centers for Disease Control and Prevention
- **Lorex/Sylvania SAF-7006 Volume Safe Headphones for Kids**—contains no hazardous materials, automatically keeps sound at child-safe levels, and never goes above 82 db; (Lorex and Sylvania are related companies offering the same products, like this one, simply branded by one or the other)
- **Maxell Kids Safe Headphones and Kids Safe Ear Clips**—ASHA-OSHA and NIOSH compliant, and never goes above 90 db
- **Phillips SHK 1030/27 Headband Headphones for Kids**—like the cBlue, it's design to continue fitting kids as they grow and has a lockable volume control

Another breed of headphones, often called noise-canceling headphones, is available that reduces ambient noise from the surroundings. This allows the user to block out noise the environment. According to the Society of Automotive Engineers, active noise cancellation works "by generating a cancelling anti-noise signal that is equal to, but 180 degrees out of phase with, the noise. This anti-noise is then introduced into the environment such that it matches the noise in the region of interest. The two signals then cancel each other out, effectively removing a significant portion of the noise energy from the environment."

Also on the market now are volume modifiers that keep the volume below dangerous levels, and Apple released an iPod software update in March 2006 that enables parents to set a maximum decibel level on their children's devices using a combination lock-type system. Information on this feature and other NIHL-prevention strategies can be found online at www.apple.com/sound. Further therapeutic technologies and improvements are on the way. Apple itself recently filed a patent application for a new program that monitors the listener's exposure to loud sounds through their headphones and automatically reduces the volume as needed.

Where Technology Leaves Off

Having described so many of these kid-safe listening devices, I would be remiss if I did not once again remind you that even at these so-called "safe" maximum levels, hearing damage can still occur with overuse over time. As Dr. Robert Harrison of the Toronto, Canada Hospital for Sick Children noted on the subject that young people "tend to really push their limits," and if there is a way to abuse even a device with all conceivable protections in place, an unsupervised kid will find a way to abuse it. Which is to say that no technology replaces direct parental supervision.

Audio Settings and the DreamChild Adventures Programs

Fortunately, for our purposes, the *DreamChild Adventures* programs are not used long enough or often enough to pose much of a threat to children's hearing. They're typically only used once or twice a day, and each listening only lasts a short time—until the child is asleep and you come in to shut off the program and remove the headset or earphones. Even on a "repeat play" setting, a child will usually fall asleep well-before any risk threshold is passed. As long as you continue to monitor and supervise program use, even if a rebellious child does turn the volume up too high for a short time while you are out of the room, you presumably won't be gone long enough for these levels to pose significant risk.

Competing Standards for Safe Listening

Now for those semi-authoritative standards for safe-listening I promised you. The first one is:

- **110+ db**: over one uninterrupted minute of this sort of exposure poses a risk of permanent NIHL
- **100 db**: less than 15 uninterrupted minutes of this sort of exposure is recommended
- **85 db**: gradual NIHL can be caused by prolonged periods of this sort of exposure over time

And the other, with the times given being the maximum durations one can listen to sound at a given decibel level before risking permanent hearing damage, is:

- **85 db**: 8 hours
- **88 db**: 4 hours
- **91 db**: 2 hours
- **94 db**: 1 hour
- **97 db**: 30 minutes
- **100 db**: 15 minutes
- **103 db**: 7.5 minutes
- **106 db**: less than 4 minutes
- **109 db**: less than 2 minutes
- **112 db**: less than 1 minute
- **115 db**: less than 30 seconds

Note that for any sound over 85 decibels, the acceptable duration exposure before risk of damage arises is cut in half for every additional 3 decibels. No doubt you have noticed some similarities in these two competing tables.

OTHER GUIDELINES FOR PROTECTING YOUR CHILD'S HEARING (AND YOUR OWN)

Beyond these guidelines, I offer a handful of other suggestions for protecting your child's hearing (and your own):

- Whenever buying children's toys, recreational equipment, power tools, and household appliances look for the ASHA noise rating; if there is none, call the manufacturer and request it
- Don't buy children's toys that produce loud sounds—remember, kids place their toys extremely close to their ears
- At sporting events, concerts, shows, and festivals, avoid sitting too close to the loudspeakers
- Carry around foam ear plugs or other disposable ear protectors with you anytime you go out with the kids—you'll never know when they may come in handy (noisy fast food restaurants, malls, excessively loud movie theaters, amusement parks, fairs, arcades, and the like)

Most importantly, if you ever suspect that you or your child is experiencing hearing loss, consult your doctor or an audiologist, and have your hearing tested. As with many medical concerns, early detection can make the difference between reversing the damage and discovering that the damage is irreversible. In this instance it means avoiding not only permanent hearing loss but resultant speech, learning, and developmental difficulties as well.

Appendix D
Audio Program Scripts

The scripts for the programs *are presented below* in case you would like to read them to your child as bedtime stories.

Country Friends

Hello, I'm Tom, an imaginary friend and guide on this Adventure in Relaxation.

Have you ever wondered what it would be like to leave the hustle and bustle of the city behind and spend some time in the countryside? Well, you're welcome to join me, if you'd like, on a trip to the north coast, where there are beautiful rolling hills as far as your eyes can see, covered by farms and forests. In the city, everybody's always running around like there's not enough time. But up there, time seems to move a little slower and people aren't in such a big hurry. Well, I'm ready to enjoy some of the simple pleasures in life, what about you? *Let's get in our car and go!*

Buckle up your safety belt! And here are some pillows you can use to make yourself really comfy. I love taking off on a trip to somewhere that's bound to be fun. If you want to, you can get the map out and keep track of where we're going. Well, we're on our way now, on an imaginary journey that's going to seem very real, especially if you close your eyes so you can enter the magic theater inside your mind.

Can you remember a time when you were riding in a car, calm and relaxed and your eyelids started feeling kind of heavy and you just couldn't resist letting them close? And then you laid your head back on the seat, listening to the sounds, rolling down the highway, just floating along, feeling relaxed and drifting even further into your imagination.

And thinking to yourself:

The world outside slipping gently by
Allowing me to go inside
Where pictures shine behind my eyes
And stories seem to come alive.

I'm coming in to have some fun
To gallop like the horses run
I'll make a dash and break a sweat
Run through a stream, get cool and wet.

So many things I like to do
Among the best, diving in pools
Hot summer days, swimming like seals
I love the way the water feels.

Getting dizzy, on swings and slides
Rolling on skates and bikes that glide,
Roller coasters, rolling up and down
Making me laugh, while making me frown.

The circus comes but once a year
With painted clowns and dogs so dear,
And I can hardly wait to see
The girl on the flying trapeze.

I like how race cars seem to sail
And trains fly by on metal rails,
How airplanes soar above the clouds
And cars cruise by with the music up loud.

Now I return to my own car
To travel on to places far,
And now it feels like I have dreamed
Of all these things, so real they seemed.

According to the map, soon we should see a trail up here that will lead us through a forest to a river and eventually down to the ocean. I think that may be the path up there. Let's park the car and check it out.

What a magical feeling here. And this pathway sure looks inviting. Let's go . . . and I'll bet if we just keep walking, sooner or later, we'll find the river.

This forest seems to be home to lots of birds and squirrels, and I think I hear a frog. Did you hear it? Listen to the wind. It's really starting to blow now.

Look, up ahead, the pathway opens into that meadow, where there's a farmhouse. Maybe we can find someone who can tell us if we're going the right way.

What an interesting place. Look at that old barn in back with all the animals out here in this yard . . . and, hey, I think I see someone over there at the house on that big covered porch. Let's go talk to them. Hi, we're trying to find the river and the pathway that leads down to the ocean. We were hoping you might tell us which way to go.

> You're already headed in the right direction. But before you head along, perhaps you'd like to come up on the porch and enjoy a little country hospitality. It's a great view of our lovely valley from up here. Would you care for a glass of lemonade? In these parts we treat strangers like friends and friends like family. And if you'd like to hear some country music, just make yourselves comfortable in any of these chairs.

We'd love to. We have time for a few songs.

> We have a band called *Harmony Grits* and we've been rehearsing inside for a party we're playing at tonight. Come on out everyone and introduce yourselves to some new friends.
>
> I'm Mike, the mandolin player . . .
> And I'm Fannie, the fiddler . . .
> And I'm Bugs, the bass player . . .
> I'm Daniel, the Dobro player . . .
> I'm Gus, and I play guitar . . .

Glad to meet ya. Let's hear some country music!

> The fun thing about country music is you get to do anything you wish.
>
> You can clap your hands, you can tap your feet,
> you can imagine that you are singing right along,
> you can be any of the instruments,
> you can hear them all together as a song.

EIO

Oh, ei, ei, eio, eio, eio, eio, eio, eio, eio,
Eio, eio, eio, eio, ei, ei, eio, ei, eio.
Oh, ei, ei, eio, eio, eio, eio, eio, eio, eio,
Eio, eio, eio, eio, ei, ei, eio, ei, eio.
Oh, ei, ei, eio, eio, eio, eio, eio, eio, eio,
Eio, eio, eio, eio, ei, ei, eio.
Ei, eio.
Oh, ei, ei, eio, eio, eio, eio, eio, eio, eio,
Eio, eio, eio, eio, ei, ei, eio.
Ei, eio.
Oh, ei, ei, eio, ei, eio.

Thank you, you're really good. Do you have any songs you wrote yourselves?

Yes, we have quite a few of our own tunes.

We'd love to hear a couple.

FARMER BROWN

Well sometimes the lightning storms come up
And all the rain comes down.
Well, lightning hit our neighbor's barn
And burned it to the ground.

He got all his livestock out,
But he lost all his feed,
Lucky he just plowed the field
And planted all his seeds.

And we're going to raise a barn for Farmer Brown.
We're using every pair of hands around.
Everybody's pitching in for the best barn that's ever been
Built by everybody in our town.

Well, the Johnson boys are coming out,
And so are the Mc Crees.
Sawmill has been helping out
By sawing up some trees.

Preacher came to say a prayer
To see that all goes well,
And Silas gets to help us out
And leave his jail cell.

And the picnic that the ladies will prepare
It's going to be enough to feed a bear.

And we're going to raise a barn for Farmer Brown.
We're using every pair of hands around.
Everybody's pitching in for the best barn that's ever been
Built by everybody in our town.

Well, we're not very fancy,
Just folks living on the land,
And when there's an emergency,
We all do what we can.

We've got to help each other out,
It's the way it's meant to be,
I'm always there for Farmer Brown,
He's always there for me.

Sometimes the only way you can get by
Is just pitch in together and try.

And we're going to raise a barn for Farmer Brown.
We're using every pair of hands around.
Everybody's pitching in for the best barn that's ever been
Built by everybody in our town.

We're going to raise a barn for Farmer Brown.

[FARMER BROWN, ©1987 Mike McKinley (BMI)]

That was great fun . . . thank you.

> You're very welcome. Are you about ready to be on your way now?

Yeah, we're ready to head along.

> Well, just stay on this path that goes down by the barn over there.

Oh, yeah.

> You can grab a couple of those fishin' poles leaned against it if you like. Then head on over between those two big oak trees and you'll be walkin' beside the stream before you know it. You'll find some spots that are so peaceful you'll want to sit for a spell.

We just might do that.

> We'll sing you one more song to send you on your way.

Thank you so much. You've made us feel like friends.

JUST BIDING TIME

Down by the river, just biding my time,
Fishing, down by the water near the shore.
Been a long time thinking, now I've come back home
To rest right here beside the shore.

Down by the river, just biding my time,
Fishing, down by the water near the shore.

I heard you singing, lady in the night
Singing a river lullaby
Singing to the ocean
Wandering with the stream
Singing to a time that's gone by.

Down by the river, just biding my time,
Fishing, down by the water near the shore.

Make no mistake, because we've met here times before
Down by the water near the shore.
Down by the river, just biding my time,
Fishing, down by the water near the shore.

Down by the river, just biding my time,
Fishing, down by the water near the shore.

[JUST BIDING TIME, ©1987 Jeff Baldwin (BMI)]

Those country folks sure are nice. I think we have some new friends that we can visit with anytime we wish.

This is such a pretty scene, fields of flowers swaying in the breeze. The oak trees waving their limbs like they're greeting us as we walk back into the forest. Birds chiming in, calling us down to the river, which we can now hear up ahead . . .

This is a great spot to sit for a while and experience the peacefulness of Mother Nature all around us. Here's some soft grass where we can get comfortable and maybe do a little fishing.

The sky high above is so blue and so clear
And nature is whispering, if I wish to hear.
Air drifts through the trees, caressing the leaves,
And tickles my face as it dips and it weaves.

Now filling my lungs as I breathe in the air,
Then releasing my breath, releasing all cares.
My heart is opening and love will be seen,
A magical garden where all is serene.

My mind is at peace, my thoughts drifting away,
I'm light as a feather and happy today.
My breathing is now so relaxed and at ease,
It's almost as though I am one with the breeze.

Let's walk on down the pathway and see what surprises might await us. Up ahead, over there, I see a shallow pond. Let's go and take a look.

When the wind blows across the water it creates little ripples, but when the wind calms down, the ripples disappear and the pond becomes like a great big mirror.

So let's stand beside it and see what we see,
Reflections appearing of both you and me.
As pictures dance by us the water will show
There's more to a mirror than I might now know.

I see that my nature is being revealed
And the hurts of the past are all being healed.
I'm more than I dreamed; I can see that it's true,
From visions within me, I'm learning anew.

An image is forming in which I perceive,
A friend who is with me, in this I believe.
To guide my steps when the path is unknown
Whatever may happen, my way will be shown.

Moving on now, further down the path, and enjoying every step along the way.

Can you hear the sound now of waves from up ahead? You can start to see the beach peeking through the trees. Such a beautiful scene.

Let's walk across the sparkling white sand, warm under our feet. Seagulls floating overhead, like little kites, held aloft by the afternoon breeze. Feeling happier and more relaxed with each gentle wave. On down now, to where the waves roll up onto the beach.

What a perfect place to play for a while. Maybe you could find some sea shells or drift wood, or perhaps you'd like to make a sand castle, or just sit and relax. You're free to do anything you'd like. We'll meet back here in just a minute.

Now, let's walk along the beach for a moment before you return to where you were before we started this adventure. I've really enjoyed being your imaginary friend, and I'm looking forward to doing this again with you sometime soon.

Walking on, feeling energized by the fresh ocean breeze, stretching your arms and legs as you open your eyes, and taking some of these wonderful feelings with you as you return.

Goodbye for now, my dear friend. Until we meet again.

MAGIC CARPET

*Now we are starting a wondrous journey
Into a realm of adventures in sound
A dream in which we will find ourselves flying
Upon a carpet of magic we've found.*

*Closing our eyes we are free to explore,
A world where we are not stuck on the ground
Like best of friends we're in this together
Safe and secure we are mystery bound.*

*This Magic Carpet was made for flying
To float around like a bird in the skies
Lifting off, as the front door swings open
Light as a feather and starting to rise.*

*The sounds of the road are now before me
Motorcycles and cars zooming on by
It feels as though I'm actually seeing
With visions revealed inside my mind's eye.*

*Slowly up, over houses and highways
The cars beneath us, like toys on the street
This carpet steers so well by just leaning
I could do it if I wish in my sleep.*

*What a feeling to be free like the birds
To fly high, float in circles and dip
With room galore, on the wind I will soar
I'm the master of my own ship.*

*The view from up here is so crystal clear
I see a hometown parade over there
Down to the crowd that is lining the street
The Grand Marshal up front is the Mayor.*

*Let's ride our Magic Carpet now
Up and into the sky
Adventures are awaiting us
So onward we will fly.*

*Now to a playground up ahead,
So many games to play,
My heart is filled with happiness
On such a special day.*

Ping Pong, basketball, and baseball
Times I've played, I can recall
Skating, bicycles, swimming pools
So much fun and very cool.

A model airplane in the sky
Controlled by levers I can try
Above my head it zooms around
Until I land it on the ground.

And now again I wish to fly
Onward, upward, to the sky
Soaring o'er the clouds so high
Flying like a bird am I.

Below it looks like Africa
That far we haven't gone
It's got to be a zoo I see
Elephants, apes, a swan.

Now moving up ahead I see
Arcades and games below
Let's lose our sense of time for now
Surrender to the flow.

And now I'm moving up and on
The city left behind
To countryside with farms below
And animals to find.

And now let's ride our carpet up
And onward through the sky
This journey leads to paradise
As on the wind we fly.

The trees and streams and sea below
So beautiful today
Inviting me to glide on down
To walk a path and play.

Where nature she is all around
To cast her magic spell
She speaks to me in nature's sounds
Her secrets she will tell.

My Magic Carpet follows me
Though I am walking now
And any time I wish to fly
I know that I know how.

Rays of sunlight streaming down
Warming every thing around
And watching branches as they sway
It's no surprise the trees would say:

"How beautifully we reach up toward the sky
Leaves of green held so high
The shade we make on you below
Our gift we give as on you go."

Walking on this winding path
And down toward the beach
It seems that if I listen close
That nature's here to teach.

And as I'm drifting on along
And listening to this bird's sweet song
I wonder what she wants to say
Each note she sings for me today.

"Oh how I love to fly,
feeling so free am I.

And any place that I should choose,
I can sit on a twig and have a snooze.

But for now I'll just float on by.
I'm your friend, come along, I'm your guide."

And now I hear a stream so clear
And walk until my toes draw near
She winds her way along so slow
The easy way she always flows.

And from her water
comes the sound
Of nature's voice,
a treasure found:

> "I AM THE STREAMBED PEBBLE SONG
> OF PEACEFUL LULLABIES.
> I LOVE YOU LIKE I LOVE THE RAIN
> THAT FILLS ME FROM THE SKY.
>
> AND AS I DRIFT ALONG UPON
> MY WAY TO MEET THE SEA,
> I'M HAPPY YOU HAVE COME ALONG
> TO PLAY AND FLOAT ON ME."

Now I am wondering how I might float
If I were small, there'd be this and that boat
Imagining now that I'm shrinking in size
Smaller and smaller, yet more and more wise.

And now a sturdy stick I see
Is big enough and meant for me
I'll climb aboard and sail this stream
The perfect place to float it seems.

And now my boat returns to shore
To let me off to walk some more
Feeling that I am growing tall
My normal size, no longer small.

Drawn down the pathway I'm starting to see
Colorful flowers swaying in the breeze
This one now seems to be waving at me
In fact she's now tapping upon my knee.

> "AND HOW I LOVE YOU WHEN
> YOU PICK ME BY MY WILLING STEM.
> AND INTO A POCKET I CAN TUCK
> TO BRING YOU THE VERY BEST OF LUCK."

Now hearing sounds of waves from the ocean
The liquid chorus of water in motion
Leaving the forest and into the sun
On to the seashore my feet want to run.

Gazing upon the water before me
Wave after wave rolling in from the sea
Nature's soft voice I can now understand
In the breeze, in the foam, in the sand:

"I'VE ALWAYS BEEN HERE, YES, I AM YOUR FRIEND
YOU ARE MY BELOVED, SO LOVE I WILL SEND
I'LL ALWAYS BE WITH YOU WHERE EVER YOU GO
THROUGH VOICES OF NATURE, YOUR WAY I WILL SHOW."

And now moving on across the white sand
Feeling the joy of this mystical land
Gliding sea gulls drifting on and on
Fresh ocean air and singing their song.

And as this one lands, getting snug in the sand
And closing his sleepy bird eyes
I wonder what dreams, so real to him seem
Of sailing around in the skies.

And if I want to, I can fly with such ease
If I want to, I can drift on the breeze
I've learned how to fly, I know I know how
Up, up and away, if I wish to now.

Coming to rest on this part of the shore
Where I will soon find new things to explore
Back on the sand feeling soft on my feet
I see there's a playhouse in which I can sleep.

Feeling invited to walk in the door
Welcome inscribed on an old weathered floor
Finding a bed, so cozy it seems
Waiting for me to drift into my dreams.

And out on the porch where a hammock is tied
I can swing in the breeze like birds in nests ride
I'll come back again when I'm ready for bed
Either place that I choose will feel soft on my head.

Off in the corner, a big wooden chest
Inside it, I wonder what I might find
And lifting the lid wide open I see
There are games and toys of every kind.

Now drawn outside and across the wide beach
To walk on down to where sound and sight merge
Where water and sand both swirl as they dance
To the restful rhythm of the ocean surge.

So many games to be thought of and played
While splashing around in the waves
Digging holes which the tide turns into pools
Making castles of sand with hands my tools.

Having so much fun as the sun sets down
Feeling sleepier with each ocean sound
Till I say to myself, it's time for bed
Return to my playhouse, lay down my head.

Feeling peaceful and calm, drifting to sleep
With beautiful dreams, so pleasant and sweet
This is a place that awaits me within
Where I can return, again and again.

Sweet dreams within dreams are here within.

Sweet dreams within dreams are here.

Sweet dreams within dreams.

Sweet dreams within.

Sweet dreams.

Dreams.

Dream.

Dream.

Playhouse on the Beach

What a wonderful day to play on the beach!
I'm so glad to find you here my dear friend.
Can you imagine how many things we can do?
How many games we can play?
How much fun we can have?

Oh I love the way the waves, which roll in to the sand,
Wave after wave inviting us to splash and play.
Watching the birds sailing above, playing tag in the sky.
What fun it must be to fly.

And feeling the wind that blows onto shore,
Caressing my cheeks, I've felt this before.
I'm so happy to be here with you,
There must be hundreds of things we can do.

Let's run and skip on the warm wet sand,
See the water splash as our footprints land.
And wading out into the waves,
They splash against me as I play.

The foam is white and soft and light,
Tickling my skin as bubbles disappear from sight.
And here is a surf raft, I can use
For many things that I might choose.

I can paddle out beyond the waves
And lie there drifting on.
I can watch the clouds as they drift by
And sing a sailor's song.

I can look straight down into the sea
And see some fish looking back at me.
Some are gold and some are green,
They look like little submarines.

It must be peaceful and quiet below
In an underwater world where beauty shows.
They seem so happy floating by
As on their way they go.

And as I'm floating upon the sea,
I'm warm beneath the sun.
I can't imagine anything
Being this much fun.

My raft can be a surf board, too,
As on the waves I ride.
And as the surf comes rolling in
I swoosh and then I glide.

And bringing my raft up to the shore,
So many things to be explored.
Walking along the shoreline now
And feeling strong and well.

*I see that there are treasures here
Of sparkling rocks and shells.
The pretty ones I pick them up
And save them for my shelf.*

*The ocean is a treasure hunt,
Full of nature's wealth.
And sitting now upon the beach,
Where little waves my toes can reach.*

*Digging holes which fill into pools
Finding my hands are perfect tools,
Building castles in the sand
Making here a magic land.*

*Where boys and girls can actually see
Anything they wish to be.
And now I see my Playhouse
Filled with fun for me.*

*I'll turn the lock and enter now
I've got the magic key.
And feeling invited to pass through the door
Walking across the wooden floor.*

*Here's a magic chest of toys
With games of every kind,
I wonder if I look inside
What treasures I will find.*

*Kites and dolls and TinkerToys®
Crayons and Legos®—oh, such joy!
Plastic boats and beads to string,
It seems that there is everything.*

*Frisbees®, baseballs, and Hula Hoops®,
Checkers, jacks, and shovels that scoop.
Paddleball, puzzles, and bubbles are stored,
And a hundred games I can play on the floor.*

*I'll take my choice as the sun sets down,
Feeling delighted in what I have found.
And as the night begins to come,
I'll play with toys, which are so much fun.*

And finding a bed, like my own, it seems
A cozy place where I can dream.
Feeling relaxed, it calls to me,
This is where I want to be.

I love to come here every night
It feels so good, it must be right.
And feeling good is just a start
Knowing I'm loved, deep in my heart.

Gentle waves greeting the shore
Singing their song to bring me more
Love and peace and happiness,
A precious place where I can rest.

And with each wave I'm sleepier.
As everything begins to blur
Into a dream that feels so real
Of joy and pleasure I can feel.

And now that I'm drifting slowly to sleep
With beautiful feelings I can keep,
I know that I am good inside,
I can hold my head high and walk with pride.

Drifting on and drifting down,
Like peaceful lullabies,
I find that as I go to sleep
I'm really very wise.

And with each wave, the ocean sounds
Are calling me to sleep.
I'm floating in the air, it seems,
A mattress, soft and deep.

With every breath I'm sleepier,
Floating and drifting away.
Feeling good about myself
And loving every day.

Dreams are a place where my heart can feel
The beauty inside that is real
For I am a child of spirit, indeed
Finding myself, I am surely freed.

So sleepy I feel
With my muscles relaxed,
Feeling so good
Since my cares have all passed.

Drifting along like a bird in the sky,
Easily floating without having to try.
Breezes blowing across the sea,
Softly and gently caressing me.

I love to feel the wind on my skin
And think of all the places it's been.
And watching a sailboat upon the sea
Moving along so quietly.

Oh, how I love this feeling inside.
My heart feels so good, opening wide.
The peace I have found is always here,
What I feel now will always be near.

And drifting deeper into sleep
Such beautiful feelings, I can keep.
Sleepier and sleepier with each ocean sound,
The treasure of love is what I found.

Drifting into a land made of dreams
Finding I am much more than it seems.
Feeling so drowsy, I now wish to go
To sleep in a place where good feelings grow.

Getting better and better with each passing day,
Knowing my feelings are all okay.
The people I meet will come to know
My beauty inside which I can show.

With smiles and laughter and a twinkle in my eye
There's really no reason for me to be shy.
And soon those around me will start to see
What a beautiful person I've come to be.

Sleepier and sleepier, drifting on and on,
So sleepy now that I might even yawn.
Letting go with ease as I drift away
To dreams within dreams, in which I can play.

APPENDIX E

BIBLIOGRAPHY

Most of the books in this bibliography *can be found on* amazon.com. Journal articles and other published papers may be downloaded from various websites which may be located using a simple Google search.

American Academy of Pediatrics: Media Education Committee on Public Education (1999). *Policy Statement*. Pediatrics, 104(2), 341-343.2

Bernstein, J. (2006). *10 days to a less defiant child: The breakthrough program for overcoming your child's difficult behavior*. Emeryville, CA: Marlowe & Company.

Branden, N. (2001). *The psychology of self-esteem: A revolutionary approach to self-understanding that launched a new era in modern psychology*. (Anniversary edition). San Francisco, CA: Jossey-Bass.

Carskadon, M.A. (2004). *Sleep Difficulties in Young People*. Arch Pediatr Adolesc Med, 158(6), 597-598.

Chansky, T.E. (2004). *Freeing your child from anxiety: Powerful, practical solutions to overcome your child's fears, worries, and phobias*. New York, NY: Broadway Books.

Cohen, L. (1995). *Debate about Parents' Right to Spank Causes Divisions among MDs*. Can Med Assoc J. 153, 73-5.

Cooper Marcus, C., & Barnes, M. (Eds.). (1999). *Healing gardens: Therapeutic benefits and design recommendations (Wiley series in healthcare and senior living design)*. Hoboken, NJ: Wiley.

Crespo, C.J., Smit, E., Troiano, R.P., Bartlett, S.J., Macera, C.A., Andersen, R.E. (2001). *Television Watching, Energy Intake, and Obesity in Us Children: Results from the Third National Health and Nutrition Examination Survey, 1988–1994*. Arch Pediatr Adolesc Med, 155(3), 360–365.

Dacey, J.S., & Fiore, L.B. (2001). *Your anxious child: How parents and teachers can relieve anxiety in children*. San Francisco, CA: Jossey-Bass.

DuPont Spencer, E., DuPont, R.L., & DuPont, C.M. (2003). *The anxiety cure for kids: A guide for parents.* Hoboken, NJ: Wiley.

Elias, M.J., Tobias, S.E., & Friedlander, B.S. (2000). *Emotionally intelligent parenting: How to raise a self-disciplined, responsible, socially skilled child.* New York, NY: Three Rivers Press.

Faber, A., & Mazlish, E. (2004). *Siblings without rivalry: How to help your children live together so you can live too.* New York, NY: Harper Paperbacks.

Ferber, R. (2006). *Solve your child's sleep problems: New, revised, and expanded edition.* (Rev exp ed.). Toronto, ON: Fireside Publishing.

Fligor, B., & Meinke, D. (2009, May 26). *Safe-listening Myths for Personal Music Players.* The ASHA Leader.

Fredriksen, K., Rhodes, J., Reddy, R., & Way, N. (2004). *Sleepless in Chicago: Tracking the Effects of Adolescent Sleep Loss During the Middle School Years.* Child Dev, 75, 84–95.

Gadd, J. (1998). *Spanked Children Suffer Intellectually.* Toronto, ON: The Globe and Mail, 30 July.

Giebenhain, J.E., & O'Dell, S.L. (1984). *Evaluation of a Parent Training Manual for Reducing Children's Fear of the Dark.* J Appl Behav Anal, 17(1), 121-125.

Glasser, H., & Easley, J. (1999). *Transforming the difficult child: The nurtured heart approach.* Altrincham, Cheshire, England: Nurtured Heart Publications.

Glazener, C.M.A., Evans, J.H.C., & Peto, R.E. (2006). *Alarm Interventions for Nocturnal Enuresis in Children.* Evid Based Child Health, 1(1), 9-97.

Glenn, H.S. (1988). *Spanking denounced as ineffective, harmful—Expert at 'Families Alive' urges positive discipline.* Source: Nii, J.K., Deseret News, 9 May.

Goodavage, M., & Gordon, J. (2002). *Good nights: The happy parents' guide to the family bed (and a peaceful night's sleep!).* New York, NY: St. Martin's Griffin.

Gottman, J., Declaire, J., & Goleman, D. (1998). *Raising an emotionally intelligent child.* New York, NY: Simon & Schuster.

Hallowell, E.M., & Ratey, J.J. (2005). *Delivered from distraction: Getting the most out of life with attention deficit disorder.* New York, NY: Ballantine Books.

Hayes, M. J., Roberts, S. M. and Stowe, R. (1996). *Early Childhood Co-sleeping: Parent-child and Parent-infant Nighttime Interactions.* Infant Mental Health Journal, 17, 348–357.

Hoban, T.F., & Chervin, R.D. *Sleep disorders in young children: Impact on social/emotional development and options for treatment. Commentary on France, Wiggs and Owens.* In: Tremblay, R.E., Barr, R.G., & Peters R.DeV. (Eds.). *Encyclopedia on early childhood development* [online]. Montreal, Quebec: Centre of Excellence for Early Childhood Development, 2004, 1-5.

Huebner, D., & Matthews, B. (2005). *What to do when you worry too much: A kids guide to overcoming anxiety (What to do guides for kids).* Washington, DC: Magination Press.

Humphreys, P.A., & Gevirtz, R.N. (2000). *Treatment of Recurrent Abdominal Pain: Components Analysis of Four Treatment Protocols.* J Pediatr Gastroenterol Nutr, 31, 47-51.

Huntley, T.M. (2002). *Helping children grieve: When someone they love dies.* (Revised ed.). Augsburg, Germany: Augsburg Books.

James, J.W., Friedman, R., & Matthews, L. (2002). *When children grieve: For adults to help children deal with death, divorce, pet loss, moving, and other losses.* New York, NY: Harper Paperbacks.

Johnson, J.G., Cohen, P., Kasen, S., First, M.B., & Brook, J.S. (2004). *Association Between Television Viewing and Sleep Problems During Adolescence and Early Adulthood.* Arch Pediatr Adolesc Med, 158, 562-568.

Kuo, F.E. (2001). *Coping with Poverty: Impacts of Environment and Attention in the Inner City.* Environment & Behavior, 33(1), 5-34.

Lantieri, L., & Goleman, D. (2008). *Building emotional intelligence: Techniques to cultivate inner strength in children.* Louisville, CO: Sounds True, Inc.

Last, C.G. (2005). *Help for worried kids: How your child can conquer anxiety and fear.* New York, NY: Guilford Press.

Lehrer, J. (2009). *How the City Hurts Your Brain...and What You Can Do about it.* The Boston Globe, January 2.

Lehrer, J. (2010) *How we decide.* (1 Reprint ed.). New York, NY: Mariner Books.

Lieberman, G. A., & Hoody, L. L. (1998). *Closing the Achievement Gap: Using the Environment as an Integrating Context for Learning.* San Diego, CA: State Education and Environment Roundtable.

Long, N., & Forehand, R.L. (2002). *Making divorce easier on your child: 50 effective ways to help children adjust.* New York, NY: McGraw-Hill.

Louv, R. (2008). *Last child in the woods: Saving our children from nature-deficit disorder.* (Updated and expanded ed.). Chapel Hill, NC: Algonquin Books.

MacKenzie, R.J. (2001). *Setting limits with your strong-willed child: Eliminating conflict by establishing clear, firm, and respectful boundaries.* New York, NY: Three Rivers Press.

Maizels, M., Rosebaum, D., & Keating, B. (1999). *Getting to dry: How to help your child overcome bedwetting.* Boston, MA: The Harvard Common Press.

Manassis, K.M. (1996). *Keys to parenting your anxious child.* Hauppauge, NY: Barron's Educational Series.

Mao, A., Burnham, M.M., Goodlin-Jones, B.L., Gaylor, E.E., & Anders, T.F. (2004). *A Comparison of the Sleep–wake Patterns of Cosleeping and Solitary-sleeping Infants.* Child Psychiatry Hum Dev, 35(2), 95-105.

McCann, D., Barrett, A., Cooper, A., Crumpler, D., Dalen, L., Grimshaw, K., Kitchin, E., Lok, K., Porteous, L., Prince, E., Sonuga-Barke, E., Warner, J.O., Stevenson, J. (2007). *Food Additives & Hyperactive Behavior in 3 Year Old and 8/9 Year Old Children in the Community: a Randomized, Double-blinded, Placebo Controlled Trial.* Lancet, 370(9598), 1560-1567.

McKenna, J.J., & McDade, T. (2005). *Why Babies Should Never Sleep Alone: a Review of the Co-sleeping Controversy in Relation to SIDS, Bedsharing and Breast Feeding.* Paediatr Respir Rev, 6(2), 134-152.

McKenna, J., Thoman, E. B., Anders, T. F., Sadeh, A., Schectman, V. L., & Glotzbach, S. F. (1993). *Infant-parent Co-sleeping in an Evolutionary Perspective: Implications for Understanding Infant Sleep Development and the Sudden Infant Death Syndrome.* Sleep, 16, 263-282.

Mindell, J.A. (2005). *Sleeping through the night, Revised edition: How infants, toddlers, and their parents can get a good night's sleep.* (Revised ed.). New York, NY: Harper Paperbacks.

Mindell, J.A., Kuhn, B., Lewin, D.S., Meltzer, L.J., & Sadeh, A. (2006). *Behavioral Treatment of Bedtime Problems and Night Wakings in Infants and Young Children.* Sleep, 29, 1263-1276.

Mindell, J.A., Meltzer, L.J., Carskadon, M.A., & Chervin, R.D. (2004). *Developmental aspects of sleep hygiene: Findings from the 2004 National Sleep Foundation Sleep in America Poll.* Sleep Med, 10(7), 771-779.

Mindell, J.A., & Owens, J.A. (2009). *A clinical guide to pediatric sleep: Diagnosis and management of sleep problems.* Philadelphia, PA: Lippincott Williams & Wilkins.

Mitrione, S. (2008). *Therapeutic Responses to Natural Environments: Using Gardens to Improve Health Care.* Minn Med, 91(3), 31-34.

Nakamura, S., Wind, M., Danello, M.A. (1999). *Adult Beds Are Unsafe Places for Children to Sleep.* Arch Pediat Adolesc Med, 153, 1019-1023.

National Institute of Health, National Institute on Deafness and Other Communication Disorders. (2002). *Noise-induced hearing loss* (NIH Pub. No. 97-4233). Bethesda, MD: NIDCD Information Clearinghouse.

Niskar, A.S., Kieszak, S.M., Holmes, A.E., Esteban, E., Rubin, C., & Brody, D.J. (1988-1994). *Estimated Prevalence of Noise Induced Hearing Threshold Shifts among Children 6 to 19 Years of Age: the Third National Health and Nutritional Examination Survey*. Pediatrics, 2001(108), 40–43.

Ogden, C.L., & Carroll, M.D. (2010). *Prevalence of Obesity among Children and Adolescents: United States, Trends 1963-1965 Through 2007–2008*. NCHS Health E-Stat. Hyattsville, MD: National Center for Health Statistics.

Ogden, C.L., Carroll, M.D., & Flegal, K.M. (2008). *High Body Mass Index for Age among Us Children and Adolescents*. JAMA, 299(20), 2401-2405.

Okie, S. (2005). *Fed up!: Winning the war against childhood obesity*. Washington, DC, Joseph Henry Press.

Perusse, B. (2007). *Hear Today, Gone Tomorrow*. Montreal Gazette, December 7.

Pinto Wagner, A. (2002). *What to do when your child has obsessive-compulsive disorder: Strategies and solutions*. (1 ed.). Apex, NC: Lighthouse Press.

Portnuff, C.D., & Fligor, B. (2006). *Sound Output Levels of the Ipod and Other Mp3 Players: Is There Potential Risk to Hearing?* Presentation at Noise-Induced Hearing Loss in Children at Work and Play Conference, Cincinnati, OH.

Portnuff, C.D., Fligor, B., & Arehart, K. (2009). *Teenage Use of Portable Listening Devices: a Hazard to Hearing?* Presentation at annual conference of the National Hearing Conservation Association, Atlanta, GA.

Prochnik, G. (2010). *In pursuit of silence: Listening for meaning in a world of noise*. New York, NY: Knopf Doubleday.

Rapee, R.M., Spence, S., Cobham, V., Wignall, A., & Lyneham, H. (2000). *Helping your anxious child: A step-by-step guide for parents*. Oakland, CA: New Harbinger Publications.

Rimm, S. (2002). *The effects of sibling competition*. Watertown, WI: Educational Assessment Service, Inc.

Schwartz, J.M., & Begley, S. (2003). *The mind and the brain: Neuroplasticity and the power of mental force*. New York, NY: Harper Perennial.

Seabrook, J. (1999, November 8). *Sleeping with the Baby*. The New Yorker, 56.

Simard, V., Nielsen, T.A., Tremblay, R., Boivin, M., & Montplaisir, J.Y. (2008). *Longitudinal Study of Bad Dreams in Preschool Children: Prevalence, Demographic Correlates, Risk and Protective Factors*. Sleep, 31, 62-70.

Strauss, M. (2001). *Beating the devil out of them: Corporal punishment in American families and its effect on children*. Piscataway, NJ: Transaction Publishers.

Stuart, A. (2007). *Childhood Fears and Anxieties.* http://children.webmd.com/features/childhood-fears-anxieties (retrieved October 10, 2010).

Taylor, J.F. (2006). *The survival guide for kids with ADD or ADHD.* Minneapolis, MN: Free Spirit Publishing.

Tessmer, K.A., Hagen, M., & Beecher, M. (2006). *Conquering childhood obesity for dummies.* Hoboken, NJ: Wiley.

Thompson, D.A., & Christakis, D.A. (2005). *The Association Between Television Viewing and Irregular Sleep Schedules among Children less than 3 Years of Age.* Pediatrics, 116, 851-856.

Touchette, E., Petit, D., Paquiet, J., Boivin, M., Japel, C., Tremblay, R.E., & Montplaisir, J.Y. (2005). *Factors Associated with Fragmented Sleep at Night Across Early Childhood.* Arch Pediatr Adolesc Med, 159, 242-249.

Ulrich, R. S. (2000). *Evidence Based Environmental Design for Improving Medical Outcomes.* Proceedings of the conference. Healing By Design: Building for Health Care in the 21st Century. Montreal: McGill University Health Centre, 3.1-3.10.

U.S. Department of Education. Office for Civil Rights. (2000). *Elementary and Secondary School Civil Rights Compliance Report, Fall 1994.* Ann Arbor, MI: Inter-university Consortium for Political and Social Research

U.S. Environmental Protection Agency (EPA), Office of Noise Abatement and Control. (1972). *Noise facts digest* (000R72102). Washington, DC.

Zeltzer, L.K., & Blackett Schlank, C. (2005). *Conquering your child's chronic pain: A pediatrician's guide for reclaiming a normal childhood.* New York, NY: Harper Paperbacks.

Zogby, J. (2006). *Survey of teens and adults about the use of personal electronic devices and head phones.* Submitted to American Speech-Language-Hearing Association, March 2006, © 2006 Zogby International. http://www.asha.org/uploadedFiles/about/news/atitbtot/zogby_survey2006.pdf (retrieved October 10, 2010).

Appendix F
3D AudioMagic Programs Catalogue

The *following programs* are *currently available* on CDs. For information on downloading MP3 files or ordering CDs, please visit www.3daudiomagic.com.

3Dimensional Living Sound Demonstration
Natural Sleep—Male Voice
Natural Sleep—Female Voice
Natural Relaxation I—Male Voice
Natural Relaxation I—Female Voice
Natural Relaxation II—Male Voice
Natural Relaxation II—Female Voice
Relaxation and Massage—Male Voice
Country Friends—Male Voice
Magic Carpet—Male Voice
Playhouse on the Beach—Male Voice
Playhouse on the Beach—Female Voice
Nature Walk
Nature Odyssey
Stream Walk
Rain and Thunder
Ocean
Reflections on the California Coast (DVD)

3D AudioMagic Program Descriptions

3Dimensional Living Sound Demonstration
(9 minutes)

All of the recordings in this series employ *3D Living Sound*, a remarkable breakthrough in audio technology. This free, downloadable demonstration program offers an astounding multi-dimensional listening experience in which sound seems to come from every direction—near and far, above, below, on all sides, and even in motion—an effect more lifelike than anything heard in a conventional audio recording.

The amazing realism of this sound technology will open the doors of your imagination in ways you never thought possible, and you will quickly come to appreciate one of the essential reasons that this series of therapeutic programs is so enjoyable and effective.

Rather than offer great technical detail describing how *3D Living Sound* surpasses ordinary stereo or surround sound, I urge you to listen to a brief sample. I believe you'll truly find it worth a thousand words. The only requirements are that you listen with headphones or ear buds, and that you don't listen to this or any of the other programs in the *3D Living Sound* series while driving or operating heavy machinery.

So, download the *3D Living Sound Demonstration*, sit back in a comfortable chair, allow your eyes to close, and prepare for your journey into the amazing world of *3D Living Sound*.

Natural Sleep
(43 minutes)

This state-of-the-art sleep-enhancement program for adults has been clinically proven through many years of use by doctors, hospitals, and sleep experts. Employing a number of advanced psychological and therapeutic techniques, this audio recording can help anyone fall asleep gently and easily, no matter what an individual's sleep problem may be.

Because *Natural Sleep* is recorded in *3D Living Sound*, the sounds of nature will seem to come from all around you.

As you settle comfortably down, headphones or ear buds in place, this program will transport you to an enchanting tropical island where you will find yourself surrounded by the restful sounds of birdsongs, a light breeze, and the distant surf. A soothing voice will bring you to a deep state of relaxation and then guide you along an imaginary pathway to a beautiful, secluded beach where you will be lulled to sleep by the gentle murmur of waves.

This program has been proven to help listeners achieve deep, refreshing sleep, resulting in increased vitality and mental alertness, as well as greater happiness and overall enjoyment of both sleeping and waking life.

Natural Relaxation I
(31 minutes)

This adult program has consistently proven an effective treatment for stress and anxiety. The noise, demands, and rapid pace of our urban world often deprive us of the peace we desire and deserve. We may experience muscle tension, fatigue, or poor concentration to the point it's a challenge just to unwind and fall asleep at night.

If you suffer any of these problems, or if you would simply like to enjoy a deeper sense of inner tranquility and harmony, this program may well be the answer. In four separate clinical studies, users of *Natural Relaxation I* have reported an average reduction in daily anxiety of 52% and a one-third decrease in baseline anxiety over several weeks.

The program begins on a tropical island, high on a hill, with the far-off rolling surf below. Surrounded by the restful sounds of nature, you listen as a gentle voice guides you through muscle relaxation and breathing techniques. Then you embark on a leisurely walk along a winding pathway down toward the beach. Nature comes to life through the gentle sound of wind in the trees, textures of flowing water beside you, and birds serenading you along the way.

The path emerges on an enchanted beach where you find a comfortable place to sit and listen to the gentle waves. Here you bask in feelings of relaxation and allow positive suggestions to wash through you.

Next, you are given the opportunity to imagine a situation that usually causes you to feel anxious, but you are guided instead to see yourself handling it in a relaxed manner, which helps to reprogram subconscious patterns and expectations to better deal with the situation when it arises again.

Finally, you walk along the beach, feeling more energetic and alert with each step as you return to full waking consciousness, feeling fully relaxed and refreshed, the cares of the day simply melted away.

Natural Relaxation II
(27 minutes)

This program is designed for adults but is more whimsical and entertaining than *Natural Relaxation I* and may be especially helpful for people who have difficulty concentrating. *Natural Relaxation II* begins with engaging 3D sound effects—such as encountered in a walk around the zoo and a county fair—in order to draw the listener into the experience.

Gradually, more relaxing elements are introduced, beginning with an inviting cabin in the woods—fire in the fireplace, rain on the roof, and a few distant claps of thunder. You luxuriate for a while in a warm, soothing bath, and then, after the rain subsides, go outdoors to enjoy a walk through a pleasant natural environment that seems to come alive all around you with amazing realism. Once you complete your relaxing journey, therapeutic suggestions help you return feeling fully refreshed and relaxed.

This program, like *Natural Relaxation I*, can be of special benefit for anyone who experiences anxiety or muscle tension, fatigue or irritability, or perhaps finds it difficult to unwind and fall asleep at night. But really anyone who would simply like to take a 30-minute "imagination vacation" from the hustle and bustle of daily life is more than welcome to come along.

Relaxation and Massage
(30 minutes)

This program, like *Natural Relaxation I* and *Relaxation II*, takes full advantage of 3Dimensional Living Sound technology. In addition, this particular program utilizes a breakthrough in massage therapy—the Magic Massager®—which you can purchase at www.massagewarehouse.com or www.amazon.com.

The first product of its kind, the Magic Massager® is an advanced, patented device composed of multiple layers of a special, silky fabric; it allows your hands to glide over your body friction-free, in a way you've never experienced before, and it even works through clothing! It's like receiving an oil massage without the messiness and other drawbacks of using massage oil.

This program will help you achieve a deep state of both physical and mental relaxation through the combined elements of a simple but effective guided self-massage treatment, visualizations, and relaxation techniques.

With this particular program it is best to wear your headphones with the right and left channels worn properly over your right and left ears. And if you wish to remain dressed, it is best to wear light, comfy clothing.

A soothing voice will set the scene—an enchanting tropical island, high on a hill, overlooking a sandy beach and tranquil sea. You will be immersed in a symphony of 3D nature sounds—bird songs, rustling wind in the trees, and waves rolling onto the beach below—as you are guided, step by step, through a relaxing self-massage. You will then walk down an imaginary pathway, serenaded by passing birds and the sounds of flowing water—from tiny trickles to a swiftly running stream. Finally, you will emerge on a secluded beach where gentle waves caress the shore. Here you will have some time to simply relax and enjoy the peacefulness of this scene.

This state-of-the-art program is completely unique and extremely enjoyable and effective for achieving deep mental and physical relaxation. Requiring only 30 minutes, your relaxing massage combined with the other therapeutic techniques contained in this "imagination vacation" will completely dissolve the stress of your daily life, leaving you feeling relaxed and rejuvenated.

Country Friends
(32 minutes)

Country Friends engages the imagination of even restless children through the use of *3D Living Sound*. This program offers unique benefits to children ages 4–12 struggling with nervousness, worry, sadness, fear, insecurity, anger, pain, bedtime resistance, or sleep problems. The program can be used any time of day to induce a deep sense of relaxation, and can also be used as a wind-down before bedtime. This children's relaxation program can also be used in conjunction with my other children's sleep programs, *Magic Carpet* and *Playhouse on the Beach*.

The narrator of *Country Friends* begins the story with a car trip to the countryside. After suggesting that your child close his eyes, the narrator guides him through a series of daydreams, with the imagination stirred by a medley of sounds: bike riding, skating, swings, slides, horses, cars, airplanes, a train, a circus, and so on. With your child's attention thus drawn inward, the program enters the relaxation phase as we begin walking down an imaginary pathway through an enchanted forest.

Soon, we come upon a meadow with a farmhouse where we stop for directions to the river that will lead us down to the ocean, and we are treated to some country hospitality by a bluegrass group named *Harmony Grits*. They play a traditional country tune and then three of their original songs, sending us on our way to the soothing sounds of "Down by the River." After a short walk, we sit beside the river and relax to the sounds of the water, wind, and birds.

Continuing our walk down the pathway we discover a pond where we watch images appear in its mirror-like reflection and contemplate poetic words of inspiration and comfort. We then walk further along the path, which emerges on a magical beach where your child enjoys time for imaginary play of his choice. The story concludes with the suggestion that, as he returns home, the child take with him some of the wonderful feelings he has experienced throughout the program.

Even adults have found this program enjoyable, and often quite useful for achieving deep states of relaxation themselves.

Magic Carpet
(45 minutes)

Does your child dislike going to bed? Does she experience disturbing dreams or simply feel too restless to easily fall asleep? This state-of-the-art, clinically-tested program offers a unique solution to these and other such problems.

Magic Carpet provides an enjoyable bedtime activity that also helps children ages 4–12 drift gently to sleep. The program engages the imagination of even restless children through the use of **3D Living Sound**. This technology is best appreciated when listening with headphones or ear buds, which can be removed once your child has drifted off to sleep. If this is not practical, you can also have your child enjoy the recording via small speakers placed on either side of the bed. You may enjoy listening to this program yourself and adults have even found it useful for inducing sleep.

Magic Carpet begins with calming music, after which the narrator tells a story in the form of a poem. Your child is taken on a magic-carpet ride through various scenes, her imagination stirred by a medley of sounds: cars and airplanes, a train, a carnival fun zone, and so on. With your child's attention thus drawn inward, the program becomes more relaxing as it invites her down a pathway through an enchanted forest. Various elements of nature come to life, accompanied throughout by caring and comforting words. The pathway emerges on a magical beach where your child will build sand castles and watch seagulls fly overhead. The suggestions for relaxation and sleepiness continue as your child is led to discover a playhouse containing a special bed where she may drift to sleep as the background of gently rolling waves gradually fades away.

Playhouse on the Beach
(30 minutes)

Playhouse on the Beach is a sequel to *Magic Carpet*, which I generally recommend for initial use. But if your child has a calmer disposition and doesn't require the livelier format of *Magic Carpet* to hold his attention, *Playhouse on the Beach* will certainly be appropriate. Like *Magic Carpet*, this program is designed for children ages 4–12, and it offers an enjoyable bedtime activity that also helps them easily fall asleep.

Playhouse on the Beach, like all programs in this series, makes use of **3D Living Sound** and is designed for listening with headphones or ear buds, which can be removed once your child has drifted off to sleep. If this is not practical, you can also have your child enjoy the recording via small speakers placed on either side of the bed.

Playhouse on the Beach takes place on a magical beach amidst the call of seabirds and the pleasant roll of the ocean. The narrator guides your child to play along the water's edge where he is invited to float over the surf on a raft and observe the fish below, to ride upon the waves, to gather seashells, and play in the sand. The program becomes gradually more restful, offering subtle suggestions for sleep. After a time your child comes upon a playhouse containing a chest of toys and a welcoming bed. Your child is then drawn into sleep by the slowly fading sound of waves.

Nature Walk
(45 minutes)

Nature Walk offers a symphony of beautiful nature sounds, creating an atmosphere of serenity in which the day's cares and concerns just seem to melt away.

Nature Walk begins high on a hill of an enchanting tropical island, overlooking a sandy beach. Pleasant birdsongs and the call of the distant surf set the scene. You will feel as though you are taking a leisurely stroll down a winding path through the rainforest, serenaded by the breeze and melodious textures of flowing water. In time you will emerge upon an open expanse of shoreline, where you can rest on a pristine beach and drift into an ever-deeper state of relaxation, to the tranquil sounds of gently rolling waves.

Nature Walk provides the nature sounds from the *Sleep* and *Natural Relaxation I* programs without the guiding voice. It can be of particular benefit if combined with the relaxation or sleep-inducing techniques explored on these other programs.

Nature Odyssey
(45 minutes)

Nature Odyssey offers a full range of beautiful nature sounds, creating an atmosphere of relaxation and serenity. This program begins in a cozy cabin where you are seated beside a crackling fire. Outside, the sounds of wind and light rain announce the start of a thunderstorm which, upon passing, leaves you feeling refreshed and ready to begin your walk through an enchanted rainforest. You will stroll along a pathway that winds under a canopy of rustling leaves, passing by the pleasant songs of birds nestled in the trees. Further along, you will meander alongside a lilting stream, finally emerging on an expanse of open beach where you can relax and drift away to the sounds of gently rolling waves.

Nature Odyssey is useful anytime you wish to create a serene atmosphere; you'll find it of particular benefit when combined with the relaxation or sleep-inducing techniques that you can learn from my other programs.

Stream Walk
(45 minutes)

Stream Walk takes you on a relaxing stroll along an enchanted stream, immersing you in subtle textures of flowing water accompanied by the bird songs and rustling wind in the trees overhead. As with the previously described *Nature Odyssey* program, *Stream Walk* is useful anytime you wish to create a serene atmosphere; it can be of particular benefit when combined with the relaxation or sleep-inducing techniques available on the *Sleep* or *Natural Relaxation I* programs.

Rain and Thunder
(45 minutes)

Rain and Thunder is one of my personal favorites. I've loved thunderstorms ever since I was a small child, sitting indoors by a warm fire with a mug of cocoa, listening to the patter of rain on the roof and the deep, rumbling roll of thunder in the distance. I recorded the storm you'll hear in Pecos, New Mexico, and later wove in subtle textures of wind and rain in a 24-track production.

Sit back comfortably with your eyes closed as the storm begins with gentle rain and wind. The thunder enters at first as only a distant rumble, building quite gradually, with no sudden jolting claps. The storm grows to a crescendo midway and then very slowly subsides, returning to the gentle sounds of rain, wind, and a few calling birds. As the program ends, as with the others in the series, you are left feeling deeply relaxed and refreshed.

Ocean
(45 minutes)

Ocean takes place on an expanse of open beach where the distant sound of sea birds and the gentle wash of ocean waves invites you to sit and relax, and let the cares of the day simply wash away. The program will transport you to the tropical beach where I recorded it, creating the feeling that you are actually right there in that lush, colorful, and above all tranquil natural setting.

Ocean can be of particular benefit to people who learn the techniques provided in my relaxation or sleep programs and wish to self-apply them using the background sound of waves, which many people find to be the most relaxing of all.

Although this program can be used at any time, it is ideal for use when trying to fall asleep in a noisy environment, as the soothing murmur of waves masks any disturbing sounds that might interfere with sleep.

Reflections on the California Coast (DVD)
(40 minutes)

This program is the first one completed in an upcoming series of nature DVDs with soundtracks in *3D Living Sound*. This 40-minute journey encompasses beautiful sights and sounds from Santa Barbara to Monterrey Bay. You will find yourself drawn into nature in a manner you have never experienced before, without actually being there.

On this DVD you will experience over one-hundred of California's uniquely spectacular coastal vistas, including ocean views, forests, meadows, streams, wildlife, and spring flowers. And this gorgeous canvas is brought to life through the magic of 3D Living Sound.

This DVD is best experienced if you make yourself comfortable by lying down on a couch or bed and positioning your computer screen as close to your eyes as possible (preferably within two feet). With this particular program, headphones should be worn with the right and left speakers over the appropriate ears so that the sound direction has the proper spatial orientation. As you relax into this experience, the boundary between reality and imagination will soon blur, and you will feel as though you are looking through a window, viewing scenes of virtual reality. A sense of relaxation will wash over you as you effortlessly escape from the cares and worries of everyday life.

Appendix G

Additional Resources

For an additional tool to assist you in helping your child relax or sleep, I suggest you visit the website www.magicmassager.com (or www.magicmassager.net for massage professionals), where you can learn about the *Magic Massager*®, an extremely valuable parenting tool. Its four layers of silky fabric provide a frictionless surface that allows you to administer soothing Swedish massage without the fuss and muss of massage oil, and it even works through clothing. The *Magic Massager*® offers a way to "connect" with your child in a caring manner that he will love. Many parents have found it helpful with their children for winding down at bedtime, but it can be used anytime you wish to help them relax. The sensations created by the *Magic Massager*® are much more pleasant than normal touch and communicate a feeling of caring that allows children to open up and discuss their concerns more easily. With even a quick back or foot rub you will sense your child's tensions melting away, replaced with a greatly enhanced sense of relaxation and contentment. If you wish to purchase a *Magic Massager*®, click on www.massagewarehouse.com or www.amazon.com (keyword: Magic Massager).

Appendix H

Research on the AudioMagic Programs and 3D Living Sound

In *DreamChild*™ *Adventures* in *Relaxation and Sleep,* you read 12 case studies that provided anecdotal evidence of the efficacy of my *DreamChild Adventures* 3D audio programs in helping children (and their parents and guardians) handle a broad spectrum of sleep problems, anxiety, and other emotional and behavioral problems. But there are other forms of evidence, besides anecdotal, that support the effectiveness of this technology.

While studies on the children's series have yet to be undertaken, scientific research has been conducted on several of the other AudioMagic programs.

A number of studies were briefly covered in the Introduction to this book and an additional study was mentioned in the commentary of Chapter 3 on Resistance to Reading. Below, I've included a brief overview of some of the studies conducted on the efficacy of certain AudioMagic programs and the therapeutic value of *3D Living Sound* technology in general.

These data and my clinical experience strongly suggest that individuals may be provided therapy more quickly and effectively with *3D Living Sound* technology than ordinary audio. In addition, the novelty and entertaining nature of the AudioMagic programs seems to enhance enjoyment and repetition, reinforcing the therapeutic effect.

Previous research has shown that non-threatening images of nature have reduced stress and even shortened post-operative recovery and length of hospitalization. It is therefore, I believe, reasonable to suggest that the *3D Living Sound* of nature in the AudioMagic recordings are inherently "therapeutic" and relaxing.

I

Conducted by: **Thomas Jackson, M.D. and Christopher Alsten, Ph.D.**
Studied: ***Natural Relaxation I*** **program with psychiatric and chemical dependency in-patients**

Studies were conducted on the *Natural Relaxation I* program on a number of units at both the Glendale Adventist Medical Center and New Beginnings Chemical Dependency Hospital. Each unit incorporated use of the *Natural Relaxation I* program into their daily schedule by designating a daily 30 minute listening period for all patients who complained of significant anxiety. Each patient was provided with the *Natural Relaxation I* program along with a player and headphones with which to listen.

Patients kept daily logs on which they charted anxiety/stress levels, using a subjective scale of 1–10, immediately before and after using the *Natural Relaxation I* program. The program demonstrated effectiveness in a number of settings, with average decreases in daily before and after anxiety/stress scores reported as follows: Adult Psychiatric Unit—61%, Adolescent Psychiatric Unit—52%, Geriatric Psychiatric/ Chemical Dependency Unit—54%, and Adult Chemical Dependency Unit—52%.

Although improvements in baseline anxiety/stress levels were noted, these changes would have been influenced by a number of variables and can not be attributed solely to use of the *Natural Relaxation I* program. Yet it is interesting to note that anxiety/stress levels decreased an average of 25%–43% (for the various units) over the course of hospitalization. On the two units where it was reviewed, another interesting phenomenon was observed, which was a statistically significant decrease in patients who left the hospital "a-m-a" (against medical advice) among those who used the *Natural Relaxation I* program.

II

Conducted by: **Gary Schwartz, Ph.D., Professor of Psychology, Neurology and Psychiatry, University of Arizona**
Studied: **Comparison of mono, stereo, and *3D Living Sound* using topographic EEG brain mapping**

In this study, 15 subjects listened to recordings of the ocean and various sound effects recorded in mono, stereo and *3D Living Sound*. Electroencephalographic (EEG) recordings of brain wave activity were made while subjects listened to the recordings and subjects rated each audio recording for interest and realism.

The following includes excerpts from the analysis that was performed.

- Subjects rated each tape (during the EEG session) for interest and realism. The line graph shows the results, averaged over ocean and sound effects. A three-way repeated measures analysis of variance was performed: (1) ocean/sound effects, (2) mono/stereo/3D, and (3) interest/realism. The main effect for mono/stereo/3D was highly significant ($p < 0.0006$). Subjects rated mono as lowest, stereo as moderate, and 3D as highest. There was a significant main effect for ocean/sound effects ($p < 0.039$) indicating that the sound effects tapes were rated overall as stronger (7.74). I repeated the analysis of variance for just stereo/3D (removing mono). The main effect for stereo/3D was significant ($p < 0.037$), as was the main effect for ocean/sound effects ($p < 0.012$). In a word, the tapes 'worked' with these subjects. On the whole, the subjects perceived the mono, stereo and 3D tapes differently. As expected, 3D tapes were rated as most interesting and realistic.

- The EEG data were spectral analyzed, saved as ASCII files, imported to Quattro Pro 4.0, transposed and imported to CSS 3.0, and statistically analyzed. Separate analyses of variance were performed on theta, alpha, beta 1 and beta 2, using a four-way repeated measure design: (1) ocean/sound effects, (2) stereo/3D, (3) right side/left side, and (4) site (eight sites each side).

- There were no significant effects for theta or beta 2. However, there were significant effects for alpha and beta 1.

- First, for alpha, there was a borderline significant ocean/sound effects by right/left interaction ($p < 0.059$). Alpha was generally greater for the ocean tapes compared to the sound effects tapes (across both stereo and 3D tapes), and the ocean alpha enhancement was stronger on the left side.

- Second, for alpha, there was a significant stereo/3D by right/left interaction ($p < 0.039$) and a significant stereo/3D by right/left by site interaction ($p < 0.018$). Alpha decreased in 3D compared to stereo, especially on the left, posterior side of the brain. I have plotted the alpha data subtracting the alpha for the mono data. Again, yellows, reds and whites mean alpha increased, blues and blacks mean alpha decreased. You can see that for stereo, alpha increased in the left and right temporal regions compared to mono, whereas for 3D, alpha increased in the right temporal regions but decreased in the left temporal and posterior regions compared to mono. These data suggest that the 3D tapes were more attention getting, novel and interesting compared to the stereo tapes. Note that these effects are independent of ocean and sound effects.

- Third, for beta 1, there was a trend for a stereo/3D by right/left interaction ($p < 0.068$) and a significant stereo/3D by site interaction ($p < 0.022$). Beta 1 increased in 3D compared to stereo, especially on the left, posterior side of the brain. I have again plotted the data subtracting the beta 1 for the mono data. Here yellows, reds and whites mean beta 1 increased in the left, posterior regions. These data further support the hypothesis that the 3D tapes were more attention getting, novel and interesting compared to the stereo tapes. The fact that they show up on the left side and the posterior, (rear) regions (occipital) are consistent with the idea that both verbal imagery and visual imagery were activated by the 3D tapes.

Although these results would, perhaps, be more interesting if you were able to view the referenced graph and topographic EEG maps (which will be provided upon request), the most striking feature of the graph is the fact that subjects rated the interest/realism of 3D so much higher than stereo. In fact, the difference between stereo and 3D was greater than the difference between mono and stereo.

The fact that 3D sound is much more engaging, relaxing and vivid than normal stereo may have particular significance because a correlation has been demonstrated between vividness of imagery and efficacy of therapeutic imagery techniques. It has been hypothesized that because it is more "vivid" the *3D Living Sound* enhances the psycho-physiological effects of the other techniques without being sleep inducing in and of itself.

III

Conducted by: Jon Sassin, M.D., Chairman, Department of Neurology, UCI Orange County Medical Center

Studied: *Natural Sleep* program

The following study was conducted at the UCI Medical Center's Sleep Disorders Clinic in 1983. It should be noted that the study was never completed and the following data was from an interim report with only 15 subjects, and, although quite interesting, should be considered in this context.

The patients in the study had been referred to the Sleep Disorders Clinic by their primary care physicians because of the severity of their sleep problems. Patients reported suffering from insomnia for an average of 14 years, had been taking sleeping pills an average of six years and reported an average of approximately 70 minutes to fall asleep (even with use of prescription sleep medications).

Patients were initially evaluated, at which time general information was collected and psychological testing was performed using the Profile of Mood States (POMS). The *Natural Sleep* program was then provided to the patients to assist them in the process of withdrawing from sleep medications. They were then asked to listen to the program while falling asleep at home as they gradually withdrew from their sleep medications over a two-week period. At the end of this withdrawal period they returned to the Sleep Clinic where they were evaluated to determine if they were still using any medication, psychological testing was repeated, and overnight electroencephalograph sleep lab studies (polysomnographs) were performed for two consecutive nights to determine the quality and quantity of their sleep.

The first night patients were tested without using the *Natural Sleep* program and the second night testing was done while using the program. This protocol was used in order to test the hypothesis that there would be a residual effect from listening to the program the previous two weeks because patients could learn the sleep inducing techniques, at least to some degree. (Previous clinical work had revealed that many patients "internalized" or learned the sleep inducing techniques after several weeks and afterwards could use the programs only as a "refresher" or on especially difficult nights.)

Although the number of patients was limited, the results were fairly dramatic. The average time to fall asleep decreased from a reported 70 minutes, with the use of sleep medications, to a measured time of 17 minutes after withdrawal from medications. Patients were asked to rate the effectiveness of the *Natural Sleep* program on a scale of 1–10 on how effective it was at putting them to sleep and the average score was 8, indicating very high patient satisfaction. A number of other elements were evaluated on the all-night polysomnographs, in addition to how long it took patients to fall asleep. However, a direct comparison could not be made between recordings of patient's condition while dependent on sleeping pills and after withdrawal because sleep medications distort brain waves, making reading unreliable.

We can, however, compare the two all-night recordings after two weeks' use of the *Natural Sleep* program and drug withdrawal. The first night's recording can be considered the "internalized" or learned condition (after two weeks of program use) because the program was not listened to that night, while the second night's polysomnograph recording can be considered an internalized plus a reinforced condition, because the program was listened to that night. Comparing these two nights, we can make several observations. During the second night, the amount of time awake after first falling asleep decreased as did the number of nighttime wakings. Total time asleep increased, percentage of time asleep increased, and the percentage of REM sleep (dreaming) increased. The only measure that did not seem to improve between the two nights was the average time to fall asleep, which increased from 12 to 17 minutes. Although these averages are both within the normal range, the increase is the result of just one patient taking significantly longer to fall asleep on the second night. It should be noted, however, that this patient rated the *Natural Sleep* program as a 10 on a scale of 1–10 and claimed that he could not have "kicked the drugs" without it. When this aberration is removed, all patients improved in this category as well.

The psychological data taken from the Profile of Mood States (POMS) was also quite revealing. It indicated notable improvement in the Depression/Dejection and Anger/ Hostility scales with somewhat less improvement on the Tension/Anxiety and Confusion/Bewilderment scales after only two weeks use of the Natural Sleep program. A control group of patients, not using the program, showed no change in any POMS scale. The average change on the Depression/Dejection scale for those using the programs was 17 points while a change of only four points is considered to be clinically significant improvement.

The *Natural Sleep* program has demonstrated great promise in the treatment of some of the most difficult cases of insomnia and, as the Profile of Mood States testing suggests, may also offer treatment for the large number of patients suffering from mood disorders.

IV

Conducted by: **Christopher Alsten, Ph.D.**
Funded by: **U.S. Air Force**
Studied: **3D *Natural Sleep* program as part of the Sleep Enhancement Fatigue Reduction Training (SEFRT) with U.S. Air Force pilots and shift workers**

The Air Force contracted with my company, Inner Health, Inc., to evaluate the effectiveness of our programs for improving sleep and reducing the fatigue experienced by jet-lagged Air Force pilots and air crews, along with the effect on shiftworker fatigue. The result was the Sleep Enhancement Fatigue Reduction Training (SEFRT) program, which incorporated the most recent versions of the *Natural Sleep* programs, and included a separate instruction booklet further detailing sleep enhancement and fatigue reduction techniques.

For Dr. Alsten and the research team's evaluation of the SEFRT, a group of 69 participants (45 pilots and 24 shift workers) underwent a battery of tests and wore small actigraphs around their wrists in order to measure their sleep objectively as they charted their sleep, mood levels, and fatigue levels. The pilots and aircrew members did this during a multi-day flight over several time zones and, following a three-week "training period" of listening to the various SEFRT programs every night in bed, they repeated the flight taking the same measurements.

The USAF flight crew evaluation involved a baseline trip before the SEFRT program and another identical trip after the training. Then a comparison was done between the two trips (repeated measures study). A third element, a "washout" period with white noise, was attempted as part of a subsequent active placebo trip evaluation. However, only a few aircrew members were able to schedule this third trip during the study period due to time constraints. (We believe this was exacerbated by the fact that it spread throughout the squadron that we were going to take away the "sleep training," something that worked, and replace it with "white noise" instead. Those who had used the white noise did not like it and knew it "did not work.")

In the second study, conducted this time with shiftworkers, an active placebo (a choice of white noise and several pieces of relaxing music) was provided as training material first in the repeated measures protocol. The results of this placebo "training" were evaluated and then the SEFRT Training was provided and the results of the actual training were evaluated. Although many liked the music to go to sleep this active placebo control did not have any effect while the SEFRT training had a very significant effect. Neither group was provided any additional sleep hygiene information, cognitive behavioral therapy instructions or similar information.

Among the findings:

- Numerous participants (and their spouses) provided comments to evaluators regarding the impact of the program on the quality of their sleep
- Many shiftworking program users were able to distinguish fellow program users from the control (placebo) group by their mood and energy levels
- Both aircrew members and shiftworkers reduced caffeine intake by an average of 35%
- By training's end, total stress levels were cut nearly in half in both groups
- Those participants who were hospital staff working graveyard shift and sleeping during the day showed an objective increase in hours slept per day from 5 hours and 15 minutes to 6 hours and 10 minutes
- Participants reported a 29% increase in how deeply they felt they slept, and a 78% improvement in how rested they felt after waking
- On Profile of Mood States* testing, program users showed a statistically significant improvement in nearly all of the subscales whereas the placebo group did not
- Participants showed an 18% improvement in job satisfaction and a 56% improvement in all-around self-perceived health
- Digestive complaints lessened noticeably and cardiovascular problems decreased measurably
- Participants showed an increased adaptability to and recovery from circadian disruption
- Self-reported quality-of-life measures improved
- It is likely that the program users' overall reduction in chronic fatigue resulted primarily from decreased circadian rhythm disruption and reduction in "sleep debt"

due to improvements in sleep quantity and quality along with the program's enhanced relaxation component.

What follows are some sample quotes from the study:

Air Crew

I feel better and less fatigued during the entire mission and it was easier to readjust to home time when I returned.

C-5A Pilot

I'm glad I used it. It was easy, didn't take much time and has made a real difference.

C-5A Pilot

Normally I don't have a problem getting to sleep when the mission schedule or responsibilities in the cockpit permit a nap. When I have a shift in my rest cycle (night sleep to day sleep) I automatically use the [programs] to help put me to sleep. They are very effective.

C-5A Pilot

Now when I have an early morning departure, I'm able to go to sleep at times that I wouldn't normally be able to, in preparation for the mission.

C-141 Pilot

I am still using the [programs] and have found them to help me calm down and get to sleep much faster, no matter how tired or alert I am.

KC-135 Pilot

With the training, I can get to sleep easier and sleep deeper and longer than before.

KC-10 Flight Engineer

I get more sleep during layovers and feel less stressed since going through the sleep training.

C-5A Pilot

I have memory of the first five minutes or so of the voice . . . then I'm usually asleep.

KC-10 Pilot

Only a few times in the past 8 years have I ever gone into a deep sleep in the aircraft. On the first use of the tapes I went into a deep sleep with dreams and was awakened only due to increased temperature in the aircraft cabin.

KC-10 Boom Operator

I'm never tired in the afternoon, but knowing that I was leaving on a very demanding trip at 10 pm I decided to try to get a nap. With the help of the tapes I had no trouble falling asleep.

KC-10 Boom Operator

Overall, in comparing this to previous relaxation/visualization tapes I have worked with in the past, I found this type to be quite effective.

USAF Flight Surgeon

Shiftworkers

I can sleep an extra hour after my first midshift and feel much better after my second consecutive midshift.

Air Traffic Controller

I now sleep two hours longer when I first change over to nightshifts and I don't feel as wiped out during the second night.

Air Traffic Controller

Now when I'm working nights, I get more and better sleep during the day and I don't feel as tired at work.

Air Traffic Controller

Not only am I sleeping and feeling better, especially when I change shifts, but I've noticed that everyone else on my shift that is also using the sleep program, seems to be more alert and in a better mood on the job making it easier to interact and communicate with each other.

Supervisor, Air Traffic Controller

I could really imagine the place and feel myself relax because of the 3D sound and descriptive phrases.

Air Traffic Controller

The views and conclusions above are those of the author and neither represent the official policy of the U.S. Air Force nor do they constitute an endorsement.

v

Conducted by: **Thomas Jackson, M.D.**
Studied: ***Natural Sleep* Programs**

Hospitalized psychiatric patients frequently experience significant sleep problems associated with both their illness and the stress of sleeping in an unfamiliar environment, and are often prescribed sleeping pills on an as-needed ("PRN") basis. A study to evaluate the effectiveness of the *Natural Sleep* Program to replace the use of sleeping pills was initiated at the Therapeutic Residential Center, in Downey, California—a 39-bed locked psychiatric facility. Primary diagnoses were schizophrenia, bipolar disorder, and major depression.

Staff psychiatrists continued to prescribe sedative-hypnotics, as usual, during the entire study. After an initial baseline period of 18 days the *Natural Sleep* program, along with bedside players, was made available to all patients. When patients wanted, or were instructed, to go to sleep they were required to listen to the *Natural Sleep* program before they could request sleep medication, which would then be dispensed at the nursing station. The study period lasted ten weeks (70 days), during which time there were 130 patients admitted and 136 discharged (24/30 during the baseline period).

During the baseline period an average of 7.61 (+/- 1.46) sleeping pills were dispensed per night. The total number of patients during the baseline was 64 (greater than the capacity of 39 patients because of admissions and discharges). During the first two weeks of *Natural Sleep* program usage the rate of sleeping pill consumption dropped to an average of 1.21 (+/- 1.01) per night, representing an 84% decrease. This "transition period" represented a span of time when patients were being weaned from their customary use of sleep medications. During the remainder of the study, sleeping pill usage averaged .15 per night (+/- .41; a total of eight sleeping pills consumed over 54 days; total number of patients = 145) representing a 98% decrease in sleeping pill usage in spite of the large number of discharges and admissions. One-way ANOVA indicated high significance with a *p* value of < 0.0001. No compensating increase in other potentially sedative medications was noted or any change in the percentage of diagnostic categories of admitted and discharged patients.

Patients reported that the *Natural Sleep* program was effective for both sleep onset and sleep maintenance. It was believed that compliance was high due to the desire of many patients to take an active part in their own treatment and the pleasantness of the Sleep program experience. Staff reported additional patient benefits including decreased morning drowsiness and improved mood.

VI

Conducted by: **Christopher Alsten, Ph.D.**
Studied: *3D Living Sound Nature Sound* programs

Quoted from Dr. Alsten's presentation at the 2002 International Society for Ecosystem Health Conference in Washington, D.C.:

> In response to numerous anecdotal reports of the increase in appreciation and "love" of and for nature by individuals who have been exposed to the *3D Living Sound Nature Sound* programs, we conducted a unidimensional retrospective analysis of this psychological change. We asked subjects if they noticed a shift in their appreciation of, or relationship to, nature after using the recordings which contained *3D Living Sound Nature Sound* programs. We then asked them to attempt to quantify their appreciation on a zero to 10 scale, after repeated exposure to the *3D Living Sound Nature Sound* programs and retrospectively, prior to exposure.
>
> While retrospective analyses of this type are subject to numerous psychological influences affecting the results, several individuals commented on the fact that they didn't realize that their appreciation of nature could improve so much in so little time and that if they had scored it before listening they probably would have scored themselves much higher initially and "run out of room" to show the magnitude and significance of the change.

Here are some sample quotes from participants in the study:

The 3D Sounds (of Nature) really make me want to go back out into nature. It reminds me of how much I miss it. If you would have asked me how much I appreciated nature before listening to the programs, I would have given a higher score than a "two," but I would have run out of room to indicate how much this has affected me.

Gerald F.

I noticed that I am more in tune to the smells, sights and sounds of nature than I was in the past. I notice the birds chirping more often. I am enjoying the fragrance of flowering plants more. I seem to be able to see "islands of nature" even in the midst of residential or commercial areas.

Jan W.

I like nature but I didn't get as much out of it as when I was listening to the tapes. I was able to visualize nature in the city! It was definitely more relaxing and I appreciate nature a lot more. I'm glad you asked the questions in this order or I would have had to change my starting point to get in a big enough change.

Ellen C.

I love how it focused my appreciation of nature.

Trudy R.

I've always liked nature. I found the 3D or "virtual reality" sounds of nature really calms me down and makes me feel like I'm in another place.

Norma N.

I have always been sensitive to noise, but noticed recently that I am becoming more and more appreciative of quiet, and more tuned in to birds. I am not a "birder," but I have noticed that my appreciation of birds singing has increased lately. I am tolerating the mess to have a feeder and a small birdbath outside a living room window, near the chimney where I notice they hang out in the morning. Their songs fill the living room when they sit up on the chimney!

Jane M.

I don't know if it improved my appreciation of nature, but I noticed that I hear nature sounds differently than I once did. Now I "hear" nature "in color." And when I close my eyes and listen to the recordings, it's like I'm seeing it!

Lee D.

VII

Conducted by: A. Bystritsky, MD, Professor of Psychiatry, University of California at Los Angeles (UCLA)

Studied: **3D *Living Sound* Technology with anxious patients**

In a 1999 double-blind study conducted at UCLA, Dr. Bystritsky demonstrated that the *3D Living Sound* technology, listened to over ordinary stereo headphones, enhanced several psycho-physiological responses compared to ordinary stereo in anxious patients.

VIII

Conducted by: **Peggy Lachine, RN head nurse in a Chemical Dependency Unit**
Studied: **3D *Relaxation I & II* programs**

In a 1993 single-blind pilot study, chemical dependency patients were assigned to use either the 3D *Relaxation* programs or traditional progressive muscle relaxation and imagery audiocassette programs. Those using the 3D relaxation programs showed a statistically significant cumulative decrease in anxiety within one week. And while patients assigned to traditional progressive muscle relaxation and imagery audiocassette programs also showed daily reductions in anxiety pre-usage to post-usage, this did not amount to a statistically significant cumulative improvement over this same period of time.

IX

Conducted by: **Dr. Bruce Rybarczyk, Virginia Commonwealth University**
Funded by: **National Institutes of Health**
Studied: ***Natural Sleep* programs**

In this study, two different forms of home-based, self-help therapy for insomnia were compared in a group of older adults with different comorbidities, arthritis and coronary artery disease.

- a purely text-based (book) home version of Mimeault and Morin's Cognitive Behavioral Therapy for the treatment of Insomnia (CBT-I)
- a multimedia approach that included a guidebook with traditional CBT-I instructions, weekly videos of classroom instruction, and audio (in the form of a progressive series of 3D *Natural Sleep* programs)

This followed from a review of research in multiple domains of self-help behavioral interventions which indicated that multimedia strategies are more effective than reading materials alone (Mains & Scogin, 2003) by demonstrating that using multi-modal instructional methods increases the likelihood that the material will be thoroughly reviewed and facilitates learning and subsequent enactment of behavioral changes.

Morin (2003) has argued that since insomnia has been associated with significant morbidity and quality of life effects, effective treatments should not only produce changes in sleep parameters but also other measures of daytime functioning. As such, this study measured not only a variety of sleep factors but an array of daytime mood and general health measures as well. That way, this study could also test the hypothesis that CBT-I would lead to benefits in daytime functioning as a consequence of improved sleep.

In an intention-to-treat analysis that included all participants, the *3D Living Sound* approach demonstrated statistically significant superiority in three global sleep measures–Pittsburgh Sleep Quality Index, Sleep Impairment Index, Dysfunctional Beliefs and Attitudes about Sleep–immediately after the intervention training was completed. In contrast, there were no significant differences between the two treatment groups or the primary and comorbid insomnia groups on any baseline sleep measure, however there were notable differences in the clinical significance outcomes at post-treatment.

The book group had:

- 14 clinically significant improvements
- 10 moderately clinically significant improvements
- 2 substantial improvements
- 32 no improvements

The multimedia group had:

- 16 clinically significant improvements
- 13 moderately clinically significant improvements
- 19 no improvements

When combining the three clinical improvement categories together, the multimedia group had an overall rate of 60.4% clinically significant change compared to 44.8% for book group.

The findings from the present study indicate that home treatment CBT-I is an effective treatment for both primary insomnia and comorbid insomnia in older adults, with the combined rate of clinically significant change at 52%. This suggests only a moderate decrease in treatment response compared to in-person classroom treatment, which showed a 78% clinically significant response rate using the same criteria in a comparable study. But even that small difference diminishes when one considers how much more laborious the six-week in-classroom program was over the at-home program, listening to headphones in bed at night and using the guidebook and video classes.

Furthermore, there were no differences in treatment response between primary and comorbid insomnia groups in the present study, further supporting the recent consensus among researchers that comorbid insomnia is undergirded by the same cognitive and behavioral factors as primary insomnia and therefore equally responsive to treatment. These overall findings add to the recently published studies showing high levels of efficacy for behavioral treatments that target secondary and comorbid insomnias (Currie et al., 2000; Lichstein et al., 2000; Quesnel et al., 2003; Rybarczyk et al., 2002).

What's more, in a one-year follow-up the CBT-I approach augmented with 3D Living Sound sleep programs continued to demonstrate significant superiority on these major sleep measures. In addition, more subjects using the 3D Living Sound approach showed clinical improvement one year post than subjects using Mimeault and Morin's home CBT-I.

These results were presented at the 2009 meeting of the Society of Behavioral Medicine in Montreal.

X

Conducted by: **Kathy Lee, R.N., Ph.D., University of California at San Francisco**
Studied: ***Natural Sleep*** **program during and after pregnancy**
Funded by: **National Institute of Health (NIH)**

This study conducted on pregnant women found that after the birth of their babies, those women who used a specific series of *Natural Sleep* programs in combination with Cognitive Behavioral Training for Insomnia (CBT-I) materials slept nearly one hour longer than the control group.

I would be remiss, however, in leaving out that during their third trimester of pregnancy, the women using the adult sleep programs with CBT-I slept no better than those who did not.

It would appear that sleeping late in pregnancy is a challenge for many women, for which there is still not a good solution. However, given that the *Natural Sleep* programs and CBT-I materials performed so splendidly at improving sleep during the critical postpartum period (when many women are inclined to experience a degree of depression) the apparent failing of the programs to help improve sleep in the third trimester is assumed to be the result of two factors:

- the women not yet having enough experience using the programs
- a general trend among pregnant women of less sleep disturbance in the third trimester than postpartum

There is evidence of both of these factors (particularly well-documented in the case of the latter—Lee et al., 1992, Goyal et al., 2002). The evidence of the former comes from the above-mentioned Air Force study, in which the subjects reported that it had taken them approximately four to six weeks to feel they had learned or been adequately "trained" in the program (Alsten et al., 1999).

Based on the recommendations of childbirth class instructors and other pregnancy sleep experts we reduced the length of program use in the study to four weeks in order to make it more acceptable to first-time pregnant mothers who are generally already overwhelmed with things to do. Based on the postpartum results this condensed period of program use seems effective, but perhaps an extended period of program use during the pregnancy would provide more adequate results during the pre-delivery time period.

In addition, the effect of program use may become more evident if those women who are at highest risk for prenatal sleep disturbance can first be identified.

The most significant objective improvement noted from the study was the previously mentioned additional 55 minutes in total sleep at night (postpartum). But that wasn't the only noted result or benefit. The quality of that sleep was improved as well, with fewer awakenings, lower Wake After Sleep Onset (WASO) percentage, and less time to get to sleep initially and after awakening for nursing. This last factor, the time it takes to fall asleep, is known as Sleep Onset Latency (SOL) and it is a noteworthy finding in this study as it is considered the most relevant screening question in relation to the risk for postpartum depression (Goyal et al., 2007).

One additional objective improvement found was better napping during the day, which increased the overall sleep quantity in a 24-hour period to 81 minutes.

Several subjective measures improved as well, notable decreases both in reported levels of fatigue and perceived stress in the morning, as well as improvements in adjustment.

The report on this study states: "We consider an extra hour of consolidated sleep during the postpartum period with this population to be a significant clinical success and worthy of pursuing to develop a commercially viable product to assist postpartum and potentially pregnant women in obtaining the sleep they need and deserve."

INDEX

- A -

AAP (see American Academy of Pediatrics)
abandonment, 25, 101, 103, 108
academic performance, 4, 6, 14, 36, 55-58, 66, 112, 127, 165, 179, 224-227, 229
ADD (see attention deficit disorder)
ADHD (see attention deficit hyperactivity disorder)
adolescence, 9, 56, 269
adolescent, 202, 268, 284
adverse reactions, 16, 201, 237
affection, 26-27, 80, 193
age-appropriate fears 8
aggression 36, 67, 73, 112
Air Force (see U.S. Air Force)
alertness, 56, 129, 183, 190, 203, 274
allergies, 11, 136
Alprazolam, 203
Alsten, Christopher, 16, 283, 287, 291, 295
Ambien, 204, 205
American Academy of Audiology, 241
American Academy of Pediatrics, 38, 267
American Sleep-Language-Hearing Association (ASHA), 245, 247, 268, 272
Anders, Thomas, 194, 270
anger, 7, 8, 12, 28, 29, 41, 53, 68, 72, 82, 88, 91, 99, 101, 104, 107, 115, 120-121, 139, 165, 167, 211-213, 217, 222, 225, 242, 245, 276, 287
antidepressant, 204
antihypertensive, 202
antipsychotic, 134, 157
antisocial 112
anxiety: , 3-12, 14-16, 26-28, 36, 56, 67, 68, 73, 77, 95, 96, 113, 123, 127-128, 133, 134, 136, 137, 143, 145, 154, 157, 158, 165, 167, 172, 176, 178, 184, 186, 188, 190, 193, 194, 199, 203, 211-222, 237, 267-269, 275, 276, 283, 284, 287, 293; about sleep, 10, 181; separation anxiety, 9, 15, 26, 165, 193, 194, 199, 212; separation anxiety disorder, 212
Anxiety Disorders Association of America 7
assertiveness, 77, 179
asthma, 155, 205, 207
attention deficit disorder (ADD), 144, 179, 208, 268, 272
attention deficit hyperactivity disorder (ADHD), 133, 148, 200, 204-205, 208-209, 228, 272
audio equipment, 239
AudioMagic, 5, 6, 16, 153, 224, 234, 273-274, 283
Audubon Medal, 224
authority figures, 67, 229
autogenic discharges, 16
autonomic nervous system, 14, 175
avoidance 7, 29

- B -

Baldwin, Jeff, 254
bedtime, 7, 10, 12, 13, 15, 24, 27, 29, 31, 32, 34, 36-39, 41, 50, 53, 58-61, 66, 67, 83, 88, 89, 96, 102, 104, 115, 116, 122, 152, 163, 182-190, 197, 203, 241, 262, 268-270, 273; resistance, 10, 12, 29, 36, 38, 41, 58, 59, 67, 83, 165, 184, 211, 276; routine, 27, 36, 39, 58, 184, 186, 187, 192; snacks, 186
bedwetting 4-5, 11, 67, 115-116, 122-123, 125, 133-141, 179, 270 (see also enuresis)
begging 94, 166, 191
Begley, Sharon, 222, 271
behavior: modification, 111, 121; problems, 22, 30, 66, 73, 117, 127, 134, 209
behavioral inhibition, 221
Benadryl, 203
benzodiazepines, 203, 204
Berman, Marc, 230, 269
biofeedback, 156
biophilia, 231
bipolar, 167, 178, 290
blame, 70, 139
blankets, 188, 195, 197-198
blood pressure, 126, 155, 165, 168, 173, 176, 204, 219
body mass index (BMI), 130, 253-254, 271
Boston Globe, The, 229, 269
boundaries, 42, 78, 228, 270
boys, 30, 112, 138, 252, 263
brain damage, 113, 210
Branden, Nathaniel, 179, 267
breast-feeding, 196, 199
breathing, 3, 24, 58, 91, 155, 195, 209, 212, 218, 254, 275
bribery, 49
bullying, 89, 188
Butler, Samuel, 111

- C -

caffeine, 89, 140, 186, 219, 288
Canada Hospital for Sick Children, 246
Canadian Medical Association Journal, 113
cancer, 112, 154-155
caretaker(s), 3-5, 10, 16, 24, 25, 49-50, 79, 225, 231, 233
causation, 223
Center for Health Systems and Design, 230
Centers for Disease Control and Prevention, 126, 242, 245
Chansky, Tamar E., 10, 211, 219, 221, 222, 267
Children's Hospital of Orange County, 15
cholesterol, 126, 129
chores, 49, 85, 225
Christian Science Monitor, The 224

chronic medical conditions, 207
chronic middle ear diseases, 207
circadian rhythms 38, 184-185, 188
cities, 227, 229, 230, 243
City of Hope, 151, 153
classroom, 9, 227, 293-294
clinginess, 9, 72, 199
Clinical Guide to Pediatric Sleep: Diagnosis and Management of Sleep Problems, A, 201, 270
Clonazepam, 203
Clonidine, 202, 204
Cochrane Library, 141
Codeine, 145, 150
cognitive behavioral therapy, 141, 288, 293
colic, 207
comforting, 26, 90, 91, 121, 186, 278
communication, 67, 77, 82, 89, 98, 160, 172, 241, 270
compassion, 26, 28, 139, 222
compliance, 104, 111-112, 271, 291
concentration, 24, 31, 33, 45-46, 56, 160, 203, 275
confidence, 6, 83, 90, 130, 139, 148, 152, 169-170, 176, 205, 215-216, 228
contentious behavior, 77
continuity, 71
continuous positive airway pressure (CPAP), 210
cooperation, 15, 51, 59, 227
coping skills 98
corporal punishment 111-112, 271
Country Friends, 2, 89, 95-96, 168-169, 232, 249, 276-277
co-sleeping, 9, 192-193, 195-199, 268, 270
CPSC (see U.S. Consumer Product Safety Commission)
crankiness, 115, 143
criticism, 49, 79, 98, 129, 131, 214
crying, 16, 59, 60, 64-65, 90, 91, 94, 98, 101-102, 107, 121, 144, 150, 159, 174, 191, 193-194
cuddle, 90, 117, 178, 200

- D -

danger, 7, 82, 88, 91, 211-213, 217, 222, 225, 242, 245
daytime sleep hygiene, 187-188
daytime sleepiness, 11, 36, 184, 208-209
deep abdominal breathing, 155
dependency, 15, 283-284, 293
depression, 10, 11, 56, 67-68, 82, 111-112, 127, 139, 165, 168, 173, 176, 178-179, 287, 290, 295
desensitization, 213, 242
Desmopressin, 140-141
despair, 11, 68
desserts, 127, 129
Desyrel, 204
Dexedrine, 229
diabetes, 11, 126, 138, 155, 207
diet, 118, 123, 128, 130, 139, 179, 184, 205, 209-210, 217, 219, 228

difficulty falling asleep, 29, 53, 101, 115, 135
difficulty unwinding, 21, 29, 59
difficulty waking in the morning, 11, 29, 184
Diphenhydramine, 203
discipline, 112, 268
discomfort, 7, 157, 212, 216-217, 221
disrespect, 73
disruptive behavior, 14
distraction, 218, 268
diuretics, 138
divorce, 25, 36, 66-72, 76, 89, 167, 188, 223-225, 229, 269
dizziness, 204, 212
DreamChild Adventures, 3, 5-6, 12, 14, 51, 89, 183, 216, 218, 222, 228, 231, 233-234, 237, 245-246, 283
dreams, 37, 64, 84, 85, 87, 89-90, 152, 174, 177-178, 260, 261, 264, 265, 271, 277, 289
drugs 188, 198, 201, 205
DuPont, Caroline M., 7, 215, 217, 268
DuPont, Robert L., 7, 215, 217, 268
DuPont Spencer, Elizabeth, 7, 215, 217, 268

- E -

earbuds, 242, 244-245
eardrum, 113, 244
earphones, 243-244, 246
eating disorders, 128
eating habits, 126, 128
EEG (see electroencephalograph)
efficacy, 15, 17, 201, 202, 224, 283, 285, 294
electroencephalograph, 51, 232, 284-286
Elementary and Secondary School Civil Rights Compliance Report, 112, 272
embarrassment, 51, 212, 214
emotional intelligence, 163, 224, 269
empathy, 81, 90, 96
empowering, 215-216, 218, 233
endorphins, 155, 219
entitlement, 71
enuresis, 137; nocturnal, 139, 141, 268; primary, 141; secondary, 141
environmental sleep hygiene, 187
EPA (see U.S. Environmental Protection Agency)
evidence-based child health, 141
excessive time to fall asleep, 21, 41
exercise, 39, 70, 126, 128-130, 140, 179, 186, 210, 217, 219, 227, 228
exhaustion, 83
extracurricular activities, 9, 217

- F -

Faber, Adele, 77, 268
failure, 8, 112, 138
fairness, 79-81
family bed, 194-200

fatigue, 10, 16, 204, 275-276, 287, 288, 296
favoritism, 76, 79
fear: of abandonment, 25, 101; of death, 25; fearfulness, 72
Ferber, Richard, 189-190, 193-195, 197, 202, 268
fidgety, 41, 43
fight or flight, 212, 219
fighting, 22, 24, 47, 64, 79
fitness, 130-131, 217
Fligor, Brian J., 243, 268, 271
forgetfulness, 209
friends, 12, 42, 49, 69, 75, 79, 89, 94-96, 123, 134, 136, 168-169, 171, 232, 249, 251, 253-254, 256, 276-277
frustration, 24, 26, 28, 49, 80, 81, 105, 138-139, 208

- G -

gastroesophageal reflux (GERD), 207
gastrointestinal complaints, 14
gender, 17, 76-77, 87
genetics: 220-221; genetic factors, 87; genetic predisposition, 213
genitalia, 113
Ghrelin, 127
girls, 9, 29, 54, 94, 112-113, 138, 166-167, 169, 263
Glenn, H. Stephen, 112, 268
Goodavage, Maria, 194-199, 268
Gordon, Jay, 194-199, 268
grades 31, 35, 45, 55, 57-58, 176
grief, 95, 98-99
guilt, 70, 71, 99, 108, 138, 157, 179, 194, 221
Guthrow, John Benjamin, 112

- H -

habits, 4, 24, 34, 36, 39, 56, 57, 126-128, 183-184, 187-188, 196, 205, 227, 228
Halcion, 203
hallucinations, 16
harm, 56, 58, 82, 91, 105, 113, 193, 212, 229, 245
Harmony Grits, 12, 251, 277
Harrison, Robert, 246
Harvard University, 6, 270
headaches, 67, 143, 145, 147, 149, 155, 165, 207
headphones, 44, 54, 86, 95, 107, 118, 122, 146, 148, 150, 152, 169, 172, 239, 243, 245-246, 274, 276-278, 280, 284, 293-294
headset, 122, 246
hearing impairment, 207
heartburn, 207
helpless, 9, 69, 150, 172
heredity, 137, 221
high blood pressure, 126, 155, 165, 168
hitting, 110, 112, 170
homeostasis, 185
homework, 39, 49, 169

hospital, 15, 25, 116, 117, 120, 149-152, 196, 230-231, 244, 246, 284, 288
household, 11, 39, 50, 66, 71, 76, 77, 81, 82, 138, 197-199, 247
hugs, 27, 89
humiliation, 212
humor, 98
Huntington Memorial Hospital, 151
hydration, 140
hyperactivity, 14, 133, 148, 204, 208-209
hypertension, 202, 204
hypnosis, 155-156, 175-176
hypnotics, 200, 202, 290

- I -

illness, 8, 98, 153, 154, 156, 219, 290
imagery, 3, 51, 74, 154, 155, 163, 233, 285, 293
imagination, 12, 13, 25, 87, 112, 146, 151, 154, 226, 237, 249, 274, 276-277, 280
immune system, 11, 154
impulsivity, 14, 208
inadequate sleep duration, 11, 184
independence, 196, 197, 200
Inderal, 168, 173
individuality, 77, 80, 197
infancy, 189
infection, 137, 155, 207, 230
insecurity, 7, 12, 93, 276
insomnia, 3, 37, 133, 143, 157, 165, 183, 200, 201, 203-205, 207, 286-287, 293-295
Institute of Child Health, 112
intelligence, 161, 224, 269
interventions, 15, 205, 210, 237, 268, 293
irrational, 7, 26, 72, 80
irritability, 41, 56, 204, 208, 209, 276

- J -

Jackson, Thomas, 3, 283, 290
judgment, 14, 49, 129, 131, 214, 226

- K -

Kagan, Jerome, 221
kindergarten 58, 144, 191
Kuo, Frances 231, 269

- L -

Lamictal, 168, 171, 173
*Lancet, Th*e 181, 209, 270
Last, Cynthia G., 9, 220, 269
learning difficulties, 36
learning disabilities, 77
Lehrer, Jonah 229-231, 269
leptin, 128
Lexapro, 171
lifestyle, 68, 70, 127, 130, 227

Index

lightning, 8, 252
lights, 21-24, 144, 146, 171
listening, 3, 5, 12, 13, 15, 16, 23, 33, 34, 45, 48, 54, 65, 68, 74, 75, 86, 89, 95, 96, 109, 118-120, 122-124, 147-148, 151, 159-162, 169-171, 173, 187, 191, 209, 232, 239, 242-246, 249, 258, 268, 271, 274, 277-279, 284, 286, 287, 291, 292, 294
3D Living Sound, 5, 6, 13, 14, 16, 51, 231-233, 273-274, 276-278, 280, 283-285, 291-294
Lorazepam, 203
loudness, 241, 242
low self-esteem, 7, 115, 117, 127, 139, 165, 178, 179
Lunesta, 204
Louv, Richard, 224-226, 229, 269

- M -

Magic Carpet, 12, 13, 22, 23, 32, 33, 43, 45, 47, 48, 54, 62, 74, 75, 84-86, 89, 95, 106, 118-120, 122, 135, 150-151, 153, 158-163, 168-170, 232, 256, 258, 277, 278
Magic Massager® 168-169, 281
Manassis, Katharina, 213-214, 216-217, 219, 221, 270
massage, 89, 155, 169, 276, 281
maturation, 133, 137, 157-158, 163
McKinley, Mike, 253
meals, 49, 129, 186
mealtimes, 39, 71
medication, 119, 122, 125, 133-134, 141, 150-152, 157-158, 167, 178, 188, 200-205, 210, 217, 230, 286, 291
medicine, 116, 154, 175, 205, 230, 237, 294
meditation, 12, 156, 232
Melatonin, 38
mental health, 7, 69, 112, 134-135, 220, 268
migraines, 155, 168, 173, 176
mimicking, 25, 103
Mitrione, Stephen 230-231, 270
Moore, Robin, 226
morning moodiness, 11, 35, 184
morning routine, 117
Mother-Baby Behavioral Sleep Laboratory, 195
motivation, 17, 176, 179, 226-227
mouthiness, 73
movies, 34, 70, 89, 130, 199
MRI, 56
music, 3, 13, 23, 44, 74, 86, 187, 242-244, 250-251, 268, 277, 288

- N -

National Health and Nutrition Examination Survey, 126, 267
National Institute for Occupational Safety and Health, 242, 245
National Institute of Health, 16, 270, 295
National Institute on Deafness, 241, 270
National Sleep Foundation, 57, 270

Natural Relaxation I, 15, 145, 275-276, 278-279, 283-284
Natural Relaxation II, 275
Natural Sleep, 145, 168, 274, 286-287, 290-291, 293, 295
nature, 3, 13, 26, 77, 81, 90, 99, 116, 130, 159, 163, 175, 177, 186-187, 214, 215, 220-221, 223-233, 245, 254-255, 257, 260, 269, 273-280, 283, 291-292
Nature Odyssey, 273, 279
nature sounds, 3, 187, 245, 278-279, 292
Nature Walk, 273, 278
Nature-Deficit Disorder (NDD), 224-229, 231, 269
nausea, 24, 155, 168, 204, 212
nervousness, 12, 93, 165, 276
neurochemicals, 219
neurology, 232, 284, 286
Neuro-Linguistic Programming, 3
New York Times, The, 6, 224
New Yorker, The, 5, 271
night terrors, 4, 11, 36, 67, 90, 91
nightlight, 27, 90, 140, 187, 199
nightmares, 4, 5, 11, 13, 29-31, 34-37, 58-60, 67, 83, 84, 86-91, 135, 143-145, 147, 165, 168, 174, 188, 211, 225
nighttime wakings, 11, 13, 29, 30, 36, 41, 59, 60, 63, 83, 184, 187, 190, 191, 195, 198, 287
NIHL in Children Conference, 243
NIOSH (see National Institute for Occupational Safety and Health)
NLP (see Neuro-Linguistic Programming)
nocturnal enuresis (see bedwetting, enuresis)
noise-canceling headphones, 246
noise-induced hearing loss (NIHL), 241-244, 246, 270, 271
nutrition, 126, 127, 129, 217, 267, 271
Nytol, 203

- O -

obedience, 112
obesity, 4, 6, 11, 36, 38, 115, 126, 127, 130, 179, 209-210, 224, 227, 242, 267, 271-272
Obsessive compulsive disorder (OCD), 219
obstructive sleep apnea (OSA), 11, 58, 209, 210
Occupational Safety and Health Act (OSHA), 242, 244, 245
oppositional behavior, 9, 21, 29, 48, 67, 101, 115, 119, 133, 148
outbursts, 26, 41, 80, 119, 134
overweight, 117, 118, 126, 127, 130, 133, 228

- P -

pain, 12, 16, 71, 95, 98, 99, 109, 111, 139, 143, 150, 151, 153-156, 163, 200, 207-208, 212, 215-217, 221, 230, 269, 272, 276
painkillers, 219
panic attacks, 16
panic disorder, 220
parasomnias, 36
parasympathetic nervous system, 218

300

pediatrician, 95, 139-141, 144, 188, 194, 200, 210, 272
peer pressure, 6, 39
peers, 9, 35, 38, 56-58, 66, 67, 127, 137, 195-196, 222, 228, 229
perception, 7, 26, 193, 212
phantom limb pain, 155
pharmacotherapy, 202
phobias, 220, 267
physical development, 10, 11
physician, 140, 200-203, 205
pillows, 188, 198, 249
Playhouse on the Beach, 12, 13, 54, 55, 74, 84, 85, 89, 106, 119, 120, 122, 158, 232, 261, 277-278
PODS (see Potty On Discreet Strips)
polysomnograph, 287
poor academic performance, 4, 36, 55, 57, 58, 163
poor reading skills, 48
Portnuff, Corey, 243, 271
positive reinforcement, 27, 51, 81, 104
postoperative recovery, 155
Post-Traumatic Stress Disorder (PTSD), 87, 178, 2220
Potty On Discreet Strips, 140
praise, 27, 51, 79, 131
preschool, 8, 118, 210, 271
prescription, 145, 188, 198, 201, 286
primary enuresis (see also bedwetting, enuresis)
Prochnik, George, 242, 271
programming, 3, 38, 39
progressive muscle relaxation, 155, 293
psychiatrist, 3, 214, 237
psychological factors, 220
psychologist, 76, 112, 230
psychopharmacology, 172
psychosomatic, 154
psychotherapy, 163
psychotic disorders, 16
PTSD (see Post-traumatic Stress Disorder)
punishment, 81, 111, 112, 128, 188, 192, 271

- R -

Rain and Thunder, 273, 279
Ramelteon, 204
rapid breathing, 24
rapid eye movement (see REM)
rapid heartbeat, 24, 212
reading, 4, 5, 11, 12, 17, 27, 29, 31, 34-36, 39, 41-42, 45-51, 57, 60, 88, 90, 105, 137, 148, 149, 154, 163, 165-166, 170, 186-187, 189, 223-225, 228-229, 232-233, 283, 286, 293
reality, 7, 25, 26, 97, 138, 178, 214, 216, 233, 280
reassurance, 25, 89, 90, 213
receptivity, 163, 164, 191
reckless playing, 29
recurrent abdominal pain, 154, 269
Reflections on the California Coast, 273, 280

regression, 67, 125
rejection, 8, 81, 93, 131
relaxation, 3, 5, 6, 10-16, 140, 145-147, 149-150, 152-156, 164, 168, 178, 187, 190, 191, 216-220, 222, 226, 229, 231, 233, 249, 273-281, 283, 284, 289, 290, 293
Relaxation and Massage, 276
relaxation response, 154, 217, 222
relaxation therapies, 14
REM, 3, 10, 14, 24-27, 37, 38, 46, 56, 69, 88-90, 116, 123, 137-139, 161, 170, 174, 187, 189, 192, 202-203, 209-210, 212, 229, 233, 239, 243-245, 274, 276, 287, 291; REM sleep, 88, 90, 210, 287
research, 5-7, 14-17, 56, 111, 127, 129, 137, 141, 154-155, 192-193, 195, 201, 203, 205, 209, 224, 229-231, 272, 283, 287, 293
resentment, 70, 79
resistance to reading, 4, 36, 39, 41, 48-50, 165, 223-225, 232, 283
responsibility, 79, 103, 139, 179, 202, 216
restful sleep, 11, 24, 38, 155, 158, 168, 179, 187-188, 209, 219, 227, 228
restless leg syndrome, 36
restlessness, 41, 59, 120
restorative sleep, 203, 204, 209, 224
Restoril, 203
retardation, 200, 210
reward, 27, 81
rhythm, 185, 204, 260, 288
Rimm, Sylvia, 76, 271
risks, 5, 9, 202-203, 241, 243, 245
Ritalin, 229
rocking, 101, 190, 199
Roosevelt, Franklin D., 7
Rozerem, 204

- S -

sadness, 12, 68, 72, 121, 276
safety, 25, 67, 71, 78, 141, 187, 193-194, 197-198, 201, 203-204, 226, 229, 231, 237, 242, 245, 249
school, 6, 8, 9, 21, 22, 24, 31, 34, 37, 38, 41, 43, 49, 53, 54, 57, 58, 61, 64-67, 75, 89, 93, 112, 117, 123, 127, 134-135, 140, 144-145, 147-148, 153, 166, 170, 176, 179, 188, 193, 208, 225-226, 228, 241, 268, 272
schoolwork, 61, 65
Schwartz, Gary E., 222, 232-233, 271, 284
Schwartz, Jeffrey, 214, 263
screaming, 47, 59, 64, 81, 90, 91, 94, 101, 102, 106, 144, 145
Seabrook, John, 197, 271
secondary enuresis (see bedwetting, enuresis)
security, 26, 71, 106, 194-195, 231
sedation, 203-205
sedative, 202, 203, 290-291
SEFRT, 287-288
seizures, 204, 210

self-confidence, 139, 148, 152, 170
self-esteem, 4, 7, 14, 71, 90, 112, 115, 117, 122, 124, 127, 130, 131, 133, 135, 139, 148, 165, 178, 179, 215, 223, 224, 226-228, 267,
Sennheiser, 239
sensitivity, 25, 72, 93, 220
shame, 9, 70, 108, 179, 221
shock, 65, 67, 94
short attention span, 21, 22, 29, 30, 143, 208
shortness of breath, 24, 212
sibling rivalry, 76-80, 82, 225
siblinghood, 80
side effects, 16, 111, 138, 141, 188, 202-204, 237
SIDS (see sudden infant death syndrome)
sleep, 3-7, 10-16, 21-25, 27, 29-39, 41, 42, 44, 45, 47, 53-67, 70, 72, 73, 83-91, 93, 94, 96, 98, 101, 102, 104, 107, 115-119, 122, 125, 127-129, 135-138, 140-141, 143-147, 149-156, 158, 160, 161, 165-170, 172, 174-176, 178, 179, 182-200, 215-217, 218-220, 224-229, 231, 233-234, 237, 246, 256, 260-261, 264-265, 267-272, 274-281, 283, 285-291, 293-296
sleep associations, 189-191, 199
sleep deprivation, 56, 57, 91
sleep disturbance, 10, 67, 88, 201, 295
sleep duration, 11, 36, 179, 184-185
Sleep Enhancement Fatigue Reduction Training, 287
sleep experts, 190, 193, 196, 202, 210, 274, 295
sleep hygiene, 183-184, 186-189, 202, 270, 288
sleep medication, 200-202, 210, 291
sleep onset delay, 10, 36, 184
sleep patterns, 10, 36, 38, 57, 58, 61, 88, 167, 183, 189, 191, 208
sleep training, 289
sleepiness, 11, 13, 24, 36, 182, 200, 201, 270
sleeping environment, 187
sleeplessness, 212, 217, 222
sleepover, 24, 141
sleepwalking, 36, 91
snoring, 23, 58, 209-210
socialization, 56, 77
Sominex, 203
Sonata, 204-205
sound effects, 3, 12, 13, 74, 284-285
spanking, 104, 105, 108, 111-113, 268
speakers, 170, 277-278, 280
State Education and Environmental Roundtable, 226
statistics, 15, 17, 57, 87, 126, 138, 193, 196, 241-242, 244, 271
stimulation, 6, 226, 230
stomach cramps, 143, 147
Strauss, Murray, 111-112, 271
Stream Walk, 273, 279
stress, 3, 6, 7, 12, 75, 77, 81, 82, 87, 91, 127, 137, 140, 143, 154, 163, 175, 178, 200, 212-213, 217-220, 222, 231, 275-276, 283-284, 288, 290, 296

stress response, 154, 212, 213, 217, 219, 220, 222
students, 56, 57, 112, 166, 179, 226-227, 230, 241
Sudden Infant Death Syndrome, 195, 270
sugar, 69, 127, 129, 140
sunlight, 188, 233, 258
surgery, 143, 149-151, 210, 230
sweating, 24, 91, 212
sympathetic nervous system, 218-219

- T -

teacher, 8, 24, 34, 49, 64, 65, 124, 175, 214
techniques, 3, 13-16, 27, 48, 153-156, 217-219, 234, 269, 274-276, 278-280, 285-287
technology, 3, 5, 6, 14, 38, 39, 239, 243, 246, 274, 276-277, 283, 292-293
television, 4, 24, 27, 29, 31, 34-39, 41, 42, 46, 58, 89, 116, 127, 144, 148, 187-188, 204, 223-226, 228, 267, 269, 272
Temazepam, 203
therapeutic audio, 3
therapist, 5, 31, 91, 99, 103, 119, 121, 124, 214
Thorazine, 157-158
Thoreau, Henry David, 223
Tofranil, 116, 119
touch, 32, 97, 110, 119, 136, 156, 159, 200, 224, 232, 281
toys, 14, 27, 31, 46, 47, 75, 76, 80, 146, 153, 247, 256, 260, 263, 278
trauma, 24, 67, 68, 71, 83, 87, 97, 178, 193, 194, 220
Triazolam, 203
triggers, 9, 56, 67, 211-213
trust, 67, 71, 105, 226, 229
Tryptophan, 186
TV, 6, 34-39, 42, 44-46, 48, 50, 60, 63, 75, 86, 129, 146, 154, 184-185, 187-188, 197, 217-218 148, 156, 186-187, 189-190, 199, 225-226
Tylenol, 145, 150

- U -

Ulrich, Roger S. 230, 272
understanding 6, 10, 12, 13, 26, 28, 51, 66, 87, 90, 131, 163, 215, 221, 242, 267, 270
unhappiness 115, 127
Unisom, 203
United Nations Convention on the Rights of the Child, 113
U.S. Air Force 16, 287-288, 290, 295
U.S. Consumer Product Safety Commission, 193
U.S. Department of Education 112
U.S. Environmental Protection Agency, 242, 272
University of California Irvine Medical Center 16
University of Michigan, 230
University of North Carolina, 226
urban environments 229-230

- V -

Valium, 203

302

video games 6, 50, 89, 127, 129, 130, 140, 186, 225
violence 6, 37, 78, 111-113, 133, 228
virtual reality, 178, 280
visualization 51, 153-156, 218, 220, 233, 290
volume 242-246

- W -

waking, 10, 11, 29, 30, 37, 55, 60, 83, 88-90, 116, 122, 135-136, 141, 146, 150, 152, 162, 172, 178, 184-186, 188, 190, 192, 196, 199, 209, 229, 274-275, 288
Walden, 223
Weil, Andrew, 154
Wellbutrin, 168, 171
whimpering, 90, 150, 191
whining, 53-55, 83, 84
worry, 7, 8, 12, 31, 64, 165, 166, 170-171, 176, 198-199, 217, 220-221, 244, 269, 276
worrying, 29, 33, 93, 173, 176

- X -

Xanax, 203

- Y -

yelling 53, 81
yoga 129

- Z -

Zaleplon, 204
Zogby, John, 264
Zolpidem, 204

Sage Kalmus is a freelance writer, ghostwriter and blogger with clients all over the world. He has written thousands of articles for the web, specializing in green living, alternative health, relationships and spirituality, as well as several ebooks and screenplays. He recently self-published his first novel, *Free Will Flux*, a work of metaphysical fiction, in paperback and ebook. He lives off-the-grid in the foothills of western Maine. Find him at www.SageKalmus.com.

Max Herr is a writer, editor, graphic designer, and multimedia specialist. A former photojournalist, he provides custom prepublishing services to authors, including original research and writing, editing, typography, and cover design. An expert user of Adobe Creative Suite products, he offers production of print-ready PDF, INDD, and PSD files for submission to major publishing houses and the various print-on-demand service providers. Find his profile online at Elance.com and Guru.com. You can also email him directly at mhherr@verizon.net.